甲状腺癌
Thyroid Cancer

人民卫生出版社
·北京·

版权所有，侵权必究！

图书在版编目（CIP）数据

甲状腺癌 /（美）邢明照主编；葛明华，（美）邢明照主译. —北京：人民卫生出版社，2021.12
ISBN 978-7-117-32611-7

Ⅰ.①甲… Ⅱ.①邢…②葛… Ⅲ.①甲状腺疾病—腺癌—诊疗 Ⅳ.①R736.1

中国版本图书馆 CIP 数据核字（2021）第 270555 号

| 人卫智网 | www.ipmph.com | 医学教育、学术、考试、健康，购书智慧智能综合服务平台 |
| 人卫官网 | www.pmph.com | 人卫官方资讯发布平台 |

图字：01-2019-7739 号

甲 状 腺 癌
Jiazhuangxian'ai

主　　译：葛明华　邢明照
出版发行：人民卫生出版社（中继线 010-59780011）
地　　址：北京市朝阳区潘家园南里 19 号
邮　　编：100021
E - mail：pmph @ pmph.com
购书热线：010-59787592　　010-59787584　　010-65264830
印　　刷：北京盛通印刷股份有限公司
经　　销：新华书店
开　　本：710×1000　1/16　印张：22
字　　数：383 千字
版　　次：2021 年 12 月第 1 版
印　　次：2021 年 12 月第 1 次印刷
标准书号：ISBN 978-7-117-32611-7
定　　价：198.00 元

打击盗版举报电话：010-59787491　　E-mail：WQ @ pmph.com
质量问题联系电话：010-59787234　　E-mail：zhiliang @ pmph.com

甲状腺癌
Thyroid Cancer

主　编　邢明照（Mingzhao Xing）
顾　问　Adriana G. Ioachimescu
主　译　葛明华　邢明照（Mingzhao Xing）
副主译　关海霞　吕伟明

人民卫生出版社
·北京·

Elsevier (Singapore) Pte Ltd.
3 Killiney Road#08-01 Winsland House I Singapore 239519
Tel:(65) 6349-0200 Fax:(65) 6733-1817

Thyroid Cancer, An Issue of Endocrinology and Metabolism Clinics of North America
Copyright © 2019 Elsevier Inc. All rights reserved.
ISBN-13: 978-0-323-61078-0

This translation of Thyroid Cancer, An Issue of Endocrinology and Metabolism Clinics of North America by Mingzhao Xing was undertaken by People's Medical Publishing House and is published by arrangement with Elsevier (Singapore) Pte Ltd.
Thyroid Cancer, An Issue of Endocrinology and Metabolism Clinics of North America by Mingzhao Xing 由人民卫生出版社进行翻译，并根据人民卫生出版社与爱思唯尔（新加坡）私人有限公司的协议约定出版。

《甲状腺癌》（第 2 版）（葛明华　邢明照　主译）
ISBN: 978-7-117-32611-7
Copyright ©2021 by Elsevier (Singapore) Pte Ltd. and People's Medical Publishing House.
All rights reserved. No part of this publication may be reproduced or transmitted in any form or by any means, electronic or mechanical, including photocopying, recording, or any information storage and retrieval system, without permission in writing from Elsevier (Singapore) Pte Ltd and People's Medical Publishing House.

注　意

本译本由 Elsevier (Singapore) Pte Ltd. 和人民卫生出版社完成。相关从业及研究人员必须凭借其自身经验和知识对文中描述的信息数据、方法策略、搭配组合、实验操作进行评估和使用。由于医学科学发展迅速，临床诊断和给药剂量尤其需要经过独立验证。在法律允许的最大范围内，爱思唯尔、译文的原文作者、原文编辑及原文内容提供者均不对译文或因产品责任、疏忽或其他操作造成的人身和 / 或财产伤害和 / 或损失承担责任，亦不对由于使用文中提到的方法、产品、说明或思想而导致的人身和 / 或财产伤害和 / 或损失承担责任。

Printed in China by People's Medical Publishing House under special arrangement with Elsevier (Singapore) Pte Ltd. This edition is authorized for sale in the People's Republic of China only, excluding Hong Kong SAR, Macau SAR and Taiwan. Unauthorized export of this edition is a violation of the contract.
图字：01-2019-7739 号

编　者

顾问

ADRIANA G. IOACHIMESCU, MD, PhD, FACE
Professor of Medicine (Endocrinology) and Neurosurgery, Emory University School of Medicine, Atlanta, Georgia, USA

主编

MINGZHAO XING, MD, PhD
Dean-elect, School of Medicine, Southern University of Science and Technology, Shenzhen, Guangdong, China; Professor of Medicine, Oncology, Pathology, and Cellular and Molecular Medicine, Department of Medicine, Division of Endocrinology, Diabetes, and Metabolism, Director, The Johns Hopkins Thyroid Tumor Center, Johns Hopkins School of Medicine, Baltimore, Maryland, USA

编者

EHAB S. ALAMEER, MD
Department of Surgery, Tulane University School of Medicine, New Orleans, Louisiana, USA

ANGKOON ANUWONG, MD, FRCST, FACS
Department of Surgery, Minimally Invasive and Endocrine Surgery Division, Police General Hospital, Bangkok, Thailand

SYLVIA L. ASA, MD, PhD
Professor, Department of Laboratory Medicine and Pathobiology, University of Toronto, Toronto, Ontario, Canada

SAAD AL AWWAD, MD
Department of Surgery, Tulane University School of Medicine, New Orleans, Louisiana, USA

KEITH C. BIBLE, MD, PhD
Division of Medical Oncology, Mayo Clinic, Rochester, Minnesota, USA

BERNADETTE BIONDI, MD
Associate Professor of Endocrinology, Department of Clinical Medicine and Surgery, University of Naples Federico II, Naples, Italy

JUAN P. BRITO, MD, MSc
Division of Diabetes, Endocrinology, Metabolism, and Nutrition, Department of Medicine, Knowledge and Evaluation Research Unit, Mayo Clinic, Rochester, Minnesota, USA

ASHISH V. CHINTAKUNTLAWAR, MBBS, PhD
Division of Medical Oncology, Mayo Clinic, Rochester, Minnesota, USA

DAVID S. COOPER, MD
Division of Endocrinology, Diabetes, and Metabolism, Johns Hopkins School of Medicine, Baltimore, Maryland, USA

ROSSELLA ELISEI, MD
Endocrine Unit, Department of Clinical and Experimental Medicine, University of Pisa, Pisa, Italy

AHMAD M. ELTELETY, MBBCh, MSc, MD-PhD, MRCS (ENT)
Clinical Fellow, Endocrine Head and Neck Surgery, Otolaryngology Department, Medical College of Georgia, Augusta University, Augusta, Georgia, USA; Lecturer, Otolaryngology Department, Faculty of Medicine, Cairo University, Cairo, Arab Republic of Egypt

ROBERT L. FOOTE, MD
Department of Radiation Oncology, Mayo Clinic, Rochester, Minnesota, USA

MEGHAN E. GARSTKA, MD, MS
Department of Surgery, Tulane University School of Medicine, New Orleans, Louisiana, USA

BRYAN R. HAUGEN, MD
Professor of Medicine and Pathology, Division of Endocrinology, Metabolism and Diabetes, University of Colorado School of Medicine, Aurora, Colorado, USA

IAN D. HAY, MD, PhD, FRCP
Division of Diabetes, Endocrinology, Metabolism, and Nutrition, Department of Medicine, Mayo Clinic, Rochester, Minnesota, USA

YASUHIRO ITO, MD, PhD
Department of Surgery, Kuma Hospital, Kobe, Japan

PORNPEERA JITPRATOOM, MD, FRCST
Department of Surgery, Minimally Invasive and Endocrine Surgery Division, Police General Hospital, Bangkok, Thailand

ISARIYA JONGEKKASIT, MD, FRCST
Department of Surgery, Minimally Invasive and Endocrine Surgery Division, Police General Hospital, Bangkok, Thailand

DIPTI KAMANI, MD
Department of Otolaryngology, Division of Thyroid and Parathyroid Endocrine Surgery, Massachusetts Eye and Ear Infirmary, Boston, Massachusetts, USA

EMAD KANDIL, MD, MBA
Professor, Department of Surgery, Tulane University School of Medicine, New Orleans, Louisiana, USA

JAN L. KASPERBAUER, MD
Division of Head and Neck Surgery, Mayo Clinic, Rochester, Minnesota, USA

PAUL W. LADENSON, MD
Professor of Medicine, Division of Endocrinology, Diabetes, and Metabolism, Johns Hopkins School of Medicine, Baltimore, Maryland, USA

CAROLYN MAXWELL, MD
Associate Professor of Medicine, Division of Endocrinology and Metabolism, Stony Brook University School of Medicine, Stony Brook, New York, USA

SARAH E. MAYSON, MD
Assistant Professor of Medicine, Division of Endocrinology, Metabolism and Diabetes, University of Colorado School of Medicine, Aurora, Colorado, USA

AKIRA MIYAUCHI, MD, PhD
Department of Surgery, Kuma Hospital, Kobe, Japan

CARMELO NUCERA, MD, PhD
Laboratory of Human Thyroid Cancers Preclinical and Translational Research, Division of Experimental Pathology, Department of Pathology, Cancer Research Institute (CRI), Cancer Center, Center for Vascular Biology Research (CVBR), Beth Israel Deaconess Medical Center, Harvard Medical School, Boston, Massachusetts, USA; Broad Institute of MIT and Harvard, Cambridge, Massachusetts, USA

GREGORY W. RANDOLPH, MD, FACS, FACE
Department of Otolaryngology, Division of Thyroid and Parathyroid Endocrine Surgery, Massachusetts Eye and Ear Infirmary, Boston, Massachusetts, USA

BENJAMIN R. ROMAN, MD, MSHP
Department of Surgery, Division of Head and Neck, Memorial Sloan Kettering Cancer Center, New York, New York, USA

PRASANNA SANTHANAM, MBBS, MD
Assistant Professor of Medicine, Division of Endocrinology, Diabetes, and Metabolism, Johns Hopkins School of Medicine, Baltimore, Maryland, USA

THANYAWAT SASANAKIETKUL, MD, FRCST
Department of Surgery, Minimally Invasive and Endocrine Surgery Division, Police General Hospital, Bangkok, Thailand

CAROLYN DACEY SEIB, MD, MAS
Clinical Instructor of General Surgery, University of California, San Francisco, San Francisco, California, USA

STEVEN I. SHERMAN, MD
Naguib Samaan Distinguished Professor and Department Chair, Department of Endocrine Neoplasia and Hormonal Disorders, The University of Texas MD Anderson Cancer Center, Houston, Texas, USA

JENNIFER A. SIPOS, MD
Professor of Medicine, Division of Endocrinology and Metabolism, The Ohio State University Wexner Medical Center, Columbus, Ohio, USA

JULIE ANN SOSA, MD, MA
Leon Goldman, MD Distinguished Professor of Surgery, Chair, Department of Surgery, Professor, Department of Medicine, University of California, San Francisco, San Francisco, California, USA

DAVID J. TERRIS, MD, FACS, FACE
Regents Professor of Otolaryngology and Endocrinology, Surgical Director, Otolaryngology Department, Augusta University, Thyroid and Parathyroid Center, Augusta, Georgia, USA

R. MICHAEL TUTTLE, MD
Endocrinology Service, Department of Medicine, Memorial Sloan Kettering Cancer Center, New York, New York, USA

FERNANDA VAISMAN, MD, PhD
Endocrinology Service, Instituto Nacional do Cancer, Universidade Federal do Rio de Janeiro, Rio de Janeiro, Rio de Janeiro, Brazil

VERONICA VALVO, PhD
Laboratory of Human Thyroid Cancers Preclinical and Translational Research, Division of Experimental Pathology, Department of Pathology, Cancer Research Institute (CRI), Cancer Center, Center for Vascular Biology Research (CVBR), Beth Israel Deaconess Medical Center, Harvard Medical School, Boston, Massachusetts, USA

DOUGLAS VAN NOSTRAND, MD, FACP, FACNP
Department of Nuclear Medicine, Nuclear Medicine Research, MedStar Health Research Institute and MedStar Washington Hospital Center, Washington, DC, USA

DAVID VIOLA, MD
Endocrine Unit, Department of Clinical and Experimental Medicine, University of Pisa, Pisa, Italy

LEONARD WARTOFSKY, MD, MACP
Thyroid Cancer Research Center, MedStar Health Research Institute, Washington, DC, USA

STEVEN P. WEITZMAN, MD
Associate Professor, Department of Endocrine Neoplasia and Hormonal Disorders, The University of Texas MD Anderson Cancer Center, Houston, Texas, USA

MINGZHAO XING, MD, PhD
Dean-elect, School of Medicine, Southern University of Science and Technology, Shenzhen, Guangdong, China; Professor of Medicine, Oncology, Pathology, and Cellular and Molecular Medicine, Department of Medicine, Division of Endocrinology, Diabetes, and Metabolism, Director, The Johns Hopkins Thyroid Tumor Center, Johns Hopkins School of Medicine, Baltimore, Maryland, USA

DORINA YLLI, MD, PhD
Thyroid Cancer Research Center, MedStar Health Research Institute, Washington, DC, USA

译 者

主 译
葛明华　浙江省人民医院
邢明照　南方科技大学医学院

副主译
关海霞　广东省人民医院
吕伟明　中山大学附属第一医院

译委会（以姓氏笔画为序）
　　王　宇　复旦大学附属肿瘤医院
　　叶　蕾　上海交通大学医学院附属瑞金医院
　　曲　伸　上海市第十人民医院
　　吕中伟　上海市第十人民医院
　　刘绍严　中国医学科学院肿瘤医院
　　孙　辉　吉林大学中日联谊医院
　　李　超　四川省肿瘤医院
　　李志辉　四川大学华西医院
　　杨　明　山东省肿瘤医院
　　杨安奎　中山大学附属肿瘤医院
　　宋韬韬　北京大学肿瘤医院

张　彬　北京大学肿瘤医院
张　毅　陆军军医大学西南医院
武晓泓　浙江省人民医院
林岩松　北京协和医院
郑传铭　浙江省人民医院
郑向前　天津市肿瘤医院
徐　琰　陆军特色医学中心
徐震纲　中国医学科学院肿瘤医院
殷德涛　郑州大学第一附属医院
郭朱明　中山大学附属肿瘤医院
黄　韬　华中科技大学同济医学院附属协和医院
嵇庆海　复旦大学附属肿瘤医院
程若川　昆明医科大学第一附属医院
谢　磊　浙江大学医学院附属邵逸夫医院
管庆波　山东省立医院
潘　毅　天津市肿瘤医院

译　者（以姓氏笔画为序）

王朝阳　中国医学科学院肿瘤医院
刘晓莉　吉林大学中日联谊医院
齐晓伟　陆军军医大学西南医院
孙　迪　北京协和医院
孙荣昊　四川省肿瘤医院
苏艳军　昆明医科大学第一附属医院
李　丹　上海市第十人民医院
张　琨　四川大学华西医院
陈颖乐　中山大学附属肿瘤医院

金立超 中国医学科学院肿瘤医院
周雨秋 四川省肿瘤医院
黄玥晔 上海市第十人民医院
景　斐 山东省立医院
魏　玲 山东省肿瘤医院

中文版序一

曾经,因为恶性程度低、病程发展慢,甲状腺癌在众多肿瘤中几乎没有存在感,但近十几年来,甲状腺癌在全球各国的发病率持续上升,增长速度在所有实体瘤中名列前茅。甲状腺癌已经迈进最常见的恶性肿瘤行列,并迅速成为业界关注的热点和焦点。

与其他恶性肿瘤相比,甲状腺癌患者的生存期较长,治疗以手术、放射性碘和甲状腺激素替代及抑制为主,需要长期监测。因此,甲状腺癌是典型的需要多学科合作的疾病,涉及外科学、核医学、内分泌学、肿瘤学、影像学、放射治疗学等多个学科。由于疾病的复杂性,临床上对甲状腺癌的诊治仍存在一些误区,造成了治疗不当或过度。而且,伴随的诸多问题还未解决,诸如全甲状腺切除的指征、FNA应用的标准、微小癌的治疗原则等临床热点问题,依旧是国内外争论的焦点。

Thyroid Cancer 一书主编邢明照教授为南方科技大学首任医学院院长,此前为美国约翰斯·霍普金斯(Johns Hopkins)大学医学院终身医学教授,甲状腺肿瘤中心主任,甲状腺细胞及分子研究室主任,是国际肿瘤学、病理学和细胞分子医学领域的著名专家,在甲状腺癌诊治方面具有丰富的造诣。作为一本面向医护人员的专业著作,本书包含19章,涵盖甲状腺癌的流行病学进展、分子及影像诊断、基因导向甲状腺癌风险评估与治疗及复发监测、进展性放射性碘难治性分化型甲状腺癌的药物治疗等诸多内容,对临床中甲状腺癌的最新诊治手段进行了详细介绍,理念新颖。同时,本书还展示了大量来自作者及所在单位的关于甲状腺癌诊治的真实彩色照片,直观明了,方便读者理解和借鉴。

为了国内医生能够吸取国际最新的甲状腺癌管理和患者治疗经验,中国抗癌协会甲状腺癌专业委员会主任委员葛明华教授联合本书主编邢明照教授共同作为主译,集国内甲状腺领域的诸多著名专家共同翻译并出版 *Thyroid*

Cancer 中文版，以为国内甲状腺肿瘤临床领域的同人提供更为便捷、易懂的学习方式。

我很乐于为此书作序，并衷心祝愿本书为国内甲状腺肿瘤的治疗提供最新的临床指导，为我国甲状腺癌事业作出巨大贡献。

滕卫平

中国医科大学内分泌研究所所长
中华医学会内分泌学分会名誉主任委员
2021 年 11 月

中文版序二

近年来,甲状腺肿瘤(尤其是甲状腺癌)的发病率及发病趋势呈全球化激增,甲状腺癌目前已成为全身十大高发恶性肿瘤之一,其在多个国家和地区的发病率已跃居女性恶性肿瘤的前三位。伴随着甲状腺癌发病率的不断攀升,国内外甲状腺癌临床诊疗、基础研究以及科研转化等方面也出现了快速的进展。近10余年来,甲状腺肿瘤相关的学术团体及组织在国内外相继成立,并在其领域积极制定、推广专业指南/专家共识,使得甲状腺癌在临床诊治规范及诊断水平、肿瘤治愈率方面都有了明显的提高,多学科协作诊疗的理念和应用也更加深入。

随着社会的进步、科技的发展,临床医学和基础研究也在大步向前,甲状腺肿瘤领域在临床诊断、分期、治疗甚至病理分型方面取得了长足的进展和成就。譬如:甲状腺肿瘤的分子诊断及风险评估的临床应用、AI联合超声影像对甲状腺癌的精准诊断、新版AJCC/UICC中甲状腺癌TNM分期的更新、NIFTP的重新命名及病理学鉴别、甲状腺微小癌的观察及消融治疗的理念、腺叶切除的国际化标准统一、小分子多靶点酪氨酸酶抑制剂的上市、高度选择性靶向药物临床试验的开展,等等,许多成果和进展在 *NEJM*、*JAMA Oncology* 和 *Lancet* 等世界顶级期刊上发表。医学专业总会伴随着进展与争论的共存,甲状腺肿瘤也不例外,虽然近年来的飞速发展有目共睹,但仍存在诸多问题还未解决,诸如全甲状腺切除的指征、FNA应用的标准、微小癌的治疗原则等临床热点问题依旧是国内外争论的焦点。

由邢明照教授主编的学术著作 *Thyroid Cancer* 从甲状腺癌的流行病学进展、组织分类、分子及影像诊断、临床评价及危险等级分层、多学科治疗方式及复发监测等方面全方位、全维度地进行了介绍,内容经典与新颖并重,理论与实用互补,是一部专业性较强、临床价值较高的图书,在国际上具有很大的影响力。此著作原版为英文版,为方便国内同僚的学习和阅读,中国抗癌协会甲状腺癌专业委员会主委葛明华教授联合本书主编邢明照教授作为主译，召集国内甲状腺领域的专家共同翻译并出版 Thyroid Cancer 中文版，为国内致力于甲状腺肿瘤临床及基础研究的同人提供了更为便捷、易懂的参考，对于我国甲状腺肿瘤专业医师具有重要的临床指导意义。

我非常高兴能够为此书作序并推荐给本专业同道，希望大家能在本书中有所收获，也祝愿我国甲状腺肿瘤事业不断发展、前行！

天津市人民医院院长
中国抗癌协会头颈肿瘤专业委员会主任委员
中华医学会肿瘤学分会甲状腺肿瘤专业委员会主任委员
2021 年 11 月

中文版序三

新世纪伊始,甲状腺肿瘤学迅速发展。回顾多年来的道路,对于临床医生而言,每一次进步意味着早期诊断、有效的治疗、患病率的降低,以及最终改善患者的生活质量并延长其寿命。目前,临床常用的治疗甲状腺恶性肿瘤的手段包括外科手术、内分泌治疗、化学药物治疗、三维适形放疗、I-131放疗等,其中外科手术作为最主要、最常用的方式,其相关治疗技术、治疗适应证受到广泛关注。随着国内外诸多相关指南的推出和更新,如何合理利用各种治疗技术治疗甲状腺恶性肿瘤,做到规范化、个体化、精准化,备受关注。中国的甲状腺癌防治任重而道远。

目前,以循证医学为依据,结合国情,多个学会(中华医学会内分泌学分会、外科学分会、核医学分会和中国抗癌协会头颈肿瘤专业委员会)共同制定出甲状腺结节与甲状腺癌诊治指南供临床实践参考。但在实际临床工作中,因甲状腺癌疾病的复杂性,仍有许多亟待斟酌、解决的问题。尤其在甲状腺癌的外科治疗领域,应针对不同病情而细化外科处理原则,不可一概而论。在这样的大背景下,我们由衷期待一部好的甲状腺肿瘤专业书的问世。

现任南方科技大学医学院首任院长的邢明照教授,多年磨一剑,编写出这本 *Thyroid Cancer*。邢明照教授坚持临床一线工作几十年,不断总结和发展甲状腺癌的理论并实践,在甲状腺癌领域颇有建树。*Thyroid Cancer* 作为一部国际流行的甲状腺肿瘤专著,自问世以来,颇受好评和欢迎,其中的临床观念被广泛接受和应用。其特点是不仅侧重于临床诊断和处理,具有实用性,还注入了新的概念和技术,具有前瞻性。本书用19个章节,翔实阐述了甲状腺癌诊治领域最让人们关注的方面——从经典的甲状腺癌临床评价和危险分层,到最前沿的机器人辅助术式。本书覆盖全面,图文并茂,便于理解和记忆。所以,它不仅可用于临床工作,也可作为临床教学的重要参考书,用于教授医学生和青年医师。*Thyroid Cancer* 一书能被翻译成中文版面世,实乃我国广大甲状腺肿瘤临床工作者之幸事。

  我为能为此书作序感到十分高兴！衷心祝愿此书为国内甲状腺癌的诊断和治疗提供最实用的帮助，希望我国医务工作者们能够借助这本书早日攻克甲状腺癌的难题！

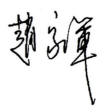

中华医学会内分泌学分会主任委员
山东第一医科大学附属省立医院院长
2021 年 11 月

中文版序四

随着国家人口老龄化不断加快,"癌症"这个词越来越频繁地出现在各种媒体中,成为大众关注的话题。甲状腺癌作为最常见的内分泌恶性肿瘤之一,发病率逐年上升,正悄然成为一种高发癌。据全国肿瘤数据登记中心测算,我国甲状腺癌以每年20%的速度持续增长,且女性发病率明显高于男性。

经过几十年的共同努力,无论是转化医学、精准医学领域还是智慧医疗或大数据医疗方面,甲状腺癌的诊治均取得了明显的进步。首先,在甲状腺癌诊断方面,单凭表象诊断疾病的传统做法已被"颠覆",从基因层面来探究疾病成为可能而且愈加重要,这表明以基因检测为代表的组学技术正越来越广泛地应用于临床诊断和治疗的各个环节。其次,在治疗方面,甲状腺癌外科技术的进步使患者术后的生活质量得到了更进一步的提升;同时,甲状腺癌内科新治疗手段的不断涌现使局部晚期或远处转移的患者获得了生存的希望。

当然,我们认识到,甲状腺癌的诊治方法依然是不太规范的,治疗过度和治疗不足问题常可闻及。而治疗过度和治疗不足所导致的不良后果往往被甲状腺癌较为良好的生物学行为和预后所掩盖,事实上,这也在一定程度上削弱了临床工作者对甲状腺癌诊治规范的重视程度。

从中国抗癌协会甲状腺癌专业委员会主委葛明华教授处得知,*Thyroid Cancer* 中文版即将出版,故欣然应邀作序。*Thyroid Cancer* 的英文原版主编为曾任美国约翰斯·霍普金斯大学医学院终身医学教授、甲状腺肿瘤中心主任、甲状腺细胞及分子研究室主任的邢明照教授,现全职担任南方科技大学医学院首任院长,是国际肿瘤学、病理学和细胞分子医学领域的著名专家,在甲状腺癌诊治方面极具造诣。该书共包括19章,在对临床甲状腺癌的最新诊治手段进行详细介绍的同时,还展示了大量作者及所在单位关于甲状腺癌诊治的真实彩色照片,直观明了。

他山之石，可以攻玉。我们相信随着 Thyroid Cancer 中文版的发布，国内同道借鉴本书的内容，吸取国际最新甲状腺癌治疗经验，将来在面对甲状腺癌的挑战时会更加从容规范，并在此领域作出更多突破。

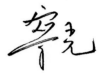

中国工程院院士
上海交通大学医学院附属瑞金医院院长
2021 年 11 月

原 著 序

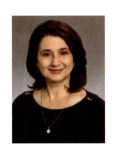

Adriana G Ioachimescu, MD, PhD, FACE
顾　问

我们可以看到，*Endocrinology and Metabolism Clinics of North America* 中的 *Thyroid Cancer* 这一分册，为近些年经历了重大变化的医学进展提供了深刻而广泛的新话题。在此，我们特别邀请到约翰斯·霍普金斯大学医学院医学、肿瘤病理学和细胞分子医学系邢明照教授作为特邀主编参与进来。邢明照教授是甲状腺肿瘤领域的杰出研究者，他的工作对甲状腺肿瘤的分子生物学和临床医学的发展有着重大影响，在基于分子层面的甲状腺肿瘤的疾病管理方面尤为突出。此外，本书的编者们有着丰富的临床背景，包含内分泌学家、外科医生、病理学家、核医学专家、肿瘤学家、基础科学家等，一同提供了相关的跨学科解决方案。

大量科学信息的积累推动了针对甲状腺癌患者的风险分层和个体化治疗方案的发展。本书为治疗此类疾病的医务工作者提供了必要的新知识、新进展。比如，本书提供了关于流行病学、组织学分类，以及用于确定甲状腺结节诊断和预后的遗传和分子标记方法。本书内容涵盖所有类型的甲状腺癌，包括乳头状癌、未分化癌，以及甲状腺髓样癌。全面分析甲状腺癌患者的临床评价与管理，包括手术选择、放射性碘治疗、甲状腺激素抑制治疗和为难治性病例提供新的治疗方案。另外，低风险乳头状甲状腺癌患者的积极监测受到了临床高度重视，本书对此进行了充分的评估。

我希望大家都有机会阅读 *Thyroid Cancer* 一书。您会发现书中的内容充实有趣，并且对您的临床实践大有裨益。在此，我再次感谢特邀主编邢明照教授对本书的贡献，也感谢其他编者们的出色贡献。此外，还要感谢爱思唯尔公司编辑工作人员的大力支持。

Adriana G. Ioachimescu, MD, PhD, FACE
Emory University School of Medicine
1365 B Clifton Road, Northeast, B6209
Atlanta, GA 30322, USA

E-mail address:
aioachi@emory.edu

原著前言

迈进甲状腺肿瘤精准诊疗的新时代

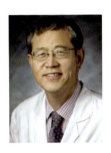

邢明照(Mingzhao Xing), MD, PhD
主　编

甲状腺癌是一种常见的内分泌恶性肿瘤。近些年来,其发病率迅速上升,累积病例数达到了前所未有的数量。绝大多数甲状腺癌患者临床预后良好。然而,另外一些患者的临床结果不佳,尽管是少数。因此,并非所有甲状腺癌患者的表现和最后的结果都是一样的。这就对临床医生提出了一项持续的挑战,即如何管理患者才会取得最佳的效果。通过最大限度地提高治疗获益,同时最大限度地减少治疗引起的负面结果,优化甲状腺癌治疗的经典理念已经演变为今天的个体化精确治疗理念。其实,运用这一简单、显而易见的概念一直是很具挑战性的。具体来说,直到今天,对原本就低风险的甲状腺癌患者的治疗过度和本性上属于侵袭性病例的治疗不足都普遍存在。受到近些年来循证医学原则和丰富的科学和临床数据的驱动,这种情况正在发生改变。今天,人们对于甲状腺癌分子层面的发病机制和临床表现的理解已远胜从前。这也为从根本上提升甲状腺肿瘤最佳诊治的准确性奠定了基础。这一巨大的进步已发生在甲状腺癌的几乎所有的临床诊疗方面,包括现代组织病理学分类、现代流行病学、临床和分子诊断、临床动态评估、基于遗传的风险分层和管理、优化设计的甲状腺切除术、精确确定颈部淋巴结清扫、美容性内镜手术、放射性碘治疗的测量选择和管理、甲状腺激素抑制治疗分层、治疗后动态监测的卫生经济学诊断策略、针对低风险甲状腺癌的适当治疗、进行性分化型甲状腺癌的新药物治疗,以及对未分化甲状腺癌和甲状腺髓样癌的特殊疾病管理等内容。

Thyroid Cancer 一书 19 章内容涵盖了以上所有话题。虽然患者的治疗是单独进行的个体,但甲状腺癌治疗过程中的所有临床领域都是系统连接的。因此,建议读者将本书作为整体进行阅读。具体而言,甲状腺癌患者的治疗是一个庞大的多步骤、系统性的管理体系,应根据疾病情况对个体患者进行精准治疗。另外,在这些步骤中的每一阶段,正如书中文章所作的广泛的讨论一样,个性化的精确疾病管理原则也应会被应用其中。

我们正在进入一个甲状腺肿瘤领域快速发展和飞跃的新时代。我很荣幸受到爱思唯尔公司邀请担任本书的主编。非常幸运能跟如此多的甲状腺肿瘤领域的杰出的国际专家和学术团队合作,有机会让这本书面世。在此,特别感谢各位专家慷慨接受邀请,为上述的每一个重要学术领域贡献的每一篇精彩绝伦的文章。我相信,这些学术贡献会在未来几年的甲状腺肿瘤领域广为应用,成为极为重要、富有价值的参考。一如既往,科学不停发展,不断地改变我们的理念,作者个人的观点偏颇也几乎无可避免。因此,建议读者在阅读和理解本书内容时,带有自己批判性的思考和认识。

邢明照(Mingzhao Xing),MD,PhD
School of Medicine
Southern University of Science and Technology
Shenzhen, Guangdong 518055, China

Department of Medicine
Johns Hopkins University School of Medicine
Baltimore, MD 21207, USA

E-mail address:
xingmz@sustech.edu.cn
mxing1@jhmi.edu

目 录

第 1 章　甲状腺癌的组织学分类 ························· 1

第 2 章　甲状腺癌流行病学研究进展 ··················· 25

第 3 章　甲状腺癌发生、发展中的编码分子 ············ 39

第 4 章　甲状腺结节临床诊断的评估 ··················· 65

第 5 章　甲状腺结节的分子诊断 ························ 91

第 6 章　分化型甲状腺癌的临床评估和风险分层 ······ 105

第 7 章　基因检测指导甲状腺癌风险评估与诊治决策 ·· 117

第 8 章　常规甲状腺切除术治疗原发性甲状腺癌 ······ 135

第 9 章　颈部淋巴结清扫在甲状腺癌手术治疗中的应用 ·· 153

第 10 章　传统机器人内镜甲状腺切除术在甲状腺癌治疗中的应用 ········ 163

第 11 章　经口内镜甲状腺癌手术 ······················ 175

第 12 章　分化型甲状腺癌的常规放射性碘治疗 ········ 193

第 13 章　甲状腺微小乳头状癌的处理 ················· 213

第 14 章　低危甲状腺乳头状微小癌的保守治疗 ⋯⋯⋯⋯⋯⋯⋯⋯⋯⋯⋯⋯⋯229

第 15 章　甲状腺癌的激素抑制治疗 ⋯⋯⋯⋯⋯⋯⋯⋯⋯⋯⋯⋯⋯⋯⋯⋯⋯⋯243

第 16 章　进展性放射性碘难治性甲状腺癌的新药治疗 ⋯⋯⋯⋯⋯⋯⋯⋯⋯255

第 17 章　分化型甲状腺癌复发的监测 ⋯⋯⋯⋯⋯⋯⋯⋯⋯⋯⋯⋯⋯⋯⋯⋯273

第 18 章　甲状腺未分化癌的诊断与治疗 ⋯⋯⋯⋯⋯⋯⋯⋯⋯⋯⋯⋯⋯⋯⋯289

第 19 章　甲状腺髓样癌的管理 ⋯⋯⋯⋯⋯⋯⋯⋯⋯⋯⋯⋯⋯⋯⋯⋯⋯⋯⋯⋯307

第1章
甲状腺癌的组织学分类

Sylvia L. Asa

关键词

- 甲状腺癌 • 分类 • 组织形态学 • 细胞学 • 基因型与表型的关系
- 预后

要点

- 在分化型甲状腺肿瘤中,根据基因型与表型的相关性可以将其分为"RAS样"滤泡状肿瘤或"BRAF样"乳头状癌。在组织形态学和表达谱方面的研究显示,"RAS样"滤泡状肿瘤分化程度更高。
- 滤泡状肿瘤缺乏非典型性核型(伴随低风险的非典型细胞学特点),提示肿瘤可能是良性的,无或仅有极低侵袭性。而伴有血管浸润则预示远处转移,提示其为侵袭性肿瘤。
- 具有乳头状结构的良性肿瘤和导致临床或亚临床甲状腺功能亢进且细胞学检查结果为良性的功能性肿瘤在TSH受体信号转导通路中具有独特的突变。
- 乳头状癌中惰性的微小癌,在欧美国家主张可以采用积极的监测(国内仍主张手术治疗为主),而一些浸润性病变需要临床干预。这些侵袭性肿瘤包括鞋钉状、高细胞和柱状亚型,会因为遗传和/或表观遗传改变而具有侵袭性。
- 伴有其他基因突变、重排和/或拷贝数变异的甲状腺癌会发生进展,转变为低分化和未分化癌。

引言

甲状腺癌具有广泛的病理学形态和生物学行为,包括最常见的惰性肿瘤,以及侵袭性强、致死性高的恶性肿瘤。在甲状腺癌的识别、诊断和预后中,病理学的应用是非常重要的。过去的10年中,甲状腺癌的分子基础研究方面取得了巨大进展,且已经证明甲状腺癌的基因型与表型关系非常紧密。但是分子研究也表明,甲状腺癌的预后不仅取决于遗传的改变。许多项研究证明,遗传和表观遗传学改变以及不良的组织病理学特征都对甲状腺癌的预后有很大的影响。

本章主要总结甲状腺滤泡细胞衍生肿瘤的组织学特征。提醒读者,还有许多其他类型的甲状腺癌,包括起源于滤泡旁C细胞、与降钙素生成有关的髓样癌,起源于甲状旁腺、胸腺和唾液腺的肿瘤,它们可能位于甲状腺内或附近,以及间质恶性肿瘤、淋巴样肿瘤和转移性病变,本章不对这些病理类型的肿瘤进行叙述。

本章讨论了滤泡细胞来源的甲状腺肿瘤的主要类型,针对其历史演变、分子相关性以及涉及组织学各成分的最新意义(包括结构、生长模式、细胞学和侵袭方式)展开,回顾了这些特征对预后的影响。对甲状腺癌组织学类型的了解的提高有助于促进细胞学筛查和诊断以及患者管理(包括积极监测,甲状腺腺叶切除术或全甲状腺切除术伴有或不伴有淋巴结清扫,放射性碘治疗或更积极的肿瘤学方法)。修订后的组织学分类产生了新的风险分层,因此,需要进一步阐明临床病理相关性,合理配置资源,权衡患者依从性以及治疗不足和治疗过度的实际风险和预期风险,从而平衡患者管理方式。

形态学分类:历史回顾

20世纪以来,甲状腺癌的分类经历了多次变化。在1953年出版的第一本《甲状腺肿瘤病理学分册》(*Armed Forces Institute of Pathology Fascicle*)中,分化型甲状腺癌的分类非常简单(表1.1):分为良性和恶性肿瘤,根据结构进行区分,每种都分为乳头状和滤泡状两种类型[1,2]。根据肿瘤侵出包膜,周围组织和/或血管的浸润等侵袭行为,病变可被诊断恶性。有趣的是,当时大多数腺瘤是滤泡状的(图1.1),而归类为"乳头状囊腺瘤"的肿瘤是第二大最常见的腺瘤类型[3]。然而,即使在非侵袭性乳头状肿瘤中也有转移性疾病的报道[4],很快就发现几乎所有具有乳头状结构的肿瘤都有可能转移。因此,是否存在真正良性的乳头状肿瘤成为一个问题[5,6]。

表 1.1 甲状腺滤泡细胞原发性肿瘤的分类(大约 1953 年)		
良性		滤泡状腺瘤
		乳头状囊腺瘤
恶性	分化	滤泡状癌
		乳头状癌
	未分化	间变性癌

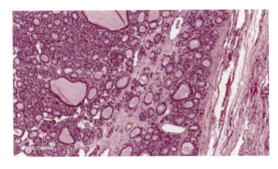

图 1.1 滤泡状腺瘤。滤泡状腺瘤是甲状腺滤泡细胞的良性肿瘤。它通常具有良好的边界并且是非侵袭性的,由滤泡组成,滤泡由单核扁平的上皮细胞覆盖,核圆且深染(苏木精-伊红染色,放大倍数 200μm)

遗憾的是,尽管有明确的临床和分子数据支持其作为功能性结节的基础(图 1.2),但乳头状腺瘤的概念已被淘汰并且没有被重新使用[2,7-11]。由于许多"乳头状癌"具有明显的滤泡状结构,使得基于结构的分类变得复杂[12-14]。因此,"乳头状和滤泡状混合型"甲状腺癌的时代到来了,尽管这些肿瘤的表现方式与经典型乳头状癌相同。

对乳头状癌的细胞学特征的认知增加了这一领域的挑战。Lindsa[14]在 1960 年认识到,与染色质的透明和边集相关的特征性核增大造成了"毛玻璃样外观"和不规则的核轮廓(图 1.3),他报道了在具有滤泡结构且发生淋巴结转移的肿瘤中发生了相同的核变化。这种异型性核由于与卡通人物小孤儿安妮(Annie)的眼睛相似而被 Nancy Warner 命名为"孤儿安妮眼核(Orphan Annie eye nuclei)"[15]。尽管事实上核透明有时在甲状腺中可能被看作人工假象[16,17],但核异型性却极为重要。1977 年,Chen 和 Rosai 的论文中再次强调了这一点,并普及了"乳头状癌的滤泡亚型"的术语[18],该亚型成为甲状腺癌的主要类型。

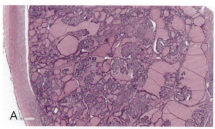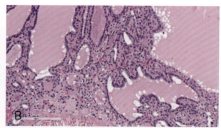

图 1.2 乳头状腺瘤。活跃的滤泡上皮性良性肿瘤的特征是乳头状结构,与乳头状癌杂乱的乳头不同。这些肿瘤具有完整的乳头状结构,但它们有组织地排列在滤泡内,并且具有明显的向心性(A)(苏木精-伊红染色,放大倍数 700μm)。乳头内层的细胞核很拥挤,但仍然是圆形的、相对均匀的,具有基本方向性。在细胞表面形成明显的扇形胶质(B)(苏木精-伊红染色,放大倍数 200μm)

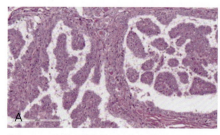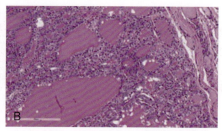

图 1.3 分化型甲状腺癌中的核异型性。乳头状癌的特征是具有一系列核特征(A)(苏木精-伊红染色,放大倍数 200μm),包括增大、伸长、拥挤和重叠,染色质边集造成的核浆透明以及可形成不规则核沟,可见为线性凹槽或形成核内假包涵体有多个微核仁。在滤泡样肿瘤中,核异型性不明显。通常细胞核拥挤、重叠和伸长不明显,但核仍有染色质透明、边集和突出,常表现为多个核仁和核形状不规则(B)(苏木精-伊红染色,放大倍数 200μm)

最初在 20 世纪 80 年代,分化较差的甲状腺癌被认为罕见但侵袭性高的甲状腺癌,其不像未分化癌一样分化低或迅速致死[19,20](表 1.2)[21]。在随后的几十年中,也出现了新的乳头状癌变异体,比传统的甲状腺乳头状癌(papillary thyroid carcinoma,PTC)更具侵略性,这些亚型包括高细胞亚型[22-25]、极少见的柱状细胞亚型[26,27],以及新发现的钉状细胞亚型[28-30]。这些亚型大多是在分化癌中产生的,其少数与未分化癌去分化相关,为甲状腺癌进行性去分化的概念铺平了道路[31]。

到 2004 年,世界卫生组织(World Health Organization,WHO)关于内分泌肿瘤[32]的书中将所有显示为"独特核特征"的肿瘤归类为乳头状癌变异体[32](表 1.3)。这些核特征在三维重建中得到了很好的描绘[33],并将核膜成分 emerin 蛋白进行染色,突出显示了核形态[34,35]。自此,结构变得不那么重要了,并且浸润对于诊断乳头状癌不是必需条件,因此它对恶性的诊断不再那么重要。越来越多的滤泡样肿瘤被重新分类为乳头状癌,滤泡癌的发生率也相应下降[36]。

表 1.2 滤泡细胞衍生的原发性甲状腺肿瘤的分类(1992年)		
良性肿瘤		滤泡样腺瘤
		• 经典型
		• 变异型
恶性肿瘤	分化型	滤泡癌
		乳头状癌
		• 经典型
		• 变异型
	低分化	岛状癌
		其他
	未分化	未分化癌

Rosai J, Carcangiu ML, DeLellis RA. Tumors of the thyroid gland.atlas of tumor pathology, Third Series, Fascicle 5.Washington, DC: Armed Forces Institute of Pathology; 1992.

表 1.3 滤泡细胞起源的原发性甲状腺癌的分类(2004年)		
良性		甲状腺滤泡状癌
		• 多种变异
		透明小梁瘤
恶性	高分化	乳头状癌
		• 多种变异
		滤泡状癌
		• 微小浸润
		• 广泛浸润
	低分化	低分化癌
	未分化	未分化癌

DeLellis RA, Lloyd RV, Heitz PU, et al. Pathology and genetics of tumours of endocrine organs. Lyon (France): IARC Press; 2004.

然而，滤泡亚型甲状腺乳头状癌（follicular variant papillary thyroid carcinoma，FVPTC）的诊断标准是目前病理学研究中最具争议的问题之一，在观察者内部和观察者之间都存在明显差异[37-40]。2016年，已有研究提出对核异型认识和分级的共识[41]。此外，在不同的疾病中也可见到相同的核异型性，如甲状腺炎也可有异型性[42]，这一现象常见于甲状腺早期活检中[43]。

目前，关于甲状腺癌的浸润分类并没有形成统一的规范，且这一方面在文献中也存在较大争议。当浸润范围广泛时不难评估。而由于一些因素，范围很小的浸润很难评估[44]。评估浸润的一个重要决定因素是观察的程度：被膜组织越多，切片越多，越容易发现微小的浸润。另一个争议是将病变归类为侵袭性病变所必需的浸润程度：是否需要为全层浸润，或者浸润到包膜内就归类为浸润。再有，因为绝大多数患者都会进行术前活检，真正的浸润与活检后的伪影很难区分[43]。

滤泡状癌的诊断完全依赖于识别强侵袭性，而乳头状癌的侵袭力相对较弱，因为它们通常较少侵犯血管和转移至局部区域淋巴结，而侵袭性滤泡癌通常侵犯血管，血行转移，并引起远处转移。因此，人们开始相信乳头状癌是所有癌症中惰性程度最高的，而滤泡癌更具侵袭性。

随着研究甲状腺癌的分子工具的出现，尤其是基因改变和基因表达谱的出现，为了解甲状腺癌的形态提供了机会，从而产生了挑战这些概念的新思想。

分子遗传学的影响：基因型与表型的相关性

早在1987年，科学家们在PTC中就发现了基因突变。*RET/PTC*致癌基因的确定为染色体重排产生融合蛋白导致细胞转化提供了证据[45]。正在进行的研究通过涉及*TRK*[46]和*PAX8-PPARG*[47,48]的重排增加了新的认知。甲状腺癌与先前的头颈辐射之间的联系已被证实[49-51]，日本原子弹爆炸和切尔诺贝利核灾难的幸存者提供了证据，证明辐射是这些染色体改变的基础[52-58]。然而，很明显，在散发的乳头状癌中最常见的是*BRAF V600E*突变[59-62]。乳头状癌的发生涉及两条通路，一条基于散发性癌症的点突变，另一条基于辐射的基因重排[62-64]。

滤泡样病变的主要分子改变是*RAS*家族基因突变[64]；这些突变见于滤泡状甲状腺癌和甲状腺乳头状癌滤泡亚型，也见于良性滤泡状腺瘤，甚至在散发性甲状腺肿的结节中也可见到[64-75]。*RAS*突变能否预测肿瘤侵袭能力目前存在较大争议[75]，由于良性病变中经常可检出*RAS*突变，因此认为该类型突变发生在甲状腺滤泡上皮转化的早期,不能用于预测侵袭性恶性肿瘤。

TCGA 数据库分析强调了遗传改变对 PTC 的进展的重要性[76]。这项研究根据肿瘤的基因改变对其进行分类,并确定了一些新的突变和重排。Veronica Valvo 和 Carmelo Nucera 在文章《编码分子决定甲状腺癌发展和进展》中也进行了相关讨论。一个主要的发现是,该文章将 PTC 分为两类:"BRAF 样"肿瘤表现为 *BRAF V600E* 突变或重排,而"RAS 样"肿瘤则具有 *RAS* 突变。BRAF 样肿瘤包括经典型 PTC,伴弥漫性或局灶性乳头状结构,通常为浸润性生长;而 RAS 样肿瘤是边界清晰的 FVPTC。即使没有这些特殊突变或重排的肿瘤,也以其结构归入上述类别。从这些肿瘤的表达谱中我们获得了更多的见解。很明显,滤泡样病变比乳头状结构的病变更具分化性,病理学家对此并不感到惊讶。分子图谱上 FVPTC 与 FTC 具有相似性,这给 FVPTC 与 FTC 的有效区分带来了困惑。事实上,一种更简单的分类方法是认为核异型性是任何甲状腺癌的特征,而不仅仅是乳头状癌的;分化型甲状腺癌应根据其结构分类为滤泡或乳头状[77]。这将导致每种肿瘤类型的分类都将改变,大量低风险、可能没有或只有很小的侵袭力且只有核异型性的肿瘤将划为滤泡癌,滤泡癌的发病率将显著增加。

上述问题是由非侵袭性包膜内 FVPTC 的重新分类引起的,该亚型是已知的低风险亚型,应减少过度治疗。这一举措虽然在其既定目标上令人钦佩,但却导致了有人建议将此类肿瘤重新命名为具有乳头状核特征的非侵袭性滤泡状甲状腺肿瘤(non-invasive follicular thyroid neoplasm with papillary-like nuclear feature,NIFT-P)[41]。该提议强调了核异型性重要性,且当这一肿瘤突然被重新归类为"非癌"时[78],该提议也产生了混淆,尽管即使应用严格的判定标准,它们也存在转移的风险[79,80]。不过度治疗低风险甲状腺癌是至关重要的,不是只有改名这一种方法,对临床医生进行宣教和制定低风险疾病管理指南都是可以选择的方法[81]。该提议不太可能达到减少过度诊断的目的,因为 NIFT-P 的发病率不高,尤其是在美国以外[79,80,82-84]。此外,这些病变需要手术诊断,只能影响放射性碘治疗的选择。事实上,通过积极筛查发现更多的微小癌[85]并加以处理[86]是过度诊治的重要原因之一,而这种重新分类并不影响过度诊断的真正原因。

在 2017 年 WHO 的内分泌肿瘤的分类(表 1.4)[87]中,可见目前甲状腺癌分类的复杂性。肿瘤边缘多态性的增加,包括 NIFT-P 和"恶性潜能未定的肿瘤"(uncertain malignant potential,UMP),没有明确如何从可能性低但有明确转移可能的病变中辨认真正的良性病变[79,80,83]。

表 1.4
世界卫生组织 2017 年滤泡细胞来源的原发性甲状腺肿瘤分类

良性	甲状腺滤泡状腺瘤	
交界性/不确定	透明小梁瘤	
	其他囊性滤泡样肿瘤	恶性潜能未定的滤泡状肿瘤
		恶性潜能未定的高分化瘤
		NIFT-P
恶性	甲状腺乳头状癌	甲状腺乳头状癌
		滤泡状乳头状癌
		包裹型乳头状癌
		微小乳头状癌
		柱状细胞型
		嗜酸细胞型
	甲状腺滤泡腺癌	滤泡腺癌,微小浸润型
		滤泡腺癌,包裹型血管浸润型
		滤泡腺癌,广泛浸润型
	嗜酸(Hürthle)细胞肿瘤	嗜酸(Hürthle)细胞癌
	甲状腺低分化癌	
	甲状腺未分化癌	

Lloyd RV, Osamura RY, Kloppel G, et al. WHO classification of tumours of endocrine organs (4th edition). Lyon (France): IARC Press; 2017.

甲状腺癌的形态特征

尽管在过去的 70 年里发生了许多争议和变化,但不可否认的是,甲状腺癌表现出一系列与临床行为相关的形态学特征。分化良好的肿瘤具有滤泡结构,与正常甲状腺相似。当它们没有细胞核异型性(图 1.1),且没有侵犯包膜的证据(如果有包膜),或没有侵犯周围实质的证据(如果没有包膜)时,它们可能是良性的。当它们表现出核异型性和/或局部侵袭能力极小时,它们可能是低风险的癌症(图 1.4)。这些肿瘤的诊断基于完整的组织病理学检查[88],只能在手术切除后进行;良好的临床管理的学习是基于对低危患者(根据美国甲状腺协会指南[81])行甲状腺腺叶切除术的意愿,这些患者在超声或其他影像学上表现为轮廓清晰、均匀膨胀性肿块。高风险的滤泡癌识别基于更明显的侵袭性,包括多灶性、包膜和周围组织的肉眼侵犯和/或血管侵犯(图 1.5)。然而,血管侵犯目前存在争议[89,90],如果想利用这一特征来确定积极的治疗,则应要求有更有价值的研究来预测血管侵犯对预测远处转移的意义[89]。

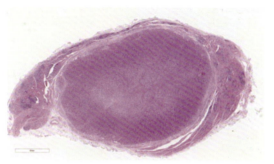

图 1.4　低风险滤泡癌。肿瘤边界清晰,包膜完整,包膜内可见浅表浸润,无广泛浸润,无血管浸润(HE 染色,放大倍数 2mm)

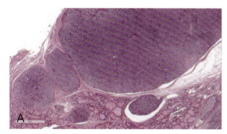 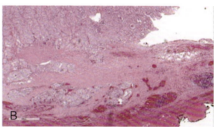

图 1.5　高风险的滤泡细胞癌。这些肿瘤具有广泛侵袭性(A)(HE 染色,放大倍数 2mm)和/或可能表现为脉管浸润(B)(HE 染色,放大倍数 500μm),提供了能够引起远处转移的证据

从分子水平上看,甲状腺乳头状癌比甲状腺滤泡样癌的分化水平更差一些,这些 BRAF 样肿瘤的乳头状结构至少具有局灶性,如果是免疫弥漫性,还具有丰富的核异型性(图 1.6)。这些乳头状结构通常是浸润性的,但也可能有边界清楚的病灶或可能是局限膨胀性的病变,甚至完全在包膜内增长。此类肿瘤多见微钙化物质,砂粒体是经典亚型 PTC 的标志。这种类型的钙化与蛋壳型的钙化形成对比,蛋壳型的钙化通常出现在任何甲状腺病灶的包膜周围。以往的研究表明,*BRAF V600E* 突变提示患者预后较差,实际上是由于该突变能够将经典型 PTC 与滤泡状 PTC 区别开[91];然而,在经典型 PTC 中,当所有其他指标(如肿瘤大小和患者人口学数据)具有可比性时,*BRAFV600E* 突变的 PTC 并不比非 *BRAF V600E* 突变的 PTC 更具侵袭性[92]。

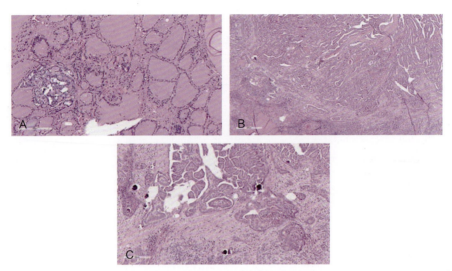

图 1.6 乳头状癌。经典乳头状癌可能是一种小而惰性的病变,可作为微小癌(A)偶然被发现(HE 染色,放大倍数 200μm),也可能是一种大的浸润性肿瘤。这些病变具有复杂乳头状结构(B)(HE 染色,放大倍数 400μm),也可能含有砂粒体(C)(HE 染色,放大倍数 200μm),同心螺环的钙化被认为是退化的乳头状突起,但实际上是肿瘤细胞破裂后的细胞质所形成的

大多数伴有 RET/PTC 重组的甲状腺癌是经典型 PTC 或其变异体[76,93],而伴有 RET/PTC3 的甲状腺癌往往是实性亚型或局灶实性型[94-96]。TRK 重组在有放射史的患者和儿童人群中更常见[46,50,55,58,97,98]。相反,最初在滤泡癌中发现的 PAX8-PPARG 重组在 FVPTC 中具有特征性[47,99]。弥漫硬化型是一种典型的 PTC,通常多发于儿童和年轻人。许多 PTC 因为间质纤维化,容易被误诊为此型;真正的弥漫性硬化型 PTC 是一种高浸润性病变,可导致甲状腺肿大,但因为没有肿块,影像检查或肉眼判断都很难确认[100-103]。虽然肿瘤形成典型的乳头状突起,但它们嵌在纤维间质内,并有通过淋巴管向整个腺体和邻近淋巴结弥散的倾向。砂粒体数量众多且分布广泛。这些病变通常不包含 BRAF V600E 突变,但有文献报道,这些病变存在基因重组,包括 RET/PTC 和 ALK 融合[104-106]。

特定亚型乳头状癌显著影响预后并具有更高的侵袭性,包括鞋钉样亚型[28-30]、高细胞亚型[22-25]、柱状细胞亚型[26,27](图 1.7)。我们主要根据细胞学的形态学标准去定义这些病变:鞋钉样细胞有与鞋钉相似的含有顶核的细胞表面突起;高细胞亚型的定义是高宽比超过 3∶1,柱状细胞被拉长,呈纺锤形,细胞核分叶,呈空泡状。这些类型的肿瘤还具有一些独

特的结构特征:高细胞型 PTC 中"履带式"滤泡拉长;柱状细胞型被认为与子宫内膜瘤相似,鞋钉细胞型有明显的水肿和/或纤维化乳头状突起,这些肿瘤常含有 BRAF V600E 突变和 BRAF 样病变[76]。此外,高细胞型 PTC 具有表观遗传改变,并借此独立出来成为一个更具侵略性的亚型[76],它们可能有 TERT 启动子突变,这样可以解释更多侵袭行为[107]。最近的研究表明,鞋钉样细胞瘤表现出较差的 TERT 和 p53 突变[108,109]。分化较差的甲状腺癌(图 1.8)表现为甲状腺正常形态的丧失,取而代之的是实巢或小梁,含有个别肿瘤细胞坏死或有丝分裂活性高[19,20,110,111]。实巢状结构与神经内分泌肿瘤的巢状结构相似,因此,它们有时被归类为"岛状癌"[19],而小梁形态在外观上更像筛状细胞。

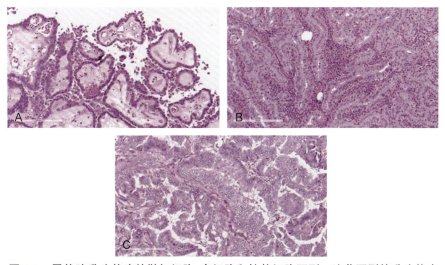

图 1.7　甲状腺乳头状癌的鞋钉细胞、高细胞和柱状细胞亚型。这些亚型的乳头状癌更具有侵袭性,除具有经典的乳头状结构之外,还因基于细胞学和一些独有的特征而被区分开来。鞋钉细胞亚型(A)的肿瘤细胞显示表面拉伸而类似于鞋钉样;还通常具有扩张的水肿乳头。高细胞亚型由拥挤拉长的细胞构成,高:宽超过 3:1(B);并形成轨道样改变。柱状细胞肿瘤具有明显拥挤和重叠的假复层细胞核以及胞浆空泡(C)(苏木精 - 伊红染色,放大倍数 200μm)

　　未分化癌是完全未分化的恶性肿瘤(图 1.9),没有证据证实其起源于甲状腺滤泡上皮;仔细观察未分化癌中,有时可以观察到局部的分化型和低分化型甲状腺癌,进而可证实未分化癌起源于分化细胞的进行性去分化[31]。当病变中缺乏局部的分化型和低分化型甲状腺癌细胞时,即可排除这一诊断,因为这一病变也可能是肉瘤或其他病变。

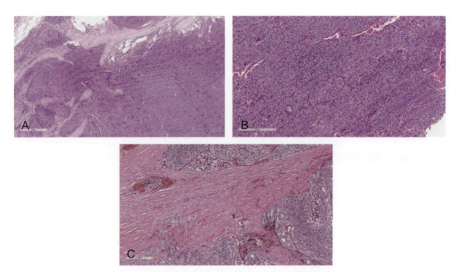

图1.8 低分化甲状腺癌。这些肿瘤比滤泡癌或乳头状癌分化差,但不到未分化癌的未分化程度。低分化甲状腺癌通常由类似于神经内分泌肿瘤的实性细胞巢和成片肿瘤细胞构成,因此又称"岛状癌"。通常呈广泛性浸润(A)(苏木精-伊红染色,放大倍数700μm),有单个肿瘤细胞坏死(B)(苏木精-伊红染色,放大倍数300μm),并通常显示血管浸润(C)(苏木精-伊红染色,放大倍数200μm)

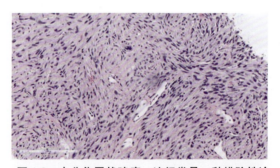

图1.9 未分化甲状腺癌。这经常是一种排除性诊断,因为这类肿瘤完全由未分化的梭形和巨细胞构成,缺乏分化相关的生物标记物;核分裂象多见且多为病理性核分裂。确诊是通过识别分化成分,从这些成分中可以证实其从甲状腺癌进展而来(苏木精-伊红染色,放大倍数200μm)

　　基于细胞学特征,诸如嗜酸性变和细胞透明变,可确定所有类型的分化型甲状腺癌的亚型。嗜酸性变和细胞透明变经常是相关的,虽然偶尔肿瘤的透明胞浆是由于糖原或脂质的累积,多数细胞透明变是与线粒体的异常有关的。关于嗜酸性变和细胞透明变可出现在传统甲状腺癌变异型中是有争议的。现在被广泛接受的是在滤泡状腺瘤、滤泡癌和乳头状癌中可以出现局灶或弥漫的嗜酸性变(图 1.10),并且在这些肿瘤中,与正常驱动改变相关的突变和重排确实已被 *GRIM19* 线粒体 DNA 的改变和突变所证实[112-118]。很明显,低分化癌同样可以具有广泛的嗜酸性改变[119-121],这也解释了这些更具侵袭性的嗜酸性恶性肿瘤被称为"Hürthle 细胞癌"(Hürthle 细胞癌是应该回避的错误的名字,因为事实上 Karl Hürthle 描述的是 C 细胞)[122]。最新研究证实了在更具侵袭性的低分化嗜酸性癌中存在线粒体基因的改变以及有意义的基因拷贝数改变[123,124]。

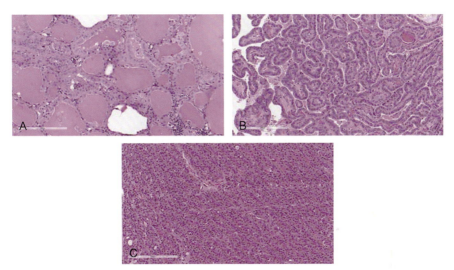

图 1.10　嗜酸细胞肿瘤。任何类型的甲状腺肿瘤中均可见到嗜酸性变,包括滤泡状腺瘤(未显示),滤泡癌或滤泡亚型乳头状癌(A),经典型乳头状癌(B),以及低分化癌(C)(苏木精 - 伊红染色,放大倍数 200μm)

预后因素

对于甲状腺医生而言,一个主要的临床目标是可否通过甲状腺肿瘤的形态学和分子特征来证实何种类型甲状腺肿瘤比其他类型肿瘤更具有侵袭性。

在分化型甲状腺癌中,已经报道了一些生物标记物、分子改变和表观遗传学特征,包括微 RNA[125]。可以预测进展的形态学特征亦是重要的[126]。临床参数,包括年龄、性别和危险因素也都具有重要相关性[127]。

被广泛接受的是肿瘤大小和生长速度是重要的临床参数,其可以将接受动态监测的经典型 PTC 中的微小癌与需要外科手术的大的浸润性癌区别开来。

微小浸润型 FTC 和包裹型 FVPTC 或 NIFT-P,甚至包括低风险的临床可检测出的经典型 PTC,普遍被认为进行甲状腺部分切除是足够的[41,128,129],而不需要全甲状腺切除或淋巴结清扫[130,131]。相反,对于具有鞋钉样、高细胞或柱状细胞型 PTC,需要更加仔细地评估来决定这些肿瘤是否有甲状腺外侵犯或区域淋巴结转移。一旦乳头状癌或滤泡癌显示有明确的血管浸润,则发生远处转移的可能性大大增加[89]。对任何存在局部去分化成分的肿瘤都应进行更加积极的治疗。平衡全甲状腺切除和放射性碘治疗的风险及可能的获益仍然是重要的,这需要对影响预后的大量相关因素的深刻理解。

对细胞学和筛查的影响

甲状腺肿瘤的分类和再分类导致了术前活检诊断的很多改变。很多专家从能够提供结构甚至可能的包膜信息的组织芯活检(core biopsy)转向依赖于细针穿刺抽吸(fine-needle aspiration,FNA)活检的细胞学检查;然而,这两种技术都是可以应用的[132-139]。

当核的形态是恶性肿瘤的重要特征时,细胞学对于区分良恶性病变是很有优势的。这种技术对于诊断良性甲状腺病变和识别明确的恶性肿瘤是非常卓越的。然而,甲状腺中的挑战是识别具有交界性细胞学异型性的滤泡病变。过去,甲状腺细胞学受制于多变的术语和描述性诊断。Bethesda 系统和几个其他国际合作组织开始规定甲状腺细胞学的明确分类[140-143]。这些指南提供了可以接受的敏感性和特异性的范围。然而,众所周知,这些标准在不同实验室之间是有差异的,因此推荐每个实验室提供他们的特异性的执行参数以使自己的临床医生可以在本实验室的背景下来解释这些诊断结果。

交界性肿瘤这一重新分类也带来了困惑。细胞学诊断的敏感性和特异性依赖于诊断者如何分类"正确的"诊断,即作为"金标准"的组织学最终诊断。许多实验室现在正为诊断为 NIFT-P(或 UMP)[144-147]的意义而努力研究;因为这些交界性病变,到底是因为细胞学阳性、假阳性,还是假阴性?

分子检测的应用可用来指导甲状腺结节患者的管理。主要应用于不确定细胞学诊断的病例。在某些情况下,这一手段确实很有帮助[148]。比如,明确 *BRAFV 600E* 突变可进一步确诊 PTC,然而具有显著的细胞异型性的经典型 PTC 的诊断并不困难,当组织学取样不充分而影响细胞学评估

时方能体现出 *BRAFV 600E* 突变检测的重要应用价值。相似地，*TERT* 启动子突变或其他不良事件的出现，比如 *p53* 突变或其他更具侵袭性的致癌改变，将改变原本认为的低风险疾病患者行甲状腺腺叶切除的治疗方案。目前，临床上已经有一些分子检测开展应用，包括基于突变分析，基因表达谱和表观遗传学，如微 RNA [149]。每种检测都有其优势和局限，具有明确的阳性预测值和阴性预测值。而且，额外的优势是因肿瘤发生率的不同而导致被研究的细胞学分类不同，这一特征在实验室和实验室之间有着广泛的差异。

总结

滤泡细胞起源的甲状腺癌是基于形态学和分子遗传学被很好认识的癌症谱系。这两者之间有很好的相关性。现在的分类过于复杂，需要简化来反映已被遗传学证实的早期的观点。

基本上，良性病变可以是滤泡状或乳头状，后者表现为"热结节"。高分化甲状腺癌是极低风险的，像 NIFT-P、UMP 或微浸润癌，它们在结构上是滤泡状的，生长方式是膨胀性的，具有一系列也可以呈侵袭性的细胞学异型性；这些病变具有极好的预后，大多数病例仅需要手术部分切除即可。一旦这些病变出现广泛浸润或血管浸润，它们将更具侵袭性并且需要全甲状腺切除作为放射性碘治疗的准备。甲状腺病理中的挑战之一是对两个决定性特征，包膜侵犯和血管浸润的准确定义和识别。乳头状癌是一种分化程度较前者略低的癌，偶有镜下病变显示缓慢生长，通常为偶然发现。这些常见的微小肿瘤的发现是"过度诊断"和"过度治疗"的重要原因。它们可以是浸润性的或边界清楚的，并且具有以砂砾体形式存在的钙化。有经验的临床医生会在临床背景下评估这些病变，当其呈明显惰性时，欧美国家建议可以保守处理（目前国内仍主张手术治疗为主）。与此相反，如果病变具有生长和/或局部播散的临床证据，需要全甲状腺切除和放射性碘的适当处理。再强调一次，存在的挑战是通过定义临床、形态学和生物标记物来区别哪些病例可以通过单独手术治愈，哪些病例有可能播散。我们已经知道甲状腺癌也可能会出现进展，进展为少见但更具侵袭性的低分化癌和未分化癌。

（潘 毅 郑向前）

参考文献

1. Warren S, Meissner WA. Tumors of the thyroid gland. Atlas of tumor pathology, Series 1, Fascicle 14. Washington, DC: Armed Forces Institute of Pathology; 1953.
2. Lyons J, Landis CA, Harsh G, et al. Two G protein oncogenes in human endocrine tumors. Science 1990;249:655–9.
3. Ackerman LV. Surgical pathology. 1st edition. St Louis (MO): C.V. Mosby; 1953.
4. Ackerman LV. Surgical pathology. 2nd edition. St Louis (MO): C.V. Mosby; 1959.
5. Meissner WA, Adler A. Papillary carcinoma of the thyroid. A study of the pathology of two hundred twenty-six cases. Arch Pathol 1958;66:518–25.
6. Meissner WA, Warren S. Tumors of the thyroid gland. atlas of tumor pathology, Series 2, Fascicle 4. Washington, DC: Armed Forces Institute of Pathology; 1969.
7. Parma J, Duprez L, van Sande J, et al. Somatic mutations in the thyrotropin receptor gene cause hyperfunctioning thyroid adenomas. Nature 1993;365:649–51.
8. Porcellini A, Ciullo I, Laviola L, et al. Novel mutations of thyrotropin receptor gene in thyroid hyperfunctioning adenomas. Rapid identification by fine needle aspiration biopsy. J Clin Endocrinol Metab 1994;79:657–61.
9. Russo D, Arturi F, Wicker R, et al. Genetic alterations in thyroid hyperfunctioning adenomas. J Clin Endocrinol Metab 1995;80:1347–51.
10. van Sande J, Parma J, Tonacchera M, et al. Genetic basis of endocrine disease. Somatic and germline mutations of the TSH receptor gene in thyroid diseases. J Clin Endocrinol Metab 1995;80:2577–85.
11. Krohn D, Fuhrer D, Holzapfel H, et al. Clonal origin of toxic thyroid nodules with constitutively activating thyrotropin receptor mutations. J Clin Endocrinol Metab 1998;83:180–4.
12. Lindsay S. Carcinoma of the thyroid gland. Springfield (IL): C.C. Thomas; 1960.
13. Lindsay S. Natural history of thyroid carcinoma. Ariz Med 1960;17:623–7.
14. Lindsay S. Carcinoma of the thyroid gland. A clinical and pathological study of 293 patients at the University of California Hospital. Springfield (IL): Charles C. Thomas; 1960.
15. DeLellis RA. Orphan Annie eye nuclei: a historical note. Am J Surg Pathol 1993;17(10):1067–8.
16. Hapke MR, Dehner LP. The optically clear nucleus. A reliable sign of papillary carcinoma of the thyroid? Am J Surg Pathol 1979;3:31–8.
17. Petrilli G, Fisogni S, Rosai J, et al. Nuclear bubbles (nuclear pseudo-pseudoinclusions): a pitfall in the interpretation of microscopic sections from the thyroid and other human organs. Am J Surg Pathol 2017;41(1):140–1.
18. Chen KTK, Rosai J. Follicular variant of thyroid papillary carcinoma: a clinicopathologic study of six cases. Am J Surg Pathol 1977;1(2):123–30.
19. Carcangiu ML, Zampi G, Rosai J. Poorly differentiated ("insular") thyroid carcinoma. A reinterpretation of Langhans' "wuchernde Struma". Am J Surg Pathol

1984;8:655–68.
20. Sakamoto A, Kasai N, Sugano H. Poorly differentiated carcinoma of the thyroid. A clinicopathologic entity for a high-risk group of papillary and follicular carcinomas. Cancer 1983;52:1849–55.
21. Rosai J, Carcangiu ML, DeLellis RA. Tumors of the thyroid gland. Atlas of tumor pathology, Third Series, Fascicle 5. Washington, DC: Armed Forces Institute of Pathology; 1992.
22. Hicks MJ, Batsakis JG. Tall cell carcinoma of the thyroid gland. Ann Otol Rhinol Laryngol 1993;102:402–3.
23. Flint A, Davenport RD, Lloyd RV. The tall cell variant of papillary carcinoma of the thyroid gland. Arch Pathol Lab Med 1991;115:169–71.
24. Akslen L, Varhaug JE. Thyroid carcinoma with mixed tall cell and columnar cell features. Am J Clin Pathol 1990;94:442–5.
25. Johnson TL, Lloyd RV, Thompson NW, et al. Prognostic implications of the tall cell variant of papillary thyroid carcinoma. Am J Surg Pathol 1988;12:22–7.
26. Wenig BM, Thompson LD, Adair CF, et al. Thyroid papillary carcinoma of columnar cell type: a clinicopathologic study of 16 cases. Cancer 1998;82(4):740–53.
27. Evans HL. Columnar-cell carcinoma of the thyroid. A report of two cases of an aggressive variant of thyroid carcinoma. Am J Clin Pathol 1986;85:77–80.
28. Asioli S, Maletta F, Pagni F, et al. Cytomorphologic and molecular features of hobnail variant of papillary thyroid carcinoma: case series and literature review. Diagn Cytopathol 2014;42(1):78–84.
29. Asioli S, Erickson LA, Sebo TJ, et al. Papillary thyroid carcinoma with prominent hobnail features: a new aggressive variant of moderately differentiated papillary carcinoma. A clinicopathologic, immunohistochemical, and molecular study of eight cases. Am J Surg Pathol 2010;34(1):44–52.
30. Motosugi U, Murata S, Nagata K, et al. Thyroid papillary carcinoma with micropapillary and hobnail growth pattern: a histological variant with intermediate malignancy? Thyroid 2009;19(5):535–7.
31. Kondo T, Ezzat S, Asa SL. Pathogenetic mechanisms in thyroid follicular-cell neoplasia. Nat Rev Cancer 2006;6(4):292–306.
32. DeLellis RA, Lloyd RV, Heitz PU, et al. Pathology and genetics of tumours of endocrine organs. Lyons (France): IARC Press; 2004.
33. Papotti M, Manazza AD, Chiarle R, et al. Confocal microscope analysis and tridimensional reconstruction of papillary thyroid carcinoma nuclei. Virchows Arch 2004;444(4):350–5.
34. Asioli S, Maletta F, Pacchioni D, et al. Cytological detection of papillary thyroid carcinomas by nuclear membrane decoration with emerin staining. Virchows Arch 2010;457(1):43–51.
35. Asioli S, Bussolati G. Emerin immunohistochemistry reveals diagnostic features of nuclear membrane arrangement in thyroid lesions. Histopathology 2009;54(5):571–9.
36. LiVolsi VA, Asa SL. The demise of follicular carcinoma of the thyroid gland. Thyroid 1994;4:233–5.
37. Hirokawa M, Carney JA, Goellner JR, et al. Observer variation of encapsulated follicular lesions of the thyroid gland. Am J Surg Pathol 2002;26(11):1508–14.

38. Lloyd RV, Erickson LA, Casey MB, et al. Observer variation in the diagnosis of follicular variant of papillary thyroid carcinoma. Am J Surg Pathol 2004;28(10): 1336–40.
39. Elsheikh TM, Asa SL, Chan JK, et al. Interobserver and intraobserver variation among experts in the diagnosis of thyroid follicular lesions with borderline nuclear features of papillary carcinoma. Am J Clin Pathol 2008;130(5):736–44.
40. Rosai J. Handling of thyroid follicular patterned lesions. Endocr Pathol 2005; 16(4):279–83.
41. Nikiforov YE, Seethala RR, Tallini G, et al. Nomenclature revision for encapsulated follicular variant of papillary thyroid carcinoma: a paradigm shift to reduce overtreatment of Indolent tumors. JAMA Oncol 2016;2(8):1023–9.
42. Chui MH, Cassol CA, Asa SL, et al. Follicular epithelial dysplasia of the thyroid: morphological and immunohistochemical characterization of a putative preneoplastic lesion to papillary thyroid carcinoma in chronic lymphocytic thyroiditis. Virchows Arch 2013;462(5):557–63.
43. LiVolsi VA, Merino MJ. Worrisome histologic alterations following fine needle aspiration of the thyroid. Pathol Annu 1994;29(2):99–120.
44. Seethala RR, Asa SL, Carty SE, et al. Protocol for the examination of specimens from patientswith carcinomas of the thyroid gland. 2014. Available at: http://www.cap.org/apps/docs/committees/cancer/cancer_protocols/2014/Thyroid_14Protocol_3100.pdf.
45. Fusco A, Grieco M, Santoro M, et al. A new oncogene in human thyroid papillary carcinomas and their lymph-nodal metastases. Nature 1987;328:170–2.
46. Bongarzone I, Vigneri P, Mariani L, et al. RET/NTRK1 rearrangements in thyroid gland tumors of the papillary carcinoma family: correlation with clinicopathological features. Clin Cancer Res 1998;4(1):223–8.
47. Kroll TG, Sarraf P, Pecciarini L, et al. PAX8-PPARgamma1 fusion oncogene in human thyroid carcinoma. Science 2000;289(5483):1357–60.
48. Castro P, Rebocho AP, Soares RJ, et al. PAX8-PPARă rearrangement is frequently detected in the follicular variant of papillary thyroid carcinoma. J Clin Endocrinol Metab 2006;91(1):213–20.
49. Robbins J, Schneider AB. Thyroid cancer following exposure to radioactive iodine. Rev Endocr Metab Disord 2000;1(3):197–203.
50. Bounacer A, Schlumberger M, Wicker R, et al. Search for NTRK1 proto-oncogene rearrangements in human thyroid tumours originated after therapeutic radiation. Br J Cancer 2000;82(2):308–14.
51. Ramljak V, Ranogajec I, Novosel I, et al. Thyroid tumour in a child previously treated for neuroblastoma. Cytopathology 2006;17(5):295–8.
52. Sampson RJ, Key CR, Buncher CR, et al. Thyroid carcinoma in Hiroshima and Nagasaki. I. Prevalence of thyroid carcinoma at autopsy. JAMA 1969;209(1): 65–70.
53. Ito T, Seyama T, Iwamoto KS, et al. In vitro irradiation is able to cause RET oncogene rearrangement. Cancer Res 1993;53(13):2940–3.
54. Nikiforov Y, Koshoffer A, Nikiforova M, et al. Chromosomal breakpoint positions sugeest a direct role for radiation in inducing illegitimate recombination between the ELE1 and RET genes in radiation-induced thyroid carcinomas. Oncogene 1999;18:6330–4.
55. Rabes HM, Demidchik EP, Sidorow JD, et al. Pattern of radiation-induced RET and NTRK1 rearrangements in 191 post-chernobyl papillary thyroid carcinomas: biological, phenotypic, and clinical implications. Clin Cancer Res 2000;6(3):

1093–103.
56. Williams D. Radiation carcinogenesis: lessons from Chernobyl. Oncogene 2008; 27(Suppl 2):S9–18.
57. Hamatani K, Mukai M, Takahashi K, et al. Rearranged anaplastic lymphoma kinase (ALK) gene in adult-onset papillary thyroid cancer amongst atomic bomb survivors. Thyroid 2012;22(11):1153–9.
58. Leeman-Neill RJ, Kelly LM, Liu P, et al. ETV6-NTRK3 is a common chromosomal rearrangement in radiation-associated thyroid cancer. Cancer 2014;120(6): 799–807.
59. Xu X, Quiros RM, Gattuso P, et al. High prevalence of BRAF gene mutation in papillary thyroid carcinomas and thyroid tumor cell lines. Cancer Res 2003; 63(15):4561–7.
60. Cohen Y, Xing M, Mambo E, et al. BRAF mutation in papillary thyroid carcinoma. J Natl Cancer Inst 2003;95(8):625–7.
61. Fukushima T, Suzuki S, Mashiko M, et al. BRAF mutations in papillary carcinomas of the thyroid. Oncogene 2003;22(41):6455–7.
62. Soares P, Trovisco V, Rocha AS, et al. BRAF mutations and RET/PTC rearrangements are alternative events in the etiopathogenesis of PTC. Oncogene 2003; 22(29):4578–80.
63. Nikiforova MN, Ciampi R, Salvatore G, et al. Low prevalence of BRAF mutations in radiation-induced thyroid tumors in contrast to sporadic papillary carcinomas. Cancer Lett 2004;209(1):1–6.
64. Giordano TJ, Kuick R, Thomas DG, et al. Molecular classification of papillary thyroid carcinoma: distinct BRAF, RAS, and RET/PTC mutation-specific gene expression profiles discovered by DNA microarray analysis. Oncogene 2005; 24(44):6646–56.
65. Suarez HG, du Villard JA, Caillou B, et al. Detection of activated *ras* oncogenes in human thyroid carcinomas. Oncogene 1988;2:403–6.
66. Lemoine NR, Mayall ES, Wyllie FS, et al. Activated *ras* oncogenes in human thyroid cancers. Cancer Res 1988;48:4459–63.
67. Lemoine NR, Mayall ES, Wyllie FS, et al. High frequency of *ras* oncogene activation in all stages of human thyroid tumorigenesis. Oncogene 1989;4:159–64.
68. Wright PA, Lemoine NR, Mayall ES, et al. Papillary and follicular thyroid carcinomas show a different pattern of *ras* oncogene mutation. Br J Cancer 1989; 60:576–7.
69. Namba H, Rubin SA, Fagin JA. Point mutations of ras oncogenes are an early event in thyroid tumorigenesis. Mol Endocrinol 1990;4:1474–9.
70. Suarez HG, du Villard JA, Severino M, et al. Presence of mutations in all three *ras* genes in human thyroid tumors. Oncogene 1990;5:565–70.
71. Namba H, Gutman RA, Matsuo K, et al. H-*ras* protooncogene mutations in human thyroid neoplasms. J Clin Endocrinol Metab 1990;71:223–9.
72. Karga H, Lee J-K, Vickery AL Jr, et al. *Ras* oncogene mutations in benign and malignant thyroid neoplasms. J Clin Endocrinol Metab 1991;73:832–6.
73. Schark C, Fulton N, Yashiro T, et al. The value of measurement of RAS oncogenes and nuclear DNA analysis in the diagnosis of Hürthle cell tumors of the thyroid. World J Surg 1992;16:745–52.
74. Ezzat S, Zheng L, Kolenda J, et al. Prevalence of activating ras mutations in morphologically characterized thyroid nodules. Thyroid 1996;6(5):409–16.

75. Garcia-Rostan G, Zhao H, Camp RL, et al. ras mutations are associated with aggressive tumor phenotypes and poor prognosis in thyroid cancer. J Clin Oncol 2003;21(17):3226–35.
76. The Cancer Genome Atlas Research Network. Integrated genomic characterization of papillary thyroid carcinoma. Cell 2014;159(3):676–90.
77. Asa SL, Giordano TJ, LiVolsi VA. Implications of the TCGA genomic characterization of papillary thyroid carcinoma for thyroid pathology: does follicular variant papillary thyroid carcinoma exist? Thyroid 2015;25(1):1–2.
78. Fagin JA, Wells SA Jr. Biologic and clinical perspectives on thyroid cancer. N Engl J Med 2016;375(11):1054–67.
79. Cho U, Mete O, Kim MH, et al. Molecular correlates and rate of lymph node metastasis of non-invasive follicular thyroid neoplasm with papillary-like nuclear features and invasive follicular variant papillary thyroid carcinoma: the impact of rigid criteria to distinguish non-invasive follicular thyroid neoplasm with papillary-like nuclear features. Mod Pathol 2017;30(6):810–25.
80. Parente DN, Kluijfhout WP, Bongers PJ, et al. Clinical Safety of renaming encapsulated follicular variant of papillary thyroid carcinoma: is NIFTP truly benign? World J Surg 2018;42(2):321–6.
81. Haugen BR, Alexander EK, Bible KC, et al. 2015 American Thyroid Association Management guidelines for adult patients with thyroid nodules and differentiated thyroid cancer: the american thyroid association guidelines task force on thyroid nodules and differentiated thyroid cancer. Thyroid 2016;26(1):1–133.
82. Bychkov A, Hirokawa M, Jung CK, et al. Low rate of noninvasive follicular thyroid neoplasm with papillary-like nuclear features in asian practice. Thyroid 2017;27(7):983–4.
83. Lloyd RV, Asa SL, LiVolsi VA, et al. The evolving diagnosis of noninvasive follicular thyroid neoplasm with papillary-like nuclear features (NIFTP). Hum Pathol 2018;74:1–4.
84. Bychkov A, Jung CK, Liu Z, et al. Noninvasive follicular thyroid neoplasm with papillary-like nuclear features in asian practice: perspectives for surgical pathology and cytopathology. Endocr Pathol 2018;29(3):276–88.
85. Ahn HS, Kim HJ, Welch HG. Korea's thyroid-cancer "epidemic"–screening and overdiagnosis. N Engl J Med 2014;371(19):1765–7.
86. Ito Y, Miyauchi A, Kudo T, et al. Trends in the implementation of active surveillance for low-risk papillary thyroid microcarcinomas at kuma hospital: gradual increase and heterogeneity in the acceptance of this new management option. Thyroid 2018;28(4):488–95.
87. Lloyd RV, Osamura RY, Kloppel G, et al. WHO classification of tumours of endocrine organs. 4th edition. Lyon (France): IARC; 2017.
88. Yamashina M. Follicular neoplasms of the thyroid. Total circumferential evaluation of the fibrous capsule. Am J Surg Pathol 1992;16:392–400.
89. Mete O, Asa SL. Pathological definition and clinical significance of vascular invasion in thyroid carcinomas of follicular epithelial derivation. Mod Pathol 2011;24(12):1545–52.
90. Wreesmann VB, Nixon IJ, Rivera M, et al. Prognostic value of vascular invasion in well-differentiated papillary thyroid carcinoma. Thyroid 2015;25(5):503–8.
91. Shi X, Liu R, Basolo F, et al. Differential clinicopathological risk and prognosis of

major papillary thyroid cancer variants. J Clin Endocrinol Metab 2016;101(1): 264-74.
92. Cheng S, Serra S, Mercado M, et al. A high-throughput proteomic approach provides distinct signatures for thyroid cancer behavior. Clin Cancer Res 2011;17(8):2385-94.
93. Lubitz CC, Economopoulos KP, Pawlak AC, et al. Hobnail variant of papillary thyroid carcinoma: an institutional case series and molecular profile. Thyroid 2014; 24(6):958-65.
94. Rhoden KJ, Johnson C, Brandao G, et al. Real-time quantitative RT-PCR identifies distinct c-RET, RET/PTC1 and RET/PTC3 expression patterns in papillary thyroid carcinoma. Lab Invest 2004;84(12):1557-70.
95. Thomas GA, Bunnell H, Cook HA, et al. High prevalence of RET/PTC rearrangements in Ukrainian and Belarussian post-Chernobyl thyroid papillary carcinomas: a strong correlation between RET/PTC3 and the solid-follicular variant. J Clin Endocrinol Metab 1999;84:4232-8.
96. Powell DJJr, Russell J, Nibu K, et al. The RET/PTC3 oncogene: metastatic solid-type papillary carcinomas in murine thyroids. Cancer Res 1998;58:5523-8.
97. Prasad ML, Vyas M, Horne MJ, et al. NTRK fusion oncogenes in pediatric papillary thyroid carcinoma in northeast United States. Cancer 2016;122(7): 1097-107.
98. Greco A, Miranda C, Pierotti MA. Rearrangements of NTRK1 gene in papillary thyroid carcinoma. Mol Cell Endocrinol 2010;321(1):44-9.
99. Armstrong MJ, Yang H, Yip L, et al. PAX8/PPARgamma rearrangement in thyroid nodules predicts follicular-pattern carcinomas, in particular the encapsulated follicular variant of papillary carcinoma. Thyroid 2014;24(9):1369-74.
100. Fujimoto Y, Obara T, Ito Y, et al. Diffuse sclerosing variant of papillary carcinoa of the thyroid. Cancer 1990;66:2306-12.
101. Soares J, Limbert E, Sobrinho-Simoes M. Diffuse sclerosing variant of papillary thyroid carcinoma. A clinicopathologic study of 10 cases. Pathol Res Pract 1989;185:200-6.
102. Carcangiu ML, Bianchi S. Diffuse sclerosing variant of papillary thyroid carcinoma: clinicopathologic study of 15 cases. Am J Surg Pathol 1989;13:1041-9.
103. Chan JKC, Tsui MS, Tse CH. Diffuse sclerosing variant of papillary carcinoma of the thyroid: a histological and immunohistochemical study of three cases. Histopathology 1987;11:191-201.
104. Pillai S, Gopalan V, Smith RA, et al. Diffuse sclerosing variant of papillary thyroid carcinoma-an update of its clinicopathological features and molecular biology. Crit Rev Oncol Hematol 2015;94(1):64-73.
105. Sheu SY, Schwertheim S, Worm K, et al. Diffuse sclerosing variant of papillary thyroid carcinoma: lack of BRAF mutation but occurrence of RET/PTC rearrangements. Mod Pathol 2007;20(7):779-87.
106. Chou A, Fraser S, Toon CW, et al. A detailed clinicopathologic study of ALK-translocated papillary thyroid carcinoma. Am J Surg Pathol 2015;39(5):652-9.
107. Dettmer MS, Schmitt A, Steinert H, et al. Tall cell papillary thyroid carcinoma: new diagnostic criteria and mutations in BRAF and TERT. Endocr Relat Cancer 2015;22(3):419-29.
108. Watutantrige-Fernando S, Vianello F, Barollo S, et al. The hobnail variant of papil-

lary thyroid carcinoma: clinical/molecular characteristics of a large monocentric series and comparison with conventional histotypes. Thyroid 2018;28(1): 96–103.
109. Cameselle-Teijeiro JM, Rodriguez-Perez I, Celestino R, et al. Hobnail variant of papillary thyroid carcinoma: clinicopathologic and molecular evidence of progression to undifferentiated carcinoma in 2 cases. Am J Surg Pathol 2017; 41(6):854–60.
110. Papotti M, Botto Micca F, Favero A, et al. Poorly differentiated thyroid carcinomas with primordial cell component. A group of aggressive lesions sharing insular, trabecular, and solid patterns. Am J Surg Pathol 1993;17:291–301.
111. Hiltzik D, Carlson DL, Tuttle RM, et al. Poorly differentiated thyroid carcinomas defined on the basis of mitosis and necrosis: a clinicopathologic study of 58 patients. Cancer 2006;106(6):1286–95.
112. Cheung CC, Ezzat S, Ramyar L, et al. Molecular basis of Hurthle cell papillary thyroid carcinoma. J Clin Endocrinol Metab 2000;85(2):878–82.
113. Maximo V, Sobrinho-Simoes M. Hurthle cell tumours of the thyroid. A review with emphasis on mitochondrial abnormalities with clinical relevance. Virchows Arch 2000;437(2):107–15.
114. Maximo V, Soares P, Lima J, et al. Mitochondrial DNA somatic mutations (point mutations and large deletions) and mitochondrial DNA variants in human thyroid pathology: a study with emphasis on Hurthle cell tumors. Am J Pathol 2002; 160(5):1857–65.
115. Chiappetta G, Toti P, Cetta F, et al. The RET/PTC oncogene is frequently activated in oncocytic thyroid tumors (Hurthle cell adenomas and carcinomas), but not in oncocytic hyperplastic lesions. J Clin Endocrinol Metab 2002;87(1): 364–9.
116. Maximo V, Botelho T, Capela J, et al. Somatic and germline mutation in GRIM-19, a dual function gene involved in mitochondrial metabolism and cell death, is linked to mitochondrion-rich (Hurthle cell) tumours of the thyroid. Br J Cancer 2005;92(10):1892–8.
117. Bonora E, Porcelli AM, Gasparre G, et al. Defective oxidative phosphorylation in thyroid oncocytic carcinoma is associated with pathogenic mitochondrial DNA mutations affecting complexes I and III. Cancer Res 2006;66(12):6087–96.
118. Gasparre G, Porcelli AM, Bonora E, et al. Disruptive mitochondrial DNA mutations in complex I subunits are markers of oncocytic phenotype in thyroid tumors. Proc Natl Acad Sci U S A 2007;104(21):9001–6.
119. Mete O, Asa SL. Oncocytes, oxyphils, Hurthle, and Askanazy cells: morphological and molecular features of oncocytic thyroid nodules. Endocr Pathol 2010; 21(1):16–24.
120. Asa SL. My approach to oncocytic tumours of the thyroid. J Clin Pathol 2004; 57(3):225–32.
121. Bai S, Baloch ZW, Samulski TD, et al. Poorly differentiated oncocytic (hurthle cell) follicular carcinoma: an institutional experience. Endocr Pathol 2015; 26(2):164–9.
122. Hurthle K. Beitrage zur Kenntiss der Secretionsvorgangs in der Schilddruse. Arch Gesamte Physiol 1894;56:1–44.
123. Gopal RK, Kubler K, Calvo SE, et al. Widespread chromosomal losses and mito-

chondrial DNA alterations as genetic drivers in hurthle cell carcinoma. Cancer Cell 2018;34(2):242–55.
124. Ganly I, Makarov V, Deraje S, et al. Integrated genomic analysis of hurthle cell cancer reveals oncogenic drivers, recurrent mitochondrial mutations, and unique chromosomal landscapes. Cancer Cell 2018;34(2):256–70.
125. Asa SL, Ezzat S. The epigenetic landscape of differentiated thyroid cancer. Mol Cell Endocrinol 2018;469:3–10.
126. Papp S, Asa SL. When thyroid carcinoma goes bad: a morphological and molecular analysis. Head Neck Pathol 2015;9(1):16–23.
127. Semrad TJ, Keegan THM, Semrad A, et al. Predictors of neck reoperation and mortality after initial total thyroidectomy for differentiated thyroid cancer. Thyroid 2018;28(9):1143–52.
128. van Heerden JA, Hay ID, Goellner JR, et al. Follicular thyroid carcinoma with capsular invasion alone: a nonthreatening malignancy. Surgery 1992;112:1130–8.
129. Goffredo P, Cheung K, Roman SA, et al. Can minimally invasive follicular thyroid cancer be approached as a benign lesion?: a population-level analysis of survival among 1,200 patients. Ann Surg Oncol 2013;20(3):767–72.
130. Hughes DT, Rosen JE, Evans DB, et al. Prophylactic central compartment neck dissection in papillary thyroid cancer and effect on locoregional recurrence. Ann Surg Oncol 2018;25(9):2526–34.
131. McHenry CR. Is prophylactic central compartment neck dissection indicated for clinically node-negative papillary thyroid cancer: the answer is dependent on how the data are interpreted and the weight given to the risks and benefits. Ann Surg Oncol 2018;25(11):3123–4.
132. Renshaw AA, Pinnar N. Comparison of thyroid fine-needle aspiration and core needle biopsy. Am J Clin Pathol 2007;128(3):370–4.
133. Strauss EB, Iovino A, Upender S. Simultaneous fine-needle aspiration and core biopsy of thyroid nodules and other superficial head and neck masses using sonographic guidance. AJR Am J Roentgenol 2008;190(6):1697–9.
134. Lieu D. Cytopathologist-performed ultrasound-guided fine-needle aspiration and core-needle biopsy: a prospective study of 500 consecutive cases. Diagn Cytopathol 2008;36(5):317–24.
135. Khoo TK, Baker CH, Hallanger-Johnson J, et al. Comparison of ultrasound-guided fine-needle aspiration biopsy with core-needle biopsy in the evaluation of thyroid nodules. Endocr Pract 2008;14(4):426–31.
136. Jung CK, Min HS, Park HJ, et al. Pathology reporting of thyroid core needle biopsy: a proposal of the Korean Endocrine Pathology Thyroid Core Needle Biopsy Study Group. J Pathol Transl Med 2015;49(4):288–99.
137. Yi KS, Kim JH, Na DG, et al. Usefulness of core needle biopsy for thyroid nodules with macrocalcifications: comparison with fine-needle aspiration. Thyroid 2015;25(6):657–64.
138. Chen BT, Jain AB, Dagis A, et al. Comparison of the efficacy and safety of ultrasound-guided core needle biopsy versus fine-needle aspiration for evaluating thyroid nodules. Endocr Pract 2015;21(2):128–35.
139. Trimboli P, Crescenzi A. Thyroid core needle biopsy: taking stock of the situation. Endocrine 2015;48(3):779–85.
140. Baloch ZW, Cibas ES, Clark DP, et al. The National Cancer Institute Thyroid fine needle aspiration state of the science conference: a summation. Cytojournal

2008;5:6.
141. Pagni F, Prada M, Goffredo P, et al. Indeterminate for malignancy' (Tir3/Thy3 in the Italian and British systems for classification) thyroid fine needle aspiration (FNA) cytology reporting: morphological criteria and clinical impact. Cytopathology 2014;25(3):170–6.
142. Pusztaszeri M, Rossi ED, Auger M, et al. The Bethesda system for reporting thyroid cytopathology: proposed modifications and updates for the second edition from an international panel. Acta Cytol 2016;60(5):399–405.
143. Satoh S, Yamashita H, Kakudo K. Thyroid cytology: the japanese system and experience at Yamashita Thyroid Hospital. J Pathol Transl Med 2017;51(6):548–54.
144. Baloch ZW, Seethala RR, Faquin WC, et al. Noninvasive follicular thyroid neoplasm with papillary-like nuclear features (NIFTP): a changing paradigm in thyroid surgical pathology and implications for thyroid cytopathology. Cancer Cytopathol 2016;124(9):616–20.
145. Poller DN, Glaysher S. Molecular pathology and thyroid FNA. Cytopathology 2017;28(6):475–81.
146. Amendoeira I, Maia T, Sobrinho-Simoes M. Non-invasive follicular thyroid neoplasm with papillary-like nuclear features (NIFTP): impact on the reclassification of thyroid nodules. Endocr Relat Cancer 2018;25(4):R247–58.
147. Bychkov A, Keelawat S, Agarwal S, et al. Impact of non-invasive follicular thyroid neoplasm with papillary-like nuclear features on the Bethesda system for reporting thyroid cytopathology: a multi-institutional study in five Asian countries. Pathol 2018;50(4):411–7.
148. Nikiforov YE, Carty SE, Chiosea SI, et al. Impact of the multi-gene ThyroSeq next-generation sequencing assay on cancer diagnosis in thyroid nodules with Atypia of undetermined significance/follicular lesion of undetermined significance cytology. Thyroid 2015;25(11):1217–23.
149. Ferris RL, Baloch Z, Bernet V, et al. American Thyroid Association statement on surgical application of molecular profiling for thyroid nodules: current impact on perioperative decision making. Thyroid 2015;25(7):760–8.

第2章
甲状腺癌流行病学研究进展

Carolyn Dacey Seib，Julie Ann Sosa

关键词

- 甲状腺癌 • 甲状腺乳头状癌 • 流行病学 • 发病率 • 环境暴露

要点

- 过去30年间,甲状腺癌的发病率不断升高,其中以新发甲状腺乳头状癌为主。
- 低风险、微小甲状腺癌发病率的升高主要是因为影像学精准诊断的进步。
- 不同大小和分期的甲状腺癌发病人数及其相关的死亡率都在增加,与发病率增加趋势是一致的。
- 环境暴露可能造成了甲状腺癌发病率的升高。
- 明确甲状腺癌的危险因素、研究风险分级的方法、探索针对晚期甲状腺癌的治疗方案、实现个体化治疗,是目前的首要任务。

引言

在美国,甲状腺癌是最常见的内分泌系统恶性肿瘤,也是发病率上升最快的肿瘤[1]。甲状腺癌在女性中更为常见,根据地理区域和人口群体调查的统计资料[2],患甲状腺癌的男女比例约为1:3,位居女性癌症的第5位[3]。与大多数恶性肿瘤相比,甲状腺癌发病年龄偏小,诊断时年龄中位数为51岁,43%的病例发生在 45~64 岁[4]。分化型甲状腺癌从甲状腺滤泡细胞衍生而来,包括甲状腺乳头状癌(papillary thyroid cancer,PTC)、滤泡性甲状腺癌(follicular thyroid cancer,FTC)和 Hürthle 细胞癌。PTC 是甲状腺癌最常见的组织学亚型,占新发病例的 90%,预后最好。甲状腺癌的 5 年生存率为 98.1%;其中未出现远处转移者 5 年生存率为 99.9%,发生远处转移者 5 年生存率为 55.5%[1]。

在过去的 30 年里,甲状腺癌在美国和世界范围内的发病率增加了 300%,主要是由于 PTC 的增加(图 2.1)[2]。是否由于对小的、危险性低的、不会引起临床症状也不需要任何治疗的 PTC 过度检查和诊断而造成 PTC 发病率增加还没有定论,所以,关于 PTC 的增加是否代表了甲状腺癌发病率的增加仍有很大争议[5,6]。因此,准确找出甲状腺癌发病率上升的危险因素,对今后的甲状腺结节的评估和甲状腺癌的治疗具有重要意义。作者所给出的数据表明,

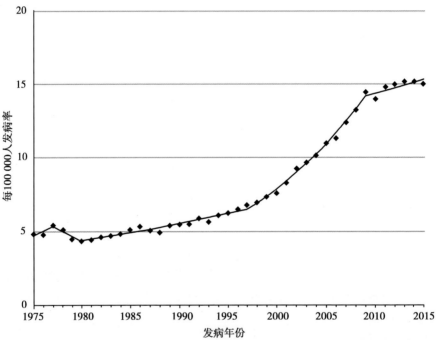

图 2.1　1975—2015 年甲状腺癌的年龄调整发病率总趋势(SEER-9 癌症登记项目)。比率为每 100 000 人,年龄调整为 2000 年美国标准人口(人口普查 P25-1130)。回归线使用 2018 年 2 月国家癌症研究所(National Cancer Institute)研发的 Joinpoint 回归程序(4.6 版本)计算

Data from Noone AM,Howlader N,Krapcho M,et al,editors.SEER cancer statistics review,1975-2015.Bethesda(MD):National Cancer Institute.2018.Available at: https://seer.cancer.gov/csr/1975_2015/,based on November 2017 SEER data submission,posted to the SEER Web site.

检出率的提高和实际病例的增加都引起了 PTC 发病率的上升。此外,他们还回顾了甲状腺癌主要危险因素以及个人易感性和环境危险因素相关性的支持性证据。

甲状腺癌的发病率
甲状腺结节

甲状腺结节是一种在影像学上有明显病损区域的良性或恶性甲状腺内病变。绝大多数的甲状腺结节是良性的,在没有辐射接触史的成人患者中恶性结节只占约 5%[7]。甲状腺结节的患病率取决于所调查的患者群体及结节的检查方法。体格检查发现的可触及甲状腺结节占 4%~7%[8],而超声检查则更为灵敏,检出度更高。Ezzat 及其同事[9]对 100 名无甲状腺疾病病史的患者进行了前瞻性研究,发现 21 名患者曾在体格检查中发现了甲状腺结节,而 67 名患者在超声检查上发现有甲状腺结节。Brander 及其同事们[10]对芬兰 253 名 19~50 岁的男性和女性进行了甲状腺结节检查和超声检查,发现 253 例中有 13 例(5.1%)甲状腺触诊结果异常,其中 5 例超声检查结果正常;69 例(27.3%)超声诊断为不少于 1 个甲状腺结节[10]。这些数据表明,作为甲状腺结节的筛查方式之一,甲状腺触诊的诊断敏感性低。甲状腺结节在年龄较大、女性、有碘缺乏史的或有电离辐射史的患者中更为常见[11-13]。Bartotta 及其同事[11]检查了 704 名无甲状腺病史的患者,发现 31% 的患者有甲状腺结节,女性(36% 有甲状腺结节)和老年患者的患病率最高,其中 60~80 岁的男性和女性中,38.5% 有甲状腺结节。Imaizumi 及其同事[14]评估了广岛和长崎原子弹爆炸幸存者的甲状腺结节患病率,其中 14% 的患者有甲状腺结节。通过与预估的辐射量相对照,研究者发现,甲状腺结节患病率与辐射暴露量有线性的剂量反应关系。同时,研究人员估计,其中 28% 的结节与接触辐射有关。由于在核事故发生 50 多年之后才进行相关分析研究,幸存者偏差可能导致研究人员对这一核暴露群体的归因危险度有所低估。

由于医学影像技术的普及和图像分辨率的提高,甲状腺结节乃至甲状腺癌的识别率逐渐增加[15]。数据显示,67% 的偶发甲状腺结节可以在颈部超声中检出[9],与此相对应,16% 可在 CT 和颈部 MRI 中检出[16],9% 可在颈动脉超声中检出[17],2% 可在 [^{18}F]- 氟代脱氧葡萄糖(^{18}F-FDG)正电子发射体层成像(PET)中检出[18]。偶发性甲状腺结节对于医生而言是一个临床挑战,因为常在伴发急性或慢性病的老年患者中被发现[22],但在没有甲状腺疾病史的普通人群中,其恶性的风险较低(恶性率为 1.6%~12.5%)[19-21]。除超声外,其他影像学手段无法准确地发现及描述甲状腺结节的恶性特征,导致临床检查和处理方式出现差异[23]。常规的头颈部影像学所检出的偶发甲状腺结节可能比文献报道中的病例更少。Uppal 及其同事[24]回顾了 2007—2012 年在同一家机构进行的超过 97 000 例头颈胸部超声、CT、FDG-PET 和 MRI,发现 387 例(0.4%)报告有偶发性甲状腺结节,其中的 163 例(42.1%)进行了甲状腺细针穿刺(FNA)活检,有 27 例被诊断为甲状腺癌(占总例数中的 0.03%,占偶发结节例数中的 7.0%)[24]。当随机选择 500 例进行 CT 扫描后,其中 10% 被检出有偶发性甲状腺结节。这表明在临床实践中,放射科医生对偶发性甲状腺结节报告的不一致性[24]。尸检研究表明,50% 或更多的成人有甲状腺结节[25]。同时,在 60 岁以上的成人中,多达 35% 的人有隐匿性甲状腺乳头状癌[26];汇总分析结果显示,隐匿性甲状腺乳头状癌患病率预计为 11%[27]。这些研究结果表明,临床上仍有大量患者有临床隐匿性的甲状腺结节和甲状腺癌,其中大部分是微小甲状腺乳头状癌(测量大小<1cm)[23]。

随着影像诊断技术的发展,FNA 的细胞病理学特征也更多地被用来诊断甲状腺结节并指导治疗。与之相对应,美国甲状腺手术的数量也在逐渐增加[28]。Sosa 及其同事[28]利用私人和公共保险的索赔数据证实,甲状腺 FNA 的使用次数从 2006—2011 年翻了 1 倍,展现出 16% 的年增长率;同时,同期甲状腺结节的手术量也增加了 31%。大量偶发性甲状腺结节患者接受了手术,其中一部分与 FNA 给出的模糊细胞学结果记录 [如意义不明的细胞非典型/滤泡样病变(Bethesda 分级Ⅲ级)或可疑滤泡性肿瘤(Bethesda 分级Ⅳ级)] 有关,然而,大多数病例的最终病理学检查是良性的。Shrestha 及其同事[29]分析了 10 年来在同一家机构所有进行甲状腺 FNA 的患者,发现 3013 名患者中有 667 名(22%)接受了手术,但是其中只有 129 名(17.1%)在术后的病理诊断中被确诊为甲状腺癌。近年来,人们越来越认识到,有必要减少诊断性甲状腺叶切除术,可通过分子检测手段对不确定的甲状腺结节进行诊断,从而减少其相关疾病的发生。

甲状腺癌的实际发病率与过度诊断

2006 年,Davies 和 Welch[15]发表了一篇关于 SEER(Surveillance, Epidemiology, and End Results)数据库数据分析的论文。结果显示,1973—2002 年,甲状腺癌的发病率增加了 2.4 倍,从 3.6/10 万增加到 8.7/10 万,而其疾病特异性死亡率保持不变。而甲状腺癌发病率的增加几乎归咎于 PTC,后者的发生率增加了

2.9 倍。在他们的研究中，1998—2002 年间的肿瘤大小的数据大多数与 PTC 有关：新诊断肿瘤中，49% 的肿瘤大小 ≤ 1cm，87% 的肿瘤 ≤ 2cm[15]。研究者把上述甲状腺癌的发病率增加归咎于对小的危险性低的肿瘤的过度诊断。这些肿瘤在临床上可能没有明显的症状，并且很多可能是监测偏倚[15]。1 年后，Kent 及其同事们[30]利用安大略省癌症登记处（Ontario Cancer Registry）提供的数据对分化型甲状腺癌的发病率进行了研究，其中包括了随机对每年度 10% 的病理报告进行再审查，并因此发表了一项基于群体的研究报告[30]。研究人员发现，1990—2001 年，DTC 的发病率稳步上升，总体每年上升 13%，其中 ≤ 2cm 的肿瘤发病率有显著上升，而 2~4cm 甚至 4cm 以上的肿瘤发病率并没有明显地增加[30]。所以 Kent 等人同意 Davies 和 Welch 的这一观点，他们认为甲状腺癌发病率的增加与小的亚临床的肿瘤检出率的增加有关，而其检出率的增加与医学影像技术的普及应用及发展有关[30]。对于过度诊断（部分原因是监测偏倚）是否会导致甲状腺癌发病率的增加，学术界一直激烈地争论；而这个问题的解决会对甲状腺结节患者和已活检证实为甲状腺癌患者的治疗有着重要意义。

监测偏倚对甲状腺癌的过度诊断的最典型的例子是韩国。该国于 1999 年制定了一项筛查常见恶性肿瘤的国家计划，同时通过收费服务来广泛筛查甲状腺癌。由于甲状腺超声检查的广泛应用，1993—2011 年，甲状腺癌的发病率增加了 15 倍，而其增长全部来源于新诊断的 PTC。大量肿瘤 ≤ 1cm 的患者接受了甲状腺全切除的手术治疗[31]，然而同期甲状腺癌的死亡率并没有增加。发病率升高的地区与进行筛查的地区在地理分布上呈现高度的关联性，这与低风险甲状腺癌的过度诊断表现一致[31]。这一现象被韩国媒体和国际科学界广泛关注，并被 Ahn 及其同事发表在了 *New England Journal of Medicine* 上[31]。2015 年的后续报道显示，韩国甲状腺癌的发病率减少了 30%，年度甲状腺手术量减少了 35%，显示患者和医生接受的"过度诊断会造成风险"的教育减少了甲状腺癌的相关筛查次数和新诊断的甲状腺癌病例数[32]。我们认为，仍需长期随访患者预后、转归等后续的长期数据，以便观察监测偏倚对韩国造成的影响。

2017 年，美国预防服务特别工作组（US Preventive Services Task Force，USPSTF）回顾分析了甲状腺癌筛查的证据，提出了 D 级的推荐，表明 USPSTF 对"颈部触诊或超声筛查无益或其危害大于益处"的观点持中立态度[33]。他们承认甲状腺癌的发病率有显著的增加，但更重要的是，分化型甲状腺癌的预后十分良好。根据工作组公布的研究结果，同期内甲状腺癌的死亡率没有随发病率升高而变化,这是他们反对筛查的证据之一[33]。并且,USPSTF 在文献回顾中没有检索到有关筛查对甲状腺癌患者预后影响的高质量随机对照试验[34]。工作组参考了 Davies 和 Welch[5,15,35] 通过对 SEER 数据库分析所得出的基于人群的观察性数据和 La Vecchia[36] 及其同事在五大洲(Five Continents)数据库中的癌症发病率数据。除此之外,结合前文提到的关于尸检研究中隐匿性 PTC 的报道以及韩国实行筛查后所引发的后果,都说明甲状腺癌的过度诊断是一个确切存在的问题[34]。并且人们担心,筛查会导致不必要的手术,并因此引起一些影响生活质量的并发症,如甲状旁腺功能减退症和喉返神经损伤等。

而反对的观点包括颈部和甲状腺评估仍然是全身体检的重要组成部分;筛查对高危患者群体(例如有辐射接触史、甲状腺癌家族史或有甲状腺恶性肿瘤相关的遗传综合征的患者群体)十分重要等[37]。此外,最新 USPSTF 的建议没有包含 SEER 数据库的发表数据,这也让"美国甲状腺癌发病率增加完全是因为过度诊断"这一主要理论饱受质疑。Enewold 及其同事[30]利用 1980—2005 年的 SEER 数据进行分析,发现不仅患小的 PTC 患者的人数显著增加,患大的晚期的 PTC 患者人数也有提高,PTC 发病率的增加中,有 50% 是由于≤1cm 的肿瘤,然而,>2cm 的肿瘤也占了 20%[38]。此外,在白人女性中,测量值>5cm 的肿瘤发病率增加了 222%[38]。如果甲状腺癌发病率的增加完全归因于过度诊断,那么其增加的发病率都应归咎于小且无临床意义的 PTC。然而,不同大小甲状腺肿瘤的确诊数量都在增加,是甲状腺癌发病率实际增加的关键。所以,如果全部归咎于过度诊断,那么就不能解释为何不同大小的甲状腺癌发病率都有增加。由于用 SEER 和 US Census 数据库的数据来评估影像诊断技术会导致其对低危险度甲状腺癌的检出率偏高,Li 及其同事[39]利用社会经济水平(socioeconomic status,SES)作为对评估影像诊断技术的辅助手段。研究发现,与低 SES 的区域相比,高 SES 区域中<4cm 的甲状腺癌发病率增加幅度增大(提示本组存在过度诊断),然而,同时两组区域中>4cm 的肿瘤发病率仍有相似且稳定的增加,表明大的甲状腺癌的发病率确有实际增加且与监测偏倚无关[39]。

最近,Lim 及其同事们[6]利用 SEER-9 癌症登记项目的数据(包含了代表 10% 美国人口的数据),结合美国国家卫生统计中心(National Center for Health Statistics)提供的死亡率,评估了甲状腺癌发病率和基于发病率的死亡率的发展趋势。研究人员发现,1974—2013 年,甲状腺癌的发病率每年增加 3.6%,其中主要是由于 PTC 的增加。研究人员同时评估了不同大小和不同分级 PTC

发病率的增加情况,包括小的局限性的肿瘤(发病率平均每年增加 4.6%)和巨大肿瘤(测量值>4cm 的肿瘤发病率平均每年增加 6.1%)[6]。此外,局部和远处转移的 PTC 在同期内也显著增加,平均每年增加 4.3% 和 2.4%。总的来说,同期基于发病率的死亡率平均每年增加 1.1%,晚期 PTC 则平均每年增加 2.9%,较小肿瘤患者的基于发病率的死亡率也在增加(≤2cm 的肿瘤平均每年增加 6.8%),表明近年来甲状腺癌的生物学特征正向更具侵袭性的方向转变。所以基于以上研究,研究人员得出结论:过度诊断并不是导致甲状腺癌发病率上升的唯一原因,并建议应重点探究造成晚期 PTC 数量增加的原因[6]。这项研究的发现将促使人们进一步探究环境暴露对甲状腺癌发病率的潜在影响,寻找针对高风险患者的跨学科诊治方案,降低日益增长的死亡率。

临床意义

根据以上数据可以得出结论,甲状腺癌发病率的增加在很大程度上归咎于监测偏倚和过度诊断。与此同时,甲状腺癌的发病率也确有增加,这值得进一步研究。认识到过度诊断的存在十分重要,这使得医生们更严谨地进行临床判断,来决定何时推荐患者进行 FNA 检查。2015 年,美国甲状腺协会出台的《成人甲状腺结节和分化型甲状腺癌患者的管理指南》中提出了有证可循的建议,临床医生应熟悉这些建议。建议中指出,不推荐对<1cm 的结节进行 FNA 检查(高危患者或有其他风险因素的患者除外,例如家族史或辐射暴露)[40]。此外,外科医生应以减少预后良好的患者的并发症为目标并及时更新观念,即:根据长期观察数据,低风险 PTC 仅行甲状腺叶切除术后疾病特异性死亡率没有明显变化[41]。晚期甲状腺癌的发病率及其疾病特异性死亡率的增加表明,甲状腺癌的生物学特征可能发生了改变(更有侵袭性),或仍有致病的危险因素未被发现。与此同时,这些研究也强调了对患者进行积极的跨学科治疗的必要性,对局部晚期和远处转移性疾病新疗法进行持续研究的重要性,以及对甲状腺癌相关的环境暴露的进一步探究的重要性。此外,还应优先寻找可以鉴别低风险与高风险甲状腺癌的标记物,以便提高对疾病的预测能力并辅助调整个性化的甲状腺癌生物治疗策略。

甲状腺癌的危险因素

造成甲状腺癌发病率实际增加的另一个可能的原因是已知甲状腺癌危险

因素的增加，包括环境暴露。因此，对已知甲状腺癌相关环境暴露和未知环境暴露的探究就显得尤为重要。甲状腺癌的已知危险因素包括：电离辐射的接触、家族史、性别、肥胖、饮酒和吸烟。除此之外，最近的研究还发现 PTC 与阻燃剂的接触相关联[42]。

电离辐射

儿童和青少年暴露于环境、诊断性及治疗性的电离辐射下是一个公认的 PTC 危险因素。切尔诺贝利事故后，在受到辐射青少年的群体开展的病例对照研究发现，青少年患甲状腺癌的风险与其接触的辐射剂量成正相关[43]。同时，暴露在广岛和长崎原子弹爆炸中的青少年中，甲状腺癌的风险与其接触的辐射剂量也成正相关[44]。暴露年龄越小，患甲状腺癌的风险越高，暴露后 15~19 年患甲状腺癌的风险达到高峰，而暴露事件后的影响持续超过 40 年[45]。应用影像学临床检查年轻患者带来的辐射对患甲状腺癌风险的影响一直受关注。一项国际研究发现，对 16 岁以下儿童使用 CT 扫描进行检查的比例是 3%~16%，其中头颈部的扫描是最常见的[46]。与此同时，成年人接触影像检查辐射的可能也在增加，其中主要是 CT 和核医学检查[44]。最近一项包括 12 篇论文中 9 个研究的 meta 分析，在对比影像学检查中所受的辐射与患甲状腺癌风险的关系后得出，CT 和口腔科 X 射线总辐射量的增加与患甲状腺癌风险的增加有关，风险比为 1.52（95% 置信区间 1.13~2.04）[47]。然而这项 meta 分析与其他回顾性研究存在局限性，包括无法确定辐射影响患癌风险的机制，以及无法避免用影像学检查来辅助诊断。因此，在考虑应用影像学检查时，尤其是甲状腺扫描范围内时，应权衡患甲状腺癌的风险。

患甲状腺癌的风险与 21 岁之前接受治疗性辐射的剂量成正比。一项研究对 1970—1986 年在美国和加拿大接受癌症治疗的 21 岁以下患者进行了长期随访，这项队列研究结果显示，接受 20Gy 辐射量以下治疗的患者，患甲状腺癌的风险与所受辐射量成线性关系，超额相对危险度峰值为 14.6[48]。女性患者和接触辐射时年龄较小的患者患甲状腺癌的风险最高[48]。尽管治疗性或过度影像检查而受到的射线辐射应被纳入甲状腺结节患者的风险分级中，但由于 PTC 的基因谱会随着时间发生变化，目前尚不清楚这一因素是否在甲状腺癌发病率增加中起到关键作用。切尔诺贝利核事故和体外放射治疗所致 PTC 的研究中发现，这些甲状腺癌中 RET/PTC 融合基因重排的比例很大[49-51]。Romei 及其同事们[52]比较了 1996—2000 年、2001—2005 年、2006—2010 年 401 例 PTC 患者的 *BRAF V600E* 突变和 *RET/PTC* 重排比例，发现随着时间的推移，RET/PTC 重排的频率有所降低（分别为 33%、17% 和 9.8%），而 BRAF V600E 的突变频率反而增加（分别为 28%、48.9% 和 58.1%）。RET/PTC 突变的减少说明辐射诱发的甲状腺癌并不能解释 PTC 发病率的大幅度增加，这表明存在额外的未知危险因素。

患者与环境暴露

某些患者因素和环境暴露因素与甲状腺癌风险增加相关，其中部分因素可能与甲状腺癌发病率增加有关。加拿大的一项大型病例对照研究发现，有甲状腺癌家族史的一级亲属有 10 倍的风险罹患甲状腺非髓样癌[53]。瑞典一项人群研究的数据表明，如果父母有甲状腺癌病史，则其 PTC 标准化发病比（standardized incidence ratio，SIR）为 3.2；兄弟姐妹有甲状腺癌病史的，SIR 为 6.2；而对于姐妹有甲状腺癌病史的人而言，其 SIR 为 11.2[54]。女性患甲状腺癌的概率是男性的 3 倍。然而，对于性别这一重要危险因素潜在机制的解释——性激素的影响，科学家们并未达成一致认识，也并未给出更多的有用信息[55]。一项包含了 14 个病例对照研究（探究与甲状腺癌相关的患者因素和环境因素）的汇总分析发现，甲状腺肿大和甲状腺功能亢进与甲状腺癌的发病率关系最为密切，并与甲状腺结节的发病率也有所关联[55]。目前，烟草的使用量与甲状腺癌发病率成剂量依赖性负相关关系。结果分析显示，与从不吸烟者相比，吸烟导致甲状腺癌发病的风险比（hazard ratio，HR）为 0.68（95% 置信区间 0.55~0.85）[56]。饮酒与患 PTC 风险之间也存在相反的关系，虽然结果并不如吸烟与患甲状腺癌风险的关系那么显著。尽管这些负相关的机制尚不清楚，但仍需进一步的研究来确定是否近期吸烟和饮酒率的下降与 PTC 发病率的增加有因果关系。

在过去的 30 年间，美国的肥胖率显著上升，与甲状腺癌发病率的趋势一致[51]。一项人群研究表明，有 39.8% 的成年人和 18.5% 的儿童患有肥胖[57]。1992—2002 年，全世界尤其是发展中国家的肥胖率增长最为迅速，而到 2006 年后，这一增长趋势趋于平稳[58]。观察研究表明，肥胖与甲状腺癌（包括 PTC、FTC 和甲状腺未分化癌）风险的增加密切相关[59]。Kitahara 及其同事[60]对 22 个来自各国的前瞻性研究进行了汇总分析，结果表明，体重指数（body mass index，BMI）越高，患甲状腺癌的风险越高［BMI 每增加 $5kg/m^2$，风险比（HR）为 1.06，95% 置信区间 1.02~1.10］，而这一结果对年轻成人而言更危险（BMI 每增加 $5kg/m^2$，HR 为 1.13，95% 置信区间 1.02~1.25）。研究人员还证明肥胖与甲状腺癌死亡率之间存在显著相关：BMI 每增加 $5kg/m^2$，

HR 为 1.29(95% 置信区间 1.07~1.55)[60]。PTC 患者的回顾性横断面研究中发现,肥胖与具有侵袭性特征的晚期甲状腺癌有关,而且在一些病例中,肥胖增加了甲状腺癌复发的风险[61-63]。肥胖和相关因素导致患甲状腺癌风险增加的机制尚不清楚,后续的实验研究可能提供更多与激素通路有关的发现[64,65]。

新的证据表明,接触特定的阻燃剂会增加 PTC 的风险。由于家具、电子产品和建筑材料防火标准的要求,阻燃剂的使用量随着时间的推移而增加,如多溴二苯醚(polybrominated diphenyl ether, PBDE)、新型的溴化和有机磷酸酯阻燃剂等,这些化合物通常存在于家庭空气的粉尘中[42]。研究证实,许多阻燃剂的化学结构与甲状腺激素相似,可以改变体内甲状腺激素的稳态,因此,目前有假说提出它们对患甲状腺癌风险会产生潜在影响[66,67]。Hoffman 及其同事[42]进行了一项病例对照研究,评估了血清中检出 27 种阻燃剂的量、家庭粉尘中检出阻燃剂的量和 PTC 发病率之间的关系。研究人员发现,接触家庭粉尘中的十溴二苯醚(decabromodiphenyl ether, BDE-209)增加了 PTC 发病率 2 倍以上,尤其是与小的低侵袭性的 PTC 有较强的相关性;而接触有机磷酸酯阻燃剂则与大的高侵袭性的肿瘤发病有关。一项早期的研究发现,血清少量的 PBDE 与甲状腺癌之间没有明显的关系[68]。然而,阻燃剂使用率和小的 PTC 发生率同时增加,有必要对两者之间的联系进一步研究,以确定接触阻燃剂对甲状腺癌发病的影响。

总结

随着甲状腺癌发病率的增加,寻找导致这一趋势发生的原因和证据对于制订更好的甲状腺癌诊治策略尤为重要。目前,基于人群的研究数据支持过度诊断在极大程度上导致 PTC 发病率增加这一观点。与此同时,PTC 的实际发病率和基于发病率的死亡率也有小幅度的增加。未来,仍需研究如何改善晚期甲状腺癌的治疗。此外,进一步调查可能引发甲状腺癌相关的患者因素和环境因素,从而消除和减少高危人群的相关接触成为优先解决的公共卫生问题。最后,改进风险分级的方法对于甲状腺癌患者选择合适和个体化的治疗方案至关重要。

(景 斐 管庆波)

参考文献

1. Surveillance Research Program NCI. Fast stats: an interactive tool for access to SEER cancer statistics. Available at: https://seer.cancer.gov/faststats. Accessed August 21, 2018.
2. Kilfoy BA, Zheng T, Holford TR, et al. International patterns and trends in thyroid cancer incidence, 1973–2002. Cancer Causes Control 2009;20(5):525–31.
3. Siegel RL, Miller KD, Jemal A. Cancer statistics, 2017. CA Cancer J Clin 2017;67(1):7–30.
4. Institute NC. SEER cancer stat facts: thyroid cancer. Available at: https://seer.cancer.gov/statfacts/html/thyro.html. Accessed August 21, 2018.
5. Davies L, Welch HG. Current thyroid cancer trends in the United States. JAMA Otolaryngol Head Neck Surg 2014;140(4):317–22.
6. Lim H, Devesa SS, Sosa JA, et al. Trends in thyroid cancer incidence and mortality in the United States, 1974-2013. JAMA 2017;317(13):1338–48.
7. Belfiore A, Giuffrida D, La Rosa GL, et al. High frequency of cancer in cold thyroid nodules occurring at young age. Acta Endocrinol (Copenh) 1989;121(2):197–202.
8. Vander JB, Gaston EA, Dawber TR. The significance of nontoxic thyroid nodules: final report of a 15-year study of the incidence of thyroid malignancy. Ann Intern Med 1968;69(3):537–40.
9. Ezzat S, Sarti DA, Cain DR, et al. Thyroid incidentalomas: prevalence by palpation and ultrasonography. Arch Intern Med 1994;154(16):1838–40.
10. Brander A, Viikinkoski P, Nickels J, et al. Thyroid gland: US screening in a random adult population. Radiology 1991;181(3):683–7.
11. Bartolotta T, Midiri M, Runza G, et al. Incidentally discovered thyroid nodules: incidence, and greyscale and colour Doppler pattern in an adult population screened by real-time compound spatial sonography. Radiol Med 2006;111(7):989–98.
12. Laurberg P, Jørgensen T, Perrild H, et al. The Danish investigation on iodine intake and thyroid disease, DanThyr: status and perspectives. Eur J Endocrinol 2006;155(2):219–28.
13. Schneider AB, Ron E, Lubin J, et al. Dose-response relationships for radiation-induced thyroid cancer and thyroid nodules: evidence for the prolonged effects of radiation on the thyroid. J Clin Endocrinol Metab 1993;77(2):362–9.
14. Imaizumi M, Tominaga T, Neriishi K, et al. Radiation dose-response relationships for thyroid nodules and autoimmune thyroid diseases in Hiroshima and Nagasaki atomic bomb survivors 55-58 years after radiation exposure. JAMA 2006;295(9):1011–22.
15. Davies L, Welch HG. Increasing incidence of thyroid cancer in the United States, 1973-2002. JAMA 2006;295(18):2164–7.
16. Youserm D, Huang T, Loevner LA, et al. Clinical and economic impact of incidental thyroid lesions found with CT and MR. AJNR Am J Neuroradiol 1997;18(8):1423–8.
17. Steele SR, Martin MJ, Mullenix PS, et al. The significance of incidental thyroid abnormalities identified during carotid duplex ultrasonography. Arch Surg 2005;140(10):981–5.

18. Cohen MS, Arslan N, Dehdashti F, et al. Risk of malignancy in thyroid incidentalomas identified by fluorodeoxyglucose-positron emission tomography. Surgery 2001;130(6):941-6.
19. Smith-Bindman R, Lebda P, Feldstein VA, et al. Risk of thyroid cancer based on thyroid ultrasound imaging characteristics: results of a population-based study. JAMA Intern Med 2013;173(19):1788-95.
20. Yoon DY, Chang SK, Choi CS, et al. The prevalence and significance of incidental thyroid nodules identified on computed tomography. J Comput Assist Tomogr 2008;32(5):810-5.
21. Hoang JK, Grady AT, Nguyen XV. What to do with incidental thyroid nodules identified on imaging studies? Review of current evidence and recommendations. Curr Opin Oncol 2015;27(1):8-14.
22. Nguyen X, Choudhury KR, Eastwood J, et al. Incidental thyroid nodules on CT: evaluation of 2 risk-categorization methods for work-up of nodules. AJNR Am J Neuroradiol 2013;34(9):1812-7.
23. Grady A, Sosa J, Tanpitukpongse T, et al. Radiology reports for incidental thyroid nodules on CT and MRI: high variability across subspecialties. AJNR Am J Neuroradiol 2015;36(2):397-402.
24. Uppal A, White MG, Nagar S, et al. Benign and malignant thyroid incidentalomas are rare in routine clinical practice: a review of 97,908 imaging studies. Cancer Epidemiol Biomarkers Prev 2015;24(9):1327-31.
25. Mortensen J, Woolner LB, Bennett WA. Gross and microscopic findings in clinically normal thyroid glands. J Clin Endocrinol Metab 1955;15(10):1270-80.
26. Harach HR, Franssila KO, Wasenius VM. Occult papillary carcinoma of the thyroid. A "normal" finding in Finland. A systematic autopsy study. Cancer 1985;56(3):531-8.
27. Furuya-Kanamori L, Bell KJL, Clark J, et al. Prevalence of differentiated thyroid cancer in autopsy studies over six decades: a meta-analysis. J Clin Oncol 2016;34(30):3672-9.
28. Sosa JA, Hanna JW, Robinson KA, et al. Increases in thyroid nodule fine-needle aspirations, operations, and diagnoses of thyroid cancer in the United States. Surgery 2013;154(6):1420-7.
29. Shrestha M, Crothers BA, Burch HB. The impact of thyroid nodule size on the risk of malignancy and accuracy of fine-needle aspiration: a 10-year study from a single institution. Thyroid 2012;22(12):1251-6.
30. Kent WD, Hall SF, Isotalo PA, et al. Increased incidence of differentiated thyroid carcinoma and detection of subclinical disease. Can Med Assoc J 2007;177(11):1357-61.
31. Ahn HS, Kim HJ, Welch HG. Korea's thyroid-cancer "epidemic"—screening and overdiagnosis. N Engl J Med 2014;371(19):1765-7.
32. Ahn HS, Welch HG. South Korea's thyroid-cancer "epidemic"—turning the tide. N Engl J Med 2015;373(24):2389-90.
33. Bibbins-Domingo K, Grossman DC, Curry SJ, et al. Screening for thyroid cancer: US Preventive Services Task Force recommendation statement. JAMA 2017;317(18):1882-7.
34. Lin JS, Bowles E, Williams SB, et al. Screening for thyroid cancer: updated evidence report and systematic review for the us preventive services task force. JAMA 2017;317(18):1888-903.
35. Davies L, Welch H. Thyroid cancer survival in the united states: observational data from 1973 to 2005. Arch Otolaryngol Head Neck Surg 2010;136(5):440-4.

36. La Vecchia C, Malvezzi M, Bosetti C, et al. Thyroid cancer mortality and incidence: a global overview. Int J Cancer 2015;136(9):2187–95.
37. Sosa J, Duh Q, Doherty G. Striving for clarity about the best approach to thyroid cancer screening and treatment: is the pendulum swinging too far? JAMA Surg 2017;152(8):721–2.
38. Enewold L, Zhu K, Ron E, et al. Rising thyroid cancer incidence in the United States by demographic and tumor characteristics, 1980-2005. Cancer Epidemiol Biomarkers Prev 2009;18(3):784–91.
39. Li N, Du XL, Reitzel LR, et al. Impact of enhanced detection on the increase in thyroid cancer incidence in the United States: review of incidence trends by socioeconomic status within the surveillance, epidemiology, and end results registry, 1980–2008. Thyroid 2013;23(1):103–10.
40. HaugenBryan R, AlexanderErik K, BibleKeith C, et al. 2015 American Thyroid Association management guidelines for adult patients with thyroid nodules and differentiated thyroid cancer: the American Thyroid Association guidelines task force on thyroid nodules and differentiated thyroid cancer. Thyroid 2016;26(1):1–133.
41. Welch HG, Doherty GM. Saving thyroids — overtreatment of small papillary cancers. N Engl J Med 2018;379(4):310–2.
42. Hoffman K, Lorenzo A, Butt CM, et al. Exposure to flame retardant chemicals and occurrence and severity of papillary thyroid cancer: a case-control study. Environ Int 2017;107:235–42.
43. Cardis E, Kesminiene A, Ivanov V, et al. Risk of thyroid cancer after exposure to 131 I in childhood. J Natl Cancer Inst 2005;97(10):724–32.
44. Parker LN, Belsky JL, Yamamoto T, et al. Thyroid carcinoma after exposure to atomic radiation: a continuing survey of a fixed population, Hiroshima and Nagasaki, 1958-1971. Ann Intern Med 1974;80(5):600–4.
45. Ron E, Lubin JH, Shore RE, et al. Thyroid cancer after exposure to external radiation: a pooled analysis of seven studies. Radiat Res 1995;141(3):259–77.
46. Linet MS, pyo Kim K, Rajaraman P. Children's exposure to diagnostic medical radiation and cancer risk: epidemiologic and dosimetric considerations. Pediatr Radiol 2009;39(1).4–26.
47. Han MA, Kim JH. Diagnostic x-ray exposure and thyroid cancer risk: systematic review and meta-analysis. Thyroid 2018;28(2):220–8.
48. Bhatti P, Veiga LH, Ronckers CM, et al. Risk of second primary thyroid cancer after radiotherapy for a childhood cancer in a large cohort study: an update from the childhood cancer survivor study. Radiat Res 2010;174(6a):741–52.
49. Elisei R, Romei C, Vorontsova T, et al. RET/PTC rearrangements in thyroid nodules: studies in irradiated and not irradiated, malignant and benign thyroid lesions in children and adults. J Clin Endocrinol Metab 2001;86(7):3211–6.
50. Thomas G, Bunnell H, Cook H, et al. High prevalence of RET/PTC rearrangements in Ukrainian and Belarussian post-Chernobyl thyroid papillary carcinomas: a strong correlation between RET/PTC3 and the solid-follicular variant. J Clin Endocrinol Metab 1999;84(11):4232–8.
51. Kitahara CM, Sosa JA. The changing incidence of thyroid cancer. Nat Rev Endocrinol 2016;12(11):646.
52. Romei C, Fugazzola L, Puxeddu E, et al. Modifications in the papillary thyroid cancer gene profile over the last 15 years. J Clin Endocrinol Metab 2012;97(9):E1758–65.

53. Pal T, Vogl FD, Chappuis PO, et al. Increased risk for nonmedullary thyroid cancer in the first degree relatives of prevalent cases of nonmedullary thyroid cancer: a hospital-based study. J Clin Endocrinol Metab 2001;86(11):5307–12.
54. Hemminki K, Eng C, Chen B. Familial risks for nonmedullary thyroid cancer. J Clin Endocrinol Metab 2005;90(10):5747–53.
55. Preston-Martin S, Franceschi S, Ron E, et al. Thyroid cancer pooled analysis from 14 case–control studies: what have we learned? Cancer Causes Control 2003; 14(8):787–9.
56. Kitahara CM, Linet MS, Freeman LEB, et al. Cigarette smoking, alcohol intake, and thyroid cancer risk: a pooled analysis of five prospective studies in the United States. Cancer Causes Control 2012;23(10):1615–24.
57. Hales CM, Carroll MD, Fryar CD, et al. Prevalence of obesity among adults and youth: United States, 2015-2016. NCHS data brief, no 288. Hyattsville, MD: National Center for Health Statistics; 2017.
58. Ng M, Fleming T, Robinson M, et al. Global, regional, and national prevalence of overweight and obesity in children and adults during 1980–2013: a systematic analysis for the Global Burden of Disease Study 2013. Lancet 2014;384(9945): 766–81.
59. Schmid D, Ricci C, Behrens G, et al. Adiposity and risk of thyroid cancer: a systematic review and meta-analysis. Obes Rev 2015;16(12):1042–54.
60. Kitahara CM, McCullough ML, Franceschi S, et al. Anthropometric factors and thyroid cancer risk by histological subtype: pooled analysis of 22 prospective studies. Thyroid 2016;26(2):306–18.
61. Kim HJ, Kim NK, Choi JH, et al. Associations between body mass index and clinico-pathological characteristics of papillary thyroid cancer. Clin Endocrinol 2013; 78(1):134–40.
62. Trésallet C, Seman M, Tissier F, et al. The incidence of papillary thyroid carcinoma and outcomes in operative patients according to their body mass indices. Surgery 2014;156(5):1145–52.
63. Harari A, Endo B, Nishimoto S, et al. Risk of advanced papillary thyroid cancer in obese patients. Arch Surg 2012;147(9):805–11.
64. Pazaitou-Panayiotou K, Polyzos S, Mantzoros C. Obesity and thyroid cancer: epidemiologic associations and underlying mechanisms. Obes Rev 2013; 14(12):1006–22.
65. Malaguarnera R, Vella V, Nicolosi ML, et al. Insulin resistance: any role in the changing epidemiology of thyroid cancer? Front Endocrinol (Lausanne) 2017;8: 314.
66. Mughal BB, Demeneix BA. Endocrine disruptors: flame retardants and increased risk of thyroid cancer. Nat Rev Endocrinol 2017;13(11):627.
67. Liu S, Zhao G, Li J, et al. Association of polybrominated diphenylethers (PBDEs) and hydroxylated metabolites (OH-PBDEs) serum levels with thyroid function in thyroid cancer patients. Environ Res 2017;159:1–8.
68. Aschebrook-Kilfoy B, DellaValle CT, Purdue M, et al. Polybrominated diphenyl ethers and thyroid cancer risk in the Prostate, Colorectal, Lung, and Ovarian Cancer Screening Trial cohort. Am J Epidemiol 2015;181(11):883–8.

第3章
甲状腺癌发生、发展中的编码分子

Veronica Valvo，Caemelo Nucera

关键词

- BRAF V600E • 甲状腺癌 • hTERT • PAX8/PPRγ • CDKN2A
- RAS • 微环境

要点

- *BRAF V600E*、*RAS*、*RET/PTC* 和 *PAX8/PPARγ* 是与甲状腺肿瘤发生有关的最具特征的基因改变，引起 MAPK（MEK1/2 和 ERK1/2）和 PI3K-AKT 细胞内信号失调。
- 在过去的几年中，包括 *hTERT* 突变的其他的基因改变被报道。
- 包括不同途径在内的多种突变累积可导致甲状腺癌进展。
- 全基因组测序揭示了甲状腺癌未知的基因图谱，发现了新的基因组改变。

引言

甲状腺癌不仅是内分泌系统最常见的恶性肿瘤，而且发病率呈现逐年上升趋势[1]，一般来说，每年增加 3%[2]。基于发病率的死亡率通常较低。但是，1994—2013 年，每年增长大约 1.1%[2]。

根据细胞来源，甲状腺癌可分为两种主要的组织学类型。滤泡旁细胞或 C 细胞具有神经内分泌功能，产生并分泌降钙素激素，引起甲状腺髓样癌，占所有恶性肿瘤的一小部分（3%~5%），而绝大多数恶性肿瘤来源于负责甲状腺激素合成的滤泡细胞。滤泡细胞源性肿瘤按其分化程度分为：分化型甲状腺癌（differentiated thyroid cancer，DTC），包括乳头状甲状腺癌（papillary thyroid cancer，PTC）(80%~85%)和滤泡性甲状腺癌（follicular thyroid cancer，FTC）(10%~15%)；低分化甲状腺癌（poorly differentiated thyroid cancer，PDTC）和间变性甲状腺癌（anaplastic thyroid cancer，ATC）(1%~2%)[3]。传统的甲状腺恶性肿瘤治疗的特点是手术切除甲状腺，然后在肿瘤病灶吸收放射性碘的情况下辅助放射性碘治疗[4]。但是，甲状腺癌的复发常见，而且发生远处转移的风险也不低[4]。在过去的10年里，人们对甲状腺癌发病分子机制的认识有了很大提高，新的治疗策略不断被提出。本章阐述了滤泡来源的甲状腺癌中具有编码能力的基因（癌基因的蛋白、突变的抑癌基因）改变的主要进展。

早期甲状腺肿瘤发生的遗传改变
基因突变
BRAF

BRAF属于丝氨酸/苏氨酸激酶家族，是RAS的下游效应子。BRAF通过丝裂原活化蛋白激酶（mitogen-activated protein kinase，MAPK）途径传递信号，已知MAPK通路在促进细胞增殖和存活方面具有重要作用[5]。在生理条件下，MAPK信号有一条由ERK1/2这个主要的效应分子介导的负反馈机制[6]。2002年，位于 BRAF 基因第15外显子的T1799A点突变首次在多个人类恶性肿瘤中被发现[7]。这种错义核苷酸替换存在时，残基600由谷氨酸转变为缬氨酸，导致组成型丝氨酸/苏氨酸激酶活性失去抑制环。BRAF V600E是黑色素瘤[8]、毛细胞白血病[9]和PTC[10,11]最常见的基因改变。PDTC和ATC也高频发生 BRAF V600E（分别为33%和45%突变）[12]，但FTC中不存在该突变[13]。不太常见的 BRAF K601E 点突变也可见于滤泡性甲状腺腺瘤（follicular thyroid adenoma，FTA）[14]和PTC滤泡变体[15,16]。一般来说，具有这种突变的肿瘤显示滤泡模式和更好的临床结局[16]。

微小PTC中存在 BRAF V600E 提示其在甲状腺肿瘤的发生中发挥驱动作用[13]。事实上，BRAF V600E 的条件性表达能够诱导大鼠正常甲状腺细胞去分化和基因组不稳定性[17]。此外，在PTC中检测到 BRAF V600E 与死亡率增加[18]和较差的临床病理结果，包括侵袭性增加、复发风险增加、放射性碘缺乏及最终治疗失败，显著相关[19]。携带 BRAF V600E 突变的转基因小鼠和异种移植瘤模型证实了其在肿瘤发生和侵袭性特征发展中的重要作用[20,21]。由于这种基因改变的高度相关性，*BRAF V600E* 的克隆性一直存在争议，因为研究报告结果不一致[22,23]。来自 TCGA 基因组测序的更具决定性的证据表明 *BRAF V600E* 是 PTC 细胞中存在的一种驱动突变[10,23]。

重要的是，*BRAF V600E* 还深入参与调控微环境，促进肿瘤进展和侵袭性[24]。*BRAF V600E* 改变了 PTC 中的免疫细胞浸润，并与某些趋化因子水平升高有关[25,26]。此外，与 BRAF 野生型肿瘤相比，*BRAF V600E* PTC 更常表达高水平的免疫抑制配体程序性死亡配体 1(53% vs. 12.5%) 和人类白细胞抗原 G(41% vs. 12.5%)[27]。重要的是，RNA 测序分析发现，与 BRAF 野生型相比，*BRAF V600E* 与免疫和炎症反应基因的整体表达降低有关，从而导致一种假说：该癌基因可引起免疫逃逸[28]。此外，血管内皮生长因子 A(vascular endothelial growth factor A, VEGFA)[29]，金属蛋白酶[30]，纤连蛋白和波形蛋白[31]，转化生长因子 β(transforming growth factor beta, TGF-β)[24,32,33]，血小板反应蛋白 1(thrombospondin 1, TSP-1)[24]，p21 激活蛋白激酶[34]，均与 *BRAF V600E* 有关。可见，甲状腺肿瘤细胞与微环境的相互作用是决定肿瘤侵袭性和进展的关键。肿瘤细胞和微环境基质细胞可以通过旁分泌和自分泌信号通路相互作用，促进肿瘤进展。最近一项研究表明，肿瘤微环境周细胞通过 TSP-1/TGF-β1 轴，在保护人甲状腺癌细胞避免靶向 *BRAF V600E*(如维莫非尼)和酪氨酸激酶(如索拉菲尼)的治疗中起重要作用[35](图 3.1)。具体而言，周细胞能够分泌 TSP-1 和 TGF-β1，从而引发耐药性。BRAF WT/V600E-PTC 临床标本在周细胞中富集，TSP-1 和 TGF-β1 表达诱发微环境中的基因调控网络和通路，这对 BRAFV600E-PTC 细胞的存活至关重要。拮抗 TSP-1/TGF-β1 轴降低肿瘤细胞生长并克服耐药性[35]。拮抗这一分子通路可能是对抗 *BRAF WT/V600E*-PTC 靶向治疗耐受的一种新的治疗途径。

BRAF V600E 也可能与某些临床症状有关：在 ATC 中，不同血管生成和促炎关键因子(如 VEGFA、VEGFC、白细胞介素 -6)的产生和分泌可能导致病理特征的恶化，如恶病质(引起发病的复杂代谢改变的结果)[36]。总之，这些结果强调了肿瘤与微环境相互作用的复杂性，以及这种相互作用如何影响甲状腺癌进展和患者的预后。

RAS

RAS 是一种 G 蛋白或鸟苷 - 核苷酸结合蛋白；RAS 蛋白属于小 GTPases 家族，位于多个细胞信号通路的上游[37]。与 GTP 结合促进其激活；RAS 蛋白具有内在的水解活性，可以水解结合的 GTP 分子为 GDP，使其成为非活性状态[38]。甲状腺癌可见 *RAS* 基因突变[39-41]。三种不同密码子(12、13 和 61)点突变与下游效应子持续异常激活有关[42]。RAS 蛋白家族由三个基因组成：*HRAS*、*KRAS* 和 *NRAS*。三个突变的 *RAS* 基因均与癌症有关，包括甲状腺癌[39,43-45]。MAPK 和 PI3K（磷脂酰肌醇 -3- 激酶）-AKT 通路均受 *RAS* 调控，具有 *RAS* 突变的甲状腺肿瘤也显示 PI3K-AKT 过度活化[46,47]。有趣的是，*RAS* 突变在滤泡型甲状腺乳头状癌（FVPTC）或甲状腺滤泡样癌（FTC）比经典的甲状腺乳头状癌（CPTC）更常见[10,44,47-51]。PTC 滤泡变异体具有 *RAS* 突变[52]。然而，具有乳头状核特征的非侵袭性滤泡性甲状腺肿瘤，其不良预后的风险非常低，也表现出 *RAS* 突变[53]。*RAS* 癌基因激活可能在甲状腺肿瘤发生的早期发挥作用，在细胞不丢失分化的情况下诱导正常人甲状腺上皮细胞增殖[54,55]。有趣的是，来自转基因小鼠模型的研究证实 *KRAS* 突变体需要额外的基因改变（如 *PTEN* 缺失）才能发展为甲状腺癌，从而导致侵袭性和转移性 FTC[56]。

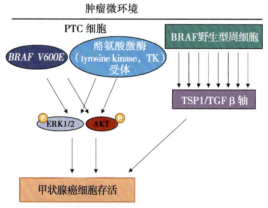

图 3.1　肿瘤微环境周细胞通过 TSP1/TGF-β1 轴促进甲状腺癌细胞存活

基因易位

RET/PTC

PTC 中最常见的基因易位是 *RET/PTC*。*RET* 基因编码跨膜 TK 受体[57]，其 3' 部分在 5' 处可与十多个其他基因融合。最常见的重排分别为 *RET/PTC1* 和 *RET/PTC3*[58,59]、核受体共激活因子 4（NCOA4，也称为 *ELE1* 或 *RFG*）和含有螺旋结构域的基因 6（*CDC6*，也称为 *H4*）[59,60]。在 *RET/PTC* 易位的情况下，融合蛋白将激酶结构域保留在 C 末端，并获得一个新的 N 末端，提供与配体无关的二聚体和组成型 TK 活性。这一易位事件的致病原因与染色体脆弱位点的共定位有关，基因组区域容易发生 DNA 断裂[61]。*RET/PTC*

发生率差异是由于甲状腺肿瘤中存在克隆或亚克隆。克隆重排是 PTC 特有的，发生率为 10%~20%[62]，而肿瘤团块中一小部分存在 *RET/PTC* 在其他甲状腺癌变异体和良性甲状腺病变中也有[63-66]。有趣的是，*RET* 融合在 PDTC 中发生率较低(6%)，但在 ATC 中不存在，显示与点突变无重叠[12]。

配对盒 8/ 增殖激活受体 γ（PAX8/PPARγ）

甲状腺癌中另一个相关的基因重排（体细胞易位）是配对盒 8（paired box 8, PAX8）和增殖激活受体 γ（proliferator activated receptor gamma, PPARγ）(PAX8/PPARγ) 的融合。PAX8 是甲状腺发育的重要转录因子[67,68]，在成熟器官中负责甲状腺特异性基因的表达[68]。相反，核激素受体 PPARγ 在甲状腺中无已知的生理作用，但被认为是巨噬细胞抗炎表型的启动子[69]和脂肪生成的主要调节因子[70]。PAX8-PPARγ 易位在 2000 年首次发现[71]，可见于 FTC（约 50%）、一小部分滤泡 PTC（1%~5%）和 FTA（2%~13%）中[72,73]。PAX8/PPARγ 与 RAS 点突变很少重叠，后者是 FTC 的另一种常见改变，可能提示肿瘤发生过程中存在不同的致病途径[39]。在 PTC 中，PAX8/PPARγ 的检测与滤泡特征密切相关：肿瘤被包裹，可能临床进展缓慢[74]。PAX8/PPARγ 具有完整的 DNA 结合域，能够靶向含原脂肪表达谱的转录因子 DNA 结合位点，并优先在这种重排的甲状腺细胞中激活[75]。在甲状腺细胞中，PAX8/PPARγ 表达可诱导 WNT/TCF 通路激活，导致肿瘤侵袭性增强并呈现进展特征，如锚定非依赖性生长[76]。

转基因小鼠模型显示，如果没有 *PTEN* 缺失等其他突变，PAX8/PPARγ (PPFP) 本身不足以诱导肿瘤发生。PPFP 和 *PTEN* 缺失联合改变的小鼠发展为转移性甲状腺癌，这与临床患者结果一致，即 PPFP 偶尔见于良性甲状腺腺瘤，而有 PPFP 的肿瘤磷酸化 AKT/ 蛋白激酶 B 表达增加[77]。小鼠模型 (PPFP × Pten⁻) Chip-seq 分析显示，结合富集于参与脂肪酸代谢、细胞周期调控和调节相关 WNT 信号的基因[78]。此外，与对照组相比，使用 PPARγ 激动剂 (吡格列酮) 治疗后，免疫细胞浸润明显增加，提示对这类甲状腺癌有潜在的治疗效果[78]（图 3.2）。

神经营养酪氨酸激酶受体

神经营养型酪氨酸激酶受体家族参与了甲状腺癌的偶发性重排。位于染色体 1q 上的 *NTRK1* 基因可以有不同的伴侣，如 *TPR*[79,80]，*TMP3*[81,82] 和 *TFG*[83]。融合蛋白具有持续性激酶活性，可促进下游通路。目前对这种基因改变的发生率仍存在争议，以前的研究显示，PTC 的发生率约为 11.8%[84]，而最近的分析显示，其患病率下降了 1%~2%[85]；同时，在年轻患者中也有较高的发病率。NTRK3/ETV6 融合只在 13% 的 PTC 滤泡变异体中发现，包括包裹变异体和浸润变异体，但在 FTA 和 FTC 中未发现[86]。NTRK3/RBPMS 是另一种融合，PTC 发生率为 1.2%[10]。重要的是，ETV6/NTRK3 融合常见（14.5%）于受辐射暴露人群（切尔诺贝利事故后 PTC）和 2% 的散发性 PTC[87]。

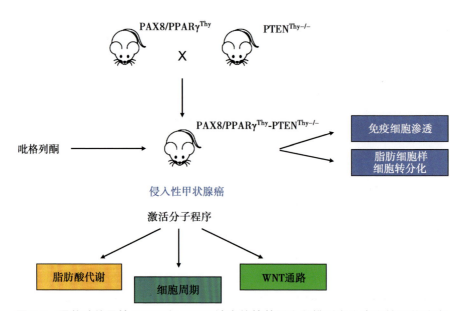

图 3.2　甲状腺特异性 PPFP 和 PTEN 缺失的转基因小鼠模型发生滤泡性甲状腺癌。在分子水平上，PPFP 弱诱导脂肪细胞 PPARγ 靶基因亚群，促进细胞周期进展，激活 WNT/TCF 通路。吡格列酮（一种与 PPFP 结合的 PPARγ 激动剂）使 PPFP 强烈激活脂肪细胞 PPARγ 靶基因，导致甲状腺癌细胞向脂肪细胞样细胞转分化。此外，吡格列酮激活的 PPFP 可以在肿瘤微环境中招募免疫细胞

纹蛋白 / 间变性淋巴瘤激酶

最近，RNAseq 分析发现了一种新的甲状腺癌基因融合，包括间变性淋巴瘤激酶（anaplastic lymphoma kinase，ALK）基因和纹状蛋白（striatin，STRN）基因[88]。这一事件是包括 2 号染色体短臂复杂重排的结果。STRN 的第 3 外显子与 ALK 的第 20 外显子的融合导致了 STRN 蛋白二聚化（通过螺旋结构域介导）和随后的 ALK 组成型激酶活性。在甲状腺癌细胞中，STRN/ALK 重排独立于 TSH 信号，可以刺激增殖，进一步诱导肿瘤转化。STRN/ALK 可见于 PTC[86,88,89]、PTC 滤泡变异体[86,88]、PDPTC 和 ATC[88]。有趣的是，STRN/ALK 融合肿瘤其他驱动突变呈阴性，表明其在甲状腺肿瘤发生中的作用，并提示其可能是该类肿瘤患者的治疗靶点。

AKAP9/BRAF

AKAP9/BRAF 是放射诱导的 PTC 中罕见的基因融合，它是通过 7q 染色体的近中心反转导致 *AKAP9* 基因外显子 1 和 8 与 *BRAF* 外显子 9 和 18 之间的框内融合。融合蛋白含有蛋白激酶结构域，缺乏 *BRAF* 自我抑制性 N 末端部分[90]。这种融合蛋白在散发 PTC 中的发生率非常低，可以认为是一种罕见事件[91,92]。这种分子融合提高了激酶活性并使 NIH3T3 细胞发生转化。

与甲状腺癌进展有关的基因改变和通路失调

甲状腺癌中发生的其他突变通常与癌症进展和肿瘤侵袭性特征有关。

WNT/β- 连环蛋白信号通路

WNT/β- 连环蛋白通路在多种细胞过程中起关键作用，如细胞生长和增殖、细胞黏附和干细胞分化。如果发生改变（如 WNT 受体突变），通常会导致人类肿瘤的组成性激活[93]。在甲状腺癌中，这一过程是由编码 β- 连环蛋白的 *CTNNB1* 基因突变引起，这种突变在 PDPTC 和 ATC 中发生率很高（接近 60%）[94-96]。其结果是生理性 β- 连环蛋白降解受损，引起其在胞质中积聚并转位进入细胞核，最终促进与肿瘤发生有关的基因转录，如细胞周期调节因子[97,98]。此外，在 DTC 中未检测到 β- 连环蛋白突变，导致该通路与侵袭性增强有关。然而，β- 连环蛋白的核异常转位和定位可能是由其他机制引起的，包括翻译后修饰[93]。众所周知，PI3K/AKT 通路通过 AKT 直接磷酸化失活 GSK3β，而 GSK3β 是 β- 连环蛋白泛素化和进一步降解的关键启动子[99]。AKT 在丝氨酸（Ser, S）552 磷酸化 β- 连环蛋白，导致 β- 连环蛋白与细胞接触解离，增强其与 14-3-3 的结合和转录活性，加强肿瘤细胞侵袭活性[100]。此外，ERK1/2 可以抑制 GSK3β，导致 β- 连环蛋白上调[101]。在甲状腺细胞中，β- 连环蛋白生理上被激活是通过 PI3K 信号通路对 TSH 和 IGF1 的应答发生的[102]，但也有研究表明 *RET/PTC* 易位和 *HRAS* 突变（而非 *BRAF*）激活了癌细胞中的 β- 连环蛋白[103-106]。人们对这种非依赖性 *BRAF V600E* 仍存在争议，因为在具有 *BRAF V600E* 的 PTC 和 ATC 细胞中发现了 β- 连环蛋白的上调[107]。然而，另一项基于免疫组织化学和微阵列分析的研究显示，*BRAF WT* 与 *BRAF V600E* PTC 中 β- 连环蛋白的上调存在差异[108]。可能需要做更多工作来理解是什么驱动了 WNT-β- 连环蛋白在生理环境中的异常激活，以及哪些分子参与了激活。

TP53

肿瘤抑制因子突变导致功能丧失和细胞周期调控子 *p53* 首次被描述为去分化甲状腺癌的一个独特特点，ATC 中发生率高达 50%~80%[109-111]。小鼠模型和靶向下一代测序的进一步分析证实了 *TP53* 改变与 ATC 较差的病理特征有关[112,113]。

TERT

2013 年，研究者在甲状腺癌中检测到两个 *TERT* 基因启动子点突变，分别为 C228T 和 C250T[114,115]。*TERT* 基因编码端粒酶复合体的逆转录酶亚基，端粒酶是一种特殊的 DNA 聚合酶，通过添加重复序列来延长染色体的端粒部分。它的表达和活性在正常细胞中通常缺失或很低，而在癌细胞中却显著增加[116]，包括侵袭性甲状腺癌[117,118]。在不同癌症中发现了 *TERT* 基因启动子突变[119-121]，确定了 E-twenty-six（ETS）转录因子的一致性结合位点。C228T 和 C250T 在 PTC 中的发生率（约 10%）低于 PDTC（40%）和 ATC（约 70%）。*TERT* 与 *BRAF* 和 *RAS* 基因突变的显著共存表明，*TERT* 的作用是一种获得性遗传改变，它使已存在驱动突变的克隆得以延长生存期，并随后导致癌症进展[114]。不同的研究证实了这一假设，显示 *TERT* 启动子突变：①在 FTC 和侵袭性 *BRAF V600E* 阳性 PTC 的发生率更高[122]，良性甲状腺病变未发现 *TERT* 突变；②与 DTC 患者较差的临床结果有关[123]；③与 *BRAF V600E* 共存对 PTC 的肿瘤侵袭性具有强大的协同作用，包括较差的临床病理特征[122,124]和较高的患者死亡率[125]；④与 *BRAF V600E*、ATC 患者年龄大和肿瘤远处转移显著相关[126]。重要的是，*BRAF V600E* 和 *TERT* 启动子突变在癌症协同共存中的分子机制最近被阐明，即 *BRAF V600E* 通过其效应子 ERK1/2 加强 *MYC* 基因表达和 FOS 磷酸化，后者促进 GA 结合蛋白 GABPB 表达。MYC 和 GABPB 都是与 *TERT* 启动子结合并触发其过表达的转录因子，在 GABPB 的作用下，*TERT* 的突变依赖于 GABPB[127]（图 3.3）。

EIF1AX

真核翻译起始因子 *EIF1AX* 首次在葡萄膜黑色素瘤中发现突变[128]，有报道称，这种基因改变在 1% 的 PTC 中，与 *BRAF* 和 *RAS* 相互排斥[10]。*EIF1AX* 突变率在 PDTC（11%）和 ATC（9%）增加且与 *RAS* 密切相关[12]。最常见的突变事件包括一个剪接突变，导致 C 末端 12- 氨基酸入框。*EIF1AX* 突变也可以预测 PDTC 的低存活率[10,12]。

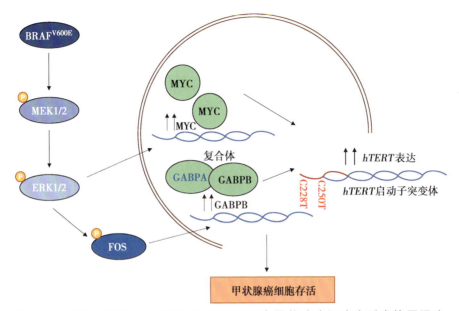

图 3.3 人 TERT 启动子突变和 BRAF V600E 在甲状腺癌细胞中诱发协同通路。BRAF V600E 通过 ERK1/2 磷酸化促进 MYC 表达和 FOS 磷酸化。FOS 是调节 GABPB 表达的转录因子。MYC 和 GABPB 都是对 TERT 启动子突变发生反应的转录因子，能够增强突变体 hTERT 表达

PI3K-AKT 通路突变和失调

PI3K 通路是由大量的蛋白质组成的，它们控制着细胞的几个过程，包括细胞增殖、存活和运动[129]。在生理条件下，PI3K 被多个跨膜 TK 受体激活的蛋白适配器募集到质膜内层。此外，一些亚型具有一个结合域，允许 RAS 激活。PI3K 磷酸化磷脂酰肌醇 -4,5- 二磷酸肌酰肌醇 -3,4,5- 三磷酸肌酰肌醇 (PIP3) 是促进 PDK1 和 AKT 等效应因子激活的第二信使。PI3K-AKT 通路伴侣携带的基因改变与甲状腺癌进展密切相关。总的来说，PI3K-AKT 信号通路在甲状腺癌形成中发挥重要作用[130]。

PTEN 是一种蛋白酪氨酸磷酸酶，与紧张素具有同源性，是一种编码蛋白和脂质磷酸酶的肿瘤抑制基因。具体来说，PTEN 抑制 PI3K-AKT 通路促进 PIP3 去磷酸化。将 PTEN 功能丧失的突变与甲状腺癌关联的第一个证据是一个来自 Cowden 综合征的研究，该综合征是一种先天性疾病，其特征是 PTEN 遗传性突变，患者对 FTA 和 FTC 高度易感[131]。随后，PTEN 作为肿瘤

抑制基因的重要性在一个杂合 PTEN1[+/−] 小鼠模型中证实,该小鼠自发发展为甲状腺癌和结肠癌[132]。然而,正如在组织特异性转基因小鼠模型中所显示的那样,甲状腺中 PTEN 完全缺失不足以引起侵袭性肿瘤,这表明为了促进甲状腺转化,额外的基因改变非常重要[133]。在人类甲状腺肿瘤中,最常见的遗传改变是 PTEN 基因的体细胞缺失(约 5%~25%),原因是 10 号染色体的杂合性缺失[134,135]。PTEN 移码突变也见于 ATC 中。此外,与 PDTC 相比,ATC 中 PTEN 突变更为频繁(15%)[12]。

PIK3CA 第 9 外显子和第 20 外显子编码 PI3K 催化亚基 p110a,在许多人类肿瘤中经常发生体细胞突变[136],包括 DTC(约 8%)[137] 和 ATC(约 25%)[138,139],与 BRAF V600E 在未分化肿瘤中发生有趣的共表达现象[12]。存在这些基因改变的情况下,激酶对其调节亚基不敏感,也不会失活[140]。在 PDTC 和 ATC 中也观察到其他 PI3K 亚基突变,但发生率较低[12]。

AKT 是 PI3K 信号的下游效应子,被 PIP3 募集,随后被 PDK1 磷酸化并被西罗莫司的靶点(mTOR)激活。AKT 是一种丝氨酸/苏氨酸激酶,有三种不同亚型,由不同基因编码,均在甲状腺组织中有规律表达,其主要差异在于调节和适应域。在转移性甲状腺癌中,AKT1 可能发生突变[141]。mTOR 是另一种丝氨酸/苏氨酸激酶,存在于两个复合物中:mTORC1(或 mTOR-raptor),由 AKT 激活,促进细胞生长和大分子生物合成;mTORC2(或 mTOR-rictor)磷酸化 AKT(如上所述),触发细胞存活过程[142]。mTOR 基因突变在 PDTC 和 ATC 中发生频率较低(分别为 1% 和 6%)[12]。总的来说,超过 50% 的 FTC 和 ATC 至少有 1 个 PI3K-AKT 通路相关的基因改变[137]。

此外,在没有突变的情况下,PI3K-AKT 信号通路可能异常活跃。FTC 中 AKT1 和 AKT2 过度表达和过度活化尤为明显[143]。AKT1 核转位还与包膜侵袭性、细胞侵袭和迁移有关[144]。在 PTEN1[+/−] 小鼠模型中,AKT1 的缺失足够抑制肿瘤发展[145],但在 PTEN1[+/−] 小鼠模型,AKT2 缺失与 AKT 的广泛作用不同,但仍能降低甲状腺肿瘤发生率[146]。

基因拷贝数变异

拷贝数变异(CNV)(包括基因扩增)是另一种重要的致癌机制[147,148]。CNV 的发生是由于染色体不稳定和非整倍性,使促进致病信号的基因获得优势[148,149]。编码多种类型 TK 受体,包括表皮生长因子受体 EGFR、PDGFRA、PDGFRB、VEGFR1、VEGFR2 等的基因,已在 FTC 和 ATC 中检测到,与磷酸化 AKT 和 ERK1/2 的激活增加有关[47]。PI3K-AKT 通路的基因也被扩增,

包括 *PIK3CA*、*PIK3CB*、*AKT1* 和 *AKT2*[47,137,139]。有趣的是，*PIK3CA* 突变与 *PIK3CA* 扩增在 DTC 中是相互排斥的[137,150]，提示 PI3K-AKT 通路的一个特异性基因改变足以促进甲状腺肿瘤发生。多种遗传改变在 ATC 中累积[47,137]，增加了转移和肿瘤进展的可能性。

在 PTC 中，CNV 包括 22 号染色体(长臂)缺失[10,146]，该区域显示了 *NF2* 和 *CHEK2* 基因序列，并报告了显著频率缺失，染色体 1q 扩增，与 *BRAF V600E* 突变相关的是 5p 和 5q 的增加[10]。*NF2* 基因编码一种肿瘤抑制蛋白，这种蛋白在细胞间接触时抑制细胞生长。*NF2* 缺失可以通过部分失活 Hippo，增强 RAS 突变体信号和 MAPK 信号，这能激活小鼠 PDTC 模型 YAP-TEAD 转录程序[151]。有转移的 *BRAF V600E*-PTC 在染色体 1q 上有 26 个基因扩增，包括在染色体 9p 上的 *MCL1*(抗凋亡基因，属于 *BCL2* 家族)和 *P16* 基因(*CDKN2A*)缺失[152]。*P16* 是细胞周期负调控子，可以削弱 G1 期 CDK4/6 复合物形成和 Rb 磷酸化[153](图 3.4)。由于这个原因，CDK4/6 抑制剂联合 *BRAF V600E* 抑制剂(维莫非尼)已经证明在具有杂合性 *BRAF V600E* 突变和 *P16* 缺失的 PTC 和 ATC 细胞强烈诱导细胞凋亡[154]。DNA 拷贝数变异 CNV 可能发生在甲状腺病变的 7 号、12 号和 17 号染色体上[155]。总体而言，侵袭性甲状腺肿瘤和 ATC 的 CNV 发生频率较高，提示其在肿瘤进展中的作用。

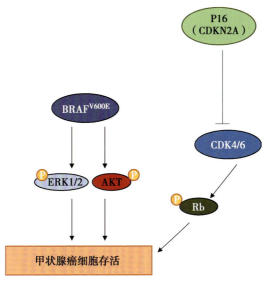

图 3.4　*BRAF V600E* 和 *P16* 缺失通过 ERK1/2 和 AKT 磷酸化、CDK4/6 活化和磷酸化失活 Rb 协同促进甲状腺肿瘤存活

NF-κB 信号通路

核因子-kappa B(nuclear factor-kappa B, NF-κB)信号在癌症发生和发展中起重要作用，为炎症和肿瘤之间提供了一种机制上的联系[156]。NF-κB 可诱导肿瘤增殖，阻断细胞凋亡，促进血管生成和侵袭[156]。多年来，人们已经知道在甲状腺癌细胞中 NF-κB 通路具有促癌作用[157-159]。更具体地说，已经证明主要发生于 NF-κB 激活的甲状腺癌变的基因改变是：*BRAF V600E* 以 MEK 非依赖模式[160]；RET/PTC3 通过 NF-κB 诱导激酶稳定[161]；PAX8/PPARγ，由于 PPARγ 蛋白丰度降低引起[162]。此外，PTEN 失活导致 PI3K-AKT 通路激活增加了 NF-κB 活性，从而加速甲状腺癌进展[163]。NF-κB 在血管生成和转移促进中的作用已经在携带 *BRAF V600E* 的 ATC 和 PDTC 小鼠模型中得到了进一步的描述，这与 IL-8 的分泌有关[164]。然而，NF-κB 抑制剂与经典化疗和放疗联合使用不足以靶向甲状腺癌细胞[165]，这表明需要进一步的研究来了解哪些患者/肿瘤可能对这种治疗靶点有反应。

RCAN1-4

RCAN1(钙调磷酸酶 1 的调控子，也称为唐氏综合征候选区域 1)基因位于 21 号染色体，有表达两个主要亚型 RCAN1-1 和 RCAN1-4 的多个转录起始位点[166]。RCAN1-4 是钙调磷酸酶的竞争性抑制剂，可以抑制钙调磷酸酶介导的脱磷酸作用和活化激活 T 细胞核转录因子(nuclear factor of activated T cells, NFAT)[167]。由于 NFAT 是一种促进 *RCAN1-4* 基因表达的转录因子，因此可以认为 RCAN1-4 是这一通路的负反馈环调节因子[168]。

有趣的是，*RCAN1* 在唐氏综合征患者中与肿瘤生长保护相关[169]，且其抑癌活性可能通过抑制 NFAT 来阻断血管生成过程(阻碍内皮细胞迁移，阻碍新生血管和肿瘤生长)实现[170-172]。

与正常组织相比，*RCAN1* 在原发肿瘤中表达增加，但在转移中表达减少，这种模式与转移抑制因子一致[173]。此外，在不同的癌细胞系(包括 FTC 细胞)中，*RCAN1* 可减少迁移并改变细胞黏附[174]。最近有报道称，RCAN1-4 在人甲状腺癌细胞系中稳定下调，可以提高细胞活力和体外侵袭能力，促进小鼠异种移植瘤模型的肿瘤生长和转移[175]。这些表型依赖于 NFE2L3(核因子，红系 2 样 3)，一种在人类甲状腺癌样本中过表达的转录因子[175]。

BRAF、*RAS*、*RET/PTC* 重叠及 MAPK 和 PI3K-AKT 间的信号通路协作

上文已讨论过 PI3K-AKT 通路的渐进突变如何加速并导致甲状腺肿瘤进展。在 DTC 中，主要致癌驱动因素（如 *BRAF*、*RAS* 和 *RET/PTC*）的基因改变是相互排斥的[10,14,176]。相反，多个基因同时突变可能是导致侵袭性甲状腺癌的机制，但仍存在争议，即 *BRAF V600E* 突变和 *RET/PTC* 易位共同导致复发性 PTC[177]，下一代测序显示 PDTC 和 ATC 的 *BRAF V600E*、*RAS* 突变和基因融合重排存在相互排他性[12]。有趣的是，据报道，可能存在同时激活 MAPK 和 PI3K 的驱动突变[47,139,141]，表明甲状腺肿瘤发生和发展的精确时间进程。因此，最常见的基因改变主要负责肿瘤的初始转化，导致肿瘤细胞进入更容易发生附加突变（继发性或伴随突变）的"癌症易发环境"。失调信号通路和异常功能蛋白质（不仅有 MAPK 和 PI3K-AKT，还包括 β- 连环蛋白、hTERT、TP53，等等）的渐进性累积和侵略性特征，如血管生成、细胞黏附、迁移、侵袭和转移，使甲状腺肿瘤向着具有最高死亡率的未分化 / 间变性肿瘤发展[178]。

甲状腺激素受体 - β：在侵袭性滤泡性甲状腺癌临床前模型中起关键作用

甲状腺激素受体是一种依赖于配体的转录因子，在甲状腺激素 T_3 作用下调节细胞生长、发育和分化。该蛋白家族完全由 *TRα* 和 *TRβ* 两个基因编码。2000 年，人们建立了携带 *TRβ* 靶向突变（TRβPV）的小鼠模型，以了解甲状腺激素抵抗综合征的分子基础，其特征是组织对甲状腺激素敏感性降低[179]。这些小鼠特点是生长受损和对甲状腺激素抵抗。数年后，据报道，*PV* 突变的小鼠纯合子（*TRβ$^{PV/PV}$*）自发发生转移性 FTC，表现出侵袭性特征，如贫血和转移[180]。后来的许多研究集中在阐明 *TRβ$^{PV/PV}$* 小鼠肿瘤发生的途径。由于 TRβPV 抑制过氧化物酶体增殖反应元件的转录活性[182]，造成 PPARγ mRNA 表达下调[181]。更重要的是，TRβPV 通过与 p85a（PI3K 的调节亚基）的相互作用，和 PI3K-AKT 通路激活建立联系，而 p85a 是众所周知的甲状腺肿瘤发生的关键调节因子[183]。如果 *PTEN* 缺失加上引起的 AKT 过度表达和过度活化及显著影响 AKT 下游靶点，包括增加 mTOR-p70S6K 信号和抑制 FOXO3a（转录因子 FOXO 叉头家族基因成员，启动促凋亡因素转录和阻遏细胞周期蛋白 D1），导致癌症进展和转移增加[163]。此外，已表明 T_3 对 β- 连环蛋白有抑制

作用。T_3 与 TRβ 结合可通过蛋白体途径诱导 β-连环蛋白在细胞内分解并降解[184]，通过与启动子中负性甲状腺激素反应元件相互作用直接抑制 *CTNNB1* 基因[185]。TRβPV 对该机制具有抗性，可以稳定 β-连环蛋白，促进肿瘤发生。$TRβ^{PV/PV}$ 小鼠模型的建立遵循以下策略：$TRβ^{PV/PV}Pten^{+/-}$ 小鼠高脂饮食显示循环瘦素水平升高，JAK2-STAT3 通路激活，转移率升高[186]。STAT3 是 cyclin D1、Myc、Bcl2 的转录因子启动子，对转移起重要作用。重要的是，使用 STAT3 选择性抑制剂可以减少血管侵犯、贫血和转移，证实了瘦素-JAK-STAT3 信号的作用[187]。而且，二甲双胍治疗高脂饮食 $TRβ^{PV/PV}$ 小鼠可以减少被膜侵袭、阻断间变和血管侵袭，但对甲状腺肿瘤生长无影响[188]。基因靶向 $TRβ^{PV/PV}$ 小鼠甲状腺上皮细胞 *KRAS*（*G12D*）突变可以发展为更具侵袭性的肿瘤，常发生间变性病灶，PAX8 表达缺失，MYC 表达上调。因此，MYC 可能成为治疗干预的潜在靶点，并提示 RAS、PI3K/AKT 和 β-连环蛋白通路之间可能存在交互通话[189]。MYC 抑制剂 JQ1 显著抑制 $TRβ^{PV/PV}$-*KRASG12D* 小鼠肿瘤生长[190]。此外，联合 JQ1 和二甲双胍治疗高脂饮食 $TRβ^{PV/PV}Pten^{+/-}$ 小鼠，可以通过降低 STAT3 减缓肿瘤生长，降低抗凋亡关键调节因子，抑制血管侵犯、细胞间变和肺转移[191]。

总结

近年来，人们对甲状腺癌分子特征（具有编码能力的主要分子改变）的认识有了显著进展。与甲状腺癌临床病理特征相关的新的遗传改变已经被发现。这些特征性基因改变揭示了 MAPK 和 PI3K/AKT 信号通路在促进甲状腺肿瘤发生、发展中的重要作用。这些结果极大地促进了精准医疗靶向治疗的发展，通过抑制这些途径中的关键基因的激活。遗憾的是，甲状腺癌中选择性耐药的问题屡屡被报道，表明为了克服肿瘤耐药需要识别新的潜在治疗靶点。最近，在对标准治疗（包括放射性碘）抵抗的难治性晚期甲状腺癌中，不同途径之间的相互作用得到了更好的印证，为早期治疗和改善预后开创了新的可能性。

（魏 玲 杨 明）

参考文献

1. Cancer Statistics Review, 1975-2015 - SEER Statistics. Available at: https://seer.cancer.gov/csr/1975_2015/. Accessed June 12, 2018.
2. Lim H, Devesa SS, Sosa JA, et al. Trends in thyroid cancer incidence and mortality in the United States, 1974-2013. JAMA 2017;317:1338.
3. Lloyd RV, Osamura RY, Klöppel G, et al. WHO classification of tumours of endocrine organs WHO classification of tumours. vol. 10. Lyon (France): IARC press; 2017.
4. Baudin E, Schlumberger M. New therapeutic approaches for metastatic thyroid carcinoma. Lancet Oncol 2007;8:148–56.
5. Fanger GR. Regulation of the MAPK family members: role of subcellular localization and architectural organization. Histol Histopathol 1999;14:887–94.
6. Kyriakis JM, App H, Zhang XF, et al. Raf-1 activates MAP kinase-kinase. Nature 1992;358:417–21.
7. Davies H, Bignell GR, Cox C, et al. Mutations of the BRAF gene in human cancer. Nature 2002;417:949–54.
8. Sosman JA, Kim KB, Schuchter L, et al. Survival in BRAF V600–mutant advanced melanoma treated with vemurafenib. N Engl J Med 2012;366:707–14.
9. Tiacci E, Trifonov V, Schiavoni G, et al. *BRAF* mutations in hairy-cell leukemia. N Engl J Med 2011;364:2305–15.
10. Cancer Genome Atlas Research Network. Integrated genomic characterization of papillary thyroid carcinoma. Cell 2014;159:676–90.
11. Cohen Y, Xing M, Mambo E, et al. BRAF mutation in papillary thyroid carcinoma. J Natl Cancer Inst 2003;95:625–7.
12. Landa I, Ibrahimpasic T, Boucai L, et al. Genomic and transcriptomic hallmarks of poorly differentiated and anaplastic thyroid cancers. J Clin Invest 2016;126:1052–66.
13. Nikiforova MN, Kimura ET, Gandhi M, et al. BRAF mutations in thyroid tumors are restricted to papillary carcinomas and anaplastic or poorly differentiated carcinomas arising from papillary carcinomas. J Clin Endocrinol Metab 2003;88:5399–404.
14. Soares P, Trovisco V, Rocha AS, et al. BRAF mutations and RET/PTC rearrangements are alternative events in the etiopathogenesis of PTC. Oncogene 2003;22:4578–80.
15. Trovisco V, Vieira de Castro I, Soares P, et al. BRAF mutations are associated with some histological types of papillary thyroid carcinoma. J Pathol 2004;202:247–51.
16. Afkhami M, Karunamurthy A, Chiosea S, et al. Histopathologic and clinical characterization of thyroid tumors carrying the BRAF(K601E) Mutation. Thyroid 2016;26:242–7.
17. Mitsutake N, Knauf JA, Mitsutake S, et al. Conditional BRAFV600E expression induces DNA synthesis, apoptosis, dedifferentiation, and chromosomal instability in thyroid PCCL3 cells. Cancer Res 2005;65:2465–73.
18. Xing M, Alzahrani AS, Carson KA, et al. Association between BRAF V600E mutation and mortality in patients with papillary thyroid cancer. JAMA 2013;309:1493.

19. Xing M, Westra WH, Tufano RP, et al. BRAF mutation predicts a poorer clinical prognosis for papillary thyroid cancer. J Clin Endocrinol Metab 2005;90:6373–9.
20. Knauf JA, Ma X, Smith EP, et al. Targeted expression of BRAF ^{V600E} in thyroid cells of transgenic mice results in papillary thyroid cancers that undergo dedifferentiation. Cancer Res 2005;65:4238–45.
21. Liu D, Liu Z, Condouris S, et al. BRAF V600E maintains proliferation, transformation, and tumorigenicity of BRAF-mutant papillary thyroid cancer cells. J Clin Endocrinol Metab 2007;92:2264–71.
22. Guerra A, Sapio MR, Marotta V, et al. The primary occurrence of BRAF(V600E) is a rare clonal event in papillary thyroid carcinoma. J Clin Endocrinol Metab 2012; 97:517–24.
23. Ghossein RA, Katabi N, Fagin JA. Immunohistochemical detection of mutated BRAF V600E supports the clonal origin of BRAF-induced thyroid cancers along the spectrum of disease progression. J Clin Endocrinol Metab 2013;98: E1414–21.
24. Nucera C, Porrello A, Antonello ZA, et al. B-Raf(V600E) and thrombospondin-1 promote thyroid cancer progression. Proc Natl Acad Sci U S A 2010;107: 10649–54.
25. Oler G, Camacho CP, Hojaij FC, et al. Gene expression profiling of papillary thyroid carcinoma identifies transcripts correlated with BRAF mutational status and lymph node metastasis. Clin Cancer Res 2008;14:4735–42.
26. Ryder M, Gild M, Hohl TM, et al. Genetic and pharmacological targeting of CSF-1/CSF-1R inhibits tumor-associated macrophages and impairs BRAF-induced thyroid cancer progression. PLoS One 2013;8:e54302.
27. Angell TE, Lechner MG, Jang JK, et al. BRAF V600E in papillary thyroid carcinoma is associated with increased programmed death ligand 1 expression and suppressive immune cell infiltration. Thyroid 2014;24:1385–93.
28. Smallridge RC, Chindris AM, Asmann YW, et al. RNA sequencing identifies multiple fusion transcripts, differentially expressed genes, and reduced expression of immune function genes in BRAF (V600E) mutant vs BRAF wild-type papillary thyroid carcinoma. J Clin Endocrinol Metab 2014;99:E338–47.
29. Jo YS, Li S, Song JH, et al. Influence of the BRAF V600E mutation on expression of vascular endothelial growth factor in papillary thyroid cancer. J Clin Endocrinol Metab 2006;91:3667–70.
30. Mesa C, Mirza M, Mitsutake N, et al. Conditional activation of RET/PTC3 and BRAFV600E in thyroid cells is associated with gene expression profiles that predict a preferential role of BRAF in extracellular matrix remodeling. Cancer Res 2006;66:6521–9.
31. Watanabe R, Hayashi Y, Sassa M, et al. Possible involvement of BRAFV600E in altered gene expression in papillary thyroid cancer. Endocr J 2009;56:407–14.
32. Riesco-Eizaguirre G, Rodríguez I, De la Vieja A, et al. The BRAFV600E oncogene induces transforming growth factor beta secretion leading to sodium iodide symporter repression and increased malignancy in thyroid cancer. Cancer Res 2009;69:8317–25.
33. Knauf JA, Sartor MA, Medvedovic M, et al. Progression of BRAF-induced thyroid cancer is associated with epithelial-mesenchymal transition requiring concomitant MAP kinase and TGFβ signaling. Oncogene 2011;30:3153–62.
34. McCarty SK, Saji M, Zhang X, et al. BRAF activates and physically interacts with PAK to regulate cell motility. Endocr Relat Cancer 2014;21:865–77.

35. Prete A, Lo AS, Sadow PM, et al. Pericytes elicit resistance to vemurafenib and sorafenib therapy in thyroid carcinoma via the TSP-1/TGFβ1 axis. Clin Cancer Res 2018. https://doi.org/10.1158/1078-0432.CCR-18-0693.
36. Husain A, Hu N, Sadow PM, et al. Expression of angiogenic switch, cachexia and inflammation factors at the crossroad in undifferentiated thyroid carcinoma with BRAF(V600E). Cancer Lett 2016;380:577–85.
37. Khosravi-Far R, Der CJ. The Ras signal transduction pathway. Cancer Metastasis Rev 1994;13:67–89.
38. Gibbs JB, Sigal IS, Poe M, et al. Intrinsic GTPase activity distinguishes normal and oncogenic ras p21 molecules. Proc Natl Acad Sci U S A 1984;81:5704–8.
39. Nikiforova MN, Lynch RA, Biddinger PW, et al. RAS point mutations and PAX8-PPAR gamma rearrangement in thyroid tumors: evidence for distinct molecular pathways in thyroid follicular carcinoma. J Clin Endocrinol Metab 2003;88:2318–26.
40. Namba H, Rubin SA, Fagin JA. Point mutations of ras oncogenes are an early event in thyroid tumorigenesis. Mol Endocrinol 1990;4:1474–9.
41. Xing M. Clinical utility of RAS mutations in thyroid cancer: a blurred picture now emerging clearer. BMC Med 2016;14:12.
42. Prior IA, Lewis PD, Mattos C. A comprehensive survey of Ras mutations in cancer. Cancer Res 2012;72:2457–67.
43. Suárez HG, Suárez HG, Du Villard JA, et al. Detection of activated ras oncogenes in human thyroid carcinomas. Oncogene 1988;2:403–6.
44. Suarez HG, du Villard JA, Severino M, et al. Presence of mutations in all three ras genes in human thyroid tumors. Oncogene 1990;5:565–70.
45. Lemoine NR, Mayall ES, Wyllie FS, et al. High frequency of ras oncogene activation in all stages of human thyroid tumorigenesis. Oncogene 1989;4:159–64.
46. Abubaker J, Jehan Z, Bavi P, et al. Clinicopathological analysis of papillary thyroid cancer with PIK3CA alterations in a Middle Eastern population. J Clin Endocrinol Metab 2008;93:611–8.
47. Liu Z, Hou P, Ji M, et al. Highly prevalent genetic alterations in receptor tyrosine kinases and phosphatidylinositol 3-kinase/akt and mitogen-activated protein kinase pathways in anaplastic and follicular thyroid cancers. J Clin Endocrinol Metab 2008;93:3106–16.
48. Esapa CT, Johnson SJ, Kendall-Taylor P, et al. Prevalence of Ras mutations in thyroid neoplasia. Clin Endocrinol (Oxf) 1999;50:529–35.
49. Manenti G, Pilotti S, Re FC, et al. Selective activation of ras oncogenes in follicular and undifferentiated thyroid carcinomas. Eur J Cancer 1994;30A:987–93.
50. Ezzat S, Zheng L, Kolenda J, et al. Prevalence of activating ras mutations in morphologically characterized thyroid nodules. Thyroid 1996;6:409–16.
51. Ellis RJ, Wang Y, Stevenson HS, et al. Genome-wide methylation patterns in papillary thyroid cancer are distinct based on histological subtype and tumor genotype. J Clin Endocrinol Metab 2014;99:E329–37.
52. Zhu Z, Gandhi M, Nikiforova MN, et al. Molecular profile and clinical-pathologic features of the follicular variant of papillary thyroid carcinoma. An unusually high prevalence of ras mutations. Am J Clin Pathol 2003;120:71–7.
53. Ferris RL, Nikiforov Y, Terris D, et al. AHNS Series: Do you know your guidelines? AHNS Endocrine Section Consensus Statement: State-of-the-art thyroid surgical recommendations in the era of noninvasive follicular thyroid neoplasm with papillary-like nuclear features. Head Neck 2018. https://doi.org/10.1002/hed.

25141.
54. Bond JA, Wyllie FS, Rowson J, et al. In vitro reconstruction of tumour initiation in a human epithelium. Oncogene 1994;9:281–90.
55. Gire V, Wynford-Thomas D. RAS oncogene activation induces proliferation in normal human thyroid epithelial cells without loss of differentiation. Oncogene 2000;19:737–44.
56. Miller KA, Yeager N, Baker K, et al. Oncogenic Kras requires simultaneous PI3K signaling to induce ERK activation and transform thyroid epithelial cells in vivo. Cancer Res 2009;69:3689–94.
57. Nikiforova MN, Stringer JR, Blough R, et al. Proximity of chromosomal loci that participate in radiation-induced rearrangements in human cells. Science 2000;290:138–41.
58. Grieco M, Santoro M, Berlingieri MT, et al. PTC is a novel rearranged form of the ret proto-oncogene and is frequently detected in vivo in human thyroid papillary carcinomas. Cell 1990;60:557–63.
59. Santoro M, Dathan NA, Berlingieri MT, et al. Molecular characterization of RET/PTC3; a novel rearranged version of the RETproto-oncogene in a human thyroid papillary carcinoma. Oncogene 1994;9:509–16.
60. Ciampi R, Nikiforov YE. RET/PTC rearrangements and BRAF mutations in thyroid tumorigenesis. Endocrinology 2007;148:936–41.
61. Gandhi M, Dillon LW, Pramanik S, et al. DNA breaks at fragile sites generate oncogenic RET/PTC rearrangements in human thyroid cells. Oncogene 2010;29:2272–80.
62. Santoro M, Carlomagno F, Hay ID, et al. Ret oncogene activation in human thyroid neoplasms is restricted to the papillary cancer subtype. J Clin Invest 1992;89:1517–22.
63. Elisei R, Romei C, Vorontsova T, et al. RET/PTC rearrangements in thyroid nodules: studies in irradiated and not irradiated, malignant and benign thyroid lesions in children and adults. J Clin Endocrinol Metab 2001;86:3211–6.
64. Chiappetta G, Toti P, Cetta F, et al. The RET/PTC oncogene is frequently activated in oncocytic thyroid tumors (Hurthle cell adenomas and carcinomas), but not in oncocytic hyperplastic lesions. J Clin Endocrinol Metab 2002;87:364–9.
65. Sapio MR, Guerra A, Marotta V, et al. High growth rate of benign thyroid nodules bearing RET/PTC rearrangements. J Clin Endocrinol Metab 2011;96:E916–9.
66. Guerra A, Sapio MR, Marotta V, et al. Prevalence of RET/PTC rearrangement in benign and malignant thyroid nodules and its clinical application. Endocr J 2011;58:31–8.
67. Macchia PE, Lapi P, Krude H, et al. PAX8 mutations associated with congenital hypothyroidism caused by thyroid dysgenesis. Nat Genet 1998;19:83–6.
68. Pasca di Magliano M, Di Lauro R, Zannini M. Pax8 has a key role in thyroid cell differentiation. Proc Natl Acad Sci U S A 2000;97:13144–9.
69. Ricote M, Li AC, Willson TM, et al. The peroxisome proliferator-activated receptor-gamma is a negative regulator of macrophage activation. Nature 1998;391:79–82.
70. Rosen ED, Sarraf P, Troy AE, et al. PPAR gamma is required for the differentiation of adipose tissue in vivo and in vitro. Mol Cell 1999;4:611–7.
71. Kroll TG, Sarraf P, Pecciarini L, et al. PAX8-PPARgamma1 fusion oncogene in human thyroid carcinoma [corrected]. Science 2000;289:1357–60.

72. Nikiforova MN, Biddinger PW, Caudill CM, et al. PAX8-PPARgamma rearrangement in thyroid tumors: RT-PCR and immunohistochemical analyses. Am J Surg Pathol 2002;26:1016–23.
73. Marques AR, Espadinha C, Catarino AL, et al. Expression of PAX8-PPAR gamma 1 rearrangements in both follicular thyroid carcinomas and adenomas. J Clin Endocrinol Metab 2002;87:3947–52.
74. Armstrong MJ, Yang H, Yip L, et al. *PAX8/PPARγ* rearrangement in thyroid nodules predicts follicular-pattern carcinomas, in particular the encapsulated follicular variant of papillary carcinoma. Thyroid 2014;24:1369–74.
75. Zhang Y, Yu J, Lee C, et al. Genomic binding and regulation of gene expression by the thyroid carcinoma-associated PAX8-PPARG fusion protein. Oncotarget 2015;6:40418–32.
76. Vu-Phan D, Grachtchouk V, Yu J, et al. The thyroid cancer PAX8-PPARG fusion protein activates Wnt/TCF-responsive cells that have a transformed phenotype. Endocr Relat Cancer 2013;20:725–39.
77. Dobson ME, Diallo-Krou E, Grachtchouk V, et al. Pioglitazone induces a proadipogenic antitumor response in mice with PAX8-PPARgamma fusion protein thyroid carcinoma. Endocrinology 2011;152:4455–65.
78. Zhang Y, Yu J, Grachtchouk V, et al. Genomic binding of PAX8-PPARG fusion protein regulates cancer-related pathways and alters the immune landscape of thyroid cancer. Oncotarget 2017;8:5761–73.
79. Greco A, Pierotti MA, Bongarzone I, et al. TRK-T1 is a novel oncogene formed by the fusion of TPR and TRK genes in human papillary thyroid carcinomas. Oncogene 1992;7:237–42.
80. Miranda C, Minoletti F, Greco A, et al. Refined localization of the human TPR gene to chromosome 1q25 by in situ hybridization. Genomics 1994;23:714–5.
81. Radice P, Sozzi G, Miozzo M, et al. The human tropomyosin gene involved in the generation of the TRK oncogene maps to chromosome 1q31. Oncogene 1991;6:2145–8.
82. Butti MG, Bongarzone I, Ferraresi G, et al. A sequence analysis of the genomic regions involved in the rearrangements between TPM3 and NTRK1 genes producing TRK oncogenes in papillary thyroid carcinomas. Genomics 1995;28:15–24.
83. Greco A, Mariani C, Miranda C, et al. The DNA rearrangement that generates the TRK-T3 oncogene involves a novel gene on chromosome 3 whose product has a potential coiled-coil domain. Mol Cell Biol 1995;15:6118–27.
84. Bongarzone I, Vigneri P, Mariani L, et al. RET/NTRK1 rearrangements in thyroid gland tumors of the papillary carcinoma family: correlation with clinicopathological features. Clin Cancer Res 1998;4:223–8.
85. Prasad ML, Vyas M, Horne MJ, et al. NTRK fusion oncogenes in pediatric papillary thyroid carcinoma in northeast United States. Cancer 2016;122:1097–107.
86. Bastos AU, de Jesus AC, Cerutti JM. ETV6-NTRK3 and STRN-ALK kinase fusions are recurrent events in papillary thyroid cancer of adult population. Eur J Endocrinol 2018;178:85–93.
87. Leeman-Neill RJ, Kelly LM, Liu P, et al. ETV6-NTRK3 is a common chromosomal rearrangement in radiation-associated thyroid cancer: *ETV6-NTRK3* Fusion in Thyroid Cancer. Cancer 2014;120:799–807.

88. Kelly LM, Barila G, Liu P, et al. Identification of the transforming STRN-ALK fusion as a potential therapeutic target in the aggressive forms of thyroid cancer. Proc Natl Acad Sci U S A 2014;111:4233–8.
89. Pérot G, Soubeyran I, Ribeiro A, et al. Identification of a recurrent STRN/ALK fusion in thyroid carcinomas. PLoS One 2014;9:e87170.
90. Ciampi R, Knauf JA, Kerler R, et al. Oncogenic AKAP9-BRAF fusion is a novel mechanism of MAPK pathway activation in thyroid cancer. J Clin Invest 2005;115:94–101.
91. Gandhi M, Evdokimova V, Nikiforov YE. Frequency of close positioning of chromosomal loci detected by FRET correlates with their participation in carcinogenic rearrangements in human cells. Genes Chromosomes Cancer 2012;51:1037–44.
92. Lee J-H, Lee ES, Kim YS, et al. BRAF mutation and AKAP9 expression in sporadic papillary thyroid carcinomas. Pathology 2006;38:201–4.
93. Clevers H, Nusse R. Wnt/β-catenin signaling and disease. Cell 2012;149:1192–205.
94. Garcia-Rostan G, Tallini G, Herrero A, et al. Frequent mutation and nuclear localization of beta-catenin in anaplastic thyroid carcinoma. Cancer Res 1999;59:1811–5.
95. Garcia-Rostan, Camp RL, Herrero A, et al. Beta-catenin dysregulation in thyroid neoplasms: down-regulation, aberrant nuclear expression, and CTNNB1 exon 3 mutations are markers for aggressive tumor phenotypes and poor prognosis. Am J Pathol 2001;158(3):987–96.
96. Ishigaki K, Namba H, Nakashima M, et al. Aberrant localization of beta-catenin correlates with overexpression of its target gene in human papillary thyroid cancer. J Clin Endocrinol Metab 2002;87:3433–40.
97. Lazzereschi D, Sambuco L, Carnovale Scalzo C, et al. Cyclin D1 and Cyclin E expression in malignant thyroid cells and in human thyroid carcinomas. Int J Cancer 1998;76:806–11.
98. Meirmanov S, Nakashima M, Kondo H, et al. Correlation of cytoplasmic beta-catenin and cyclin D1 overexpression during thyroid carcinogenesis around Semipalatinsk nuclear test site. Thyroid 2003;13:537–45.
99. Cross DA, Alessi DR, Cohen P, et al. Inhibition of glycogen synthase kinase-3 by insulin mediated by protein kinase B. Nature 1995;378:785–9.
100. Fang D, Hawke D, Zheng Y, et al. Phosphorylation of beta-catenin by AKT promotes beta-catenin transcriptional activity. J Biol Chem 2007;282:11221–9.
101. Ding Q, Xia W, Liu JC, et al. Erk associates with and primes GSK-3beta for its inactivation resulting in upregulation of beta-catenin. Mol Cell 2005;19:159–70.
102. Sastre-Perona A, Santisteban P. Wnt-independent role of β-catenin in thyroid cell proliferation and differentiation. Mol Endocrinol Baltim Md 2014;28:681–95.
103. Castellone MD, De Falco V, Rao DM, et al. The beta-catenin axis integrates multiple signals downstream from RET/papillary thyroid carcinoma leading to cell proliferation. Cancer Res 2009;69:1867–76.
104. Cassinelli G, Favini E, Degl'Innocenti D, et al. RET/PTC1-driven neoplastic transformation and proinvasive phenotype of human thyrocytes involve Met induction and beta-catenin nuclear translocation. Neoplasia 2009;11:10–21.
105. Tartari CJ, Donadoni C, Manieri E, et al. Dissection of the RET/β-catenin interaction in the TPC1 thyroid cancer cell line. Am J Cancer Res 2011;1:716–25.
106. Sastre-Perona A, Riesco-Eizaguirre G, Zaballos MA, et al. ß-catenin signaling is required for RAS-driven thyroid cancer through PI3K activation. Oncotarget 2016;7:49435–49.

107. Cho NL, Lin CI, Whang EE, et al. Sulindac reverses aberrant expression and localization of beta-catenin in papillary thyroid cancer cells with the BRAFV600E mutation. Thyroid 2010;20:615–22.
108. Cho SW, Kim YA, Sun HJ, et al. Therapeutic potential of Dickkopf-1 in wild-type BRAF papillary thyroid cancer via regulation of β-catenin/E-cadherin signaling. J Clin Endocrinol Metab 2014;99:E1641–9.
109. Ito T, Seyama T, Mizuno T, et al. Unique association of p53 mutations with undifferentiated but not with differentiated carcinomas of the thyroid gland. Cancer Res 1992;52:1369–71.
110. Fagin JA, Matsuo K, Karmakar A, et al. High prevalence of mutations of the p53 gene in poorly differentiated human thyroid carcinomas. J Clin Invest 1993;91:179–84.
111. Donghi R, Longoni A, Pilotti S, et al. Gene p53 mutations are restricted to poorly differentiated and undifferentiated carcinomas of the thyroid gland. J Clin Invest 1993;91:1753–60.
112. McFadden DG, Vernon A, Santiago PM, et al. p53 constrains progression to anaplastic thyroid carcinoma in a Braf-mutant mouse model of papillary thyroid cancer. Proc Natl Acad Sci U S A 2014;111:E1600–9.
113. Sadow PM, Dias-Santagata D, Zheng Z, et al. Identification of insertions in PTEN and TP53 in anaplastic thyroid carcinoma with angiogenic brain metastasis. Endocr Relat Cancer 2015;22:L23–8.
114. Landa I, Ganly I, Chan TA, et al. Frequent somatic TERT promoter mutations in thyroid cancer: higher prevalence in advanced forms of the disease. J Clin Endocrinol Metab 2013;98:E1562–6.
115. Liu X, Bishop J, Shan Y, et al. Highly prevalent TERT promoter mutations in aggressive thyroid cancers. Endocr Relat Cancer 2013;20:603–10.
116. Meyerson M, Counter CM, Eaton EN, et al. hEST2, the putative human telomerase catalytic subunit gene, is up-regulated in tumor cells and during immortalization. Cell 1997;90:785–95.
117. Brousset P, Chaouche N, Leprat F, et al. Telomerase activity in human thyroid carcinomas originating from the follicular cells. J Clin Endocrinol Metab 1997;82:4214–6.
118. Saji M, Xydas S, Westra WH, et al. Human telomerase reverse transcriptase (hTERT) gene expression in thyroid neoplasms. Clin Cancer Res 1999;5:1483–9.
119. Horn S, Figl A, Rachakonda PS, et al. TERT promoter mutations in familial and sporadic melanoma. Science 2013;339:959–61.
120. Huang FW, Hodis E, Xu MJ, et al. Highly recurrent TERT promoter mutations in human melanoma. Science 2013;339:957–9.
121. Vinagre J, Almeida A, Pópulo H, et al. Frequency of TERT promoter mutations in human cancers. Nat Commun 2013;4:2185.
122. Liu X, Qu S, Liu R, et al. TERT promoter mutations and their association with BRAF V600E mutation and aggressive clinicopathological characteristics of thyroid cancer. J Clin Endocrinol Metab 2014;99:E1130–6.
123. Melo M, da Rocha AG, Vinagre J, et al. TERT promoter mutations are a major indicator of poor outcome in differentiated thyroid carcinomas. J Clin Endocrinol Metab 2014;99:E754–65.
124. Xing M, Liu R, Liu X, et al. BRAF V600E and TERT promoter mutations cooperatively identify the most aggressive papillary thyroid cancer with highest recurrence. J Clin Oncol 2014;32:2718–26.

125. Liu R, Bishop J, Zhu G, et al. Mortality risk stratification by combining BRAF V600E and TERT promoter mutations in papillary thyroid cancer: genetic duet of BRAF and TERT promoter mutations in thyroid cancer mortality. JAMA Oncol 2016. https://doi.org/10.1001/jamaoncol.2016.3288.
126. Shi X, Liu R, Qu S, et al. Association of TERT promoter mutation 1,295,228 C>T with BRAF V600E mutation, older patient age, and distant metastasis in anaplastic thyroid cancer. J Clin Endocrinol Metab 2015;100:E632–7.
127. Liu R, Zhang T, Zhu G, et al. Regulation of mutant TERT by BRAF V600E/MAP kinase pathway through FOS/GABP in human cancer. Nat Commun 2018;9:579.
128. Martin M, Maßhöfer L, Temming P, et al. Exome sequencing identifies recurrent somatic mutations in EIF1AX and SF3B1 in uveal melanoma with disomy 3. Nat Genet 2013;45:933–6.
129. Cantley LC. The phosphoinositide 3-kinase pathway. Science 2002;296:1655–7.
130. Xing M. Genetic alterations in the phosphatidylinositol-3 kinase/Akt pathway in thyroid cancer. Thyroid 2010;20:697–706.
131. Liaw D, Marsh DJ, Li J, et al. Germline mutations of the PTEN gene in Cowden disease, an inherited breast and thyroid cancer syndrome. Nat Genet 1997;16:64–7.
132. Di Cristofano A, Pesce B, Cordon-Cardo C, et al. Pten is essential for embryonic development and tumour suppression. Nat Genet 1998;19:348–55.
133. Yeager N, Klein-Szanto A, Kimura S, et al. Pten loss in the mouse thyroid causes goiter and follicular adenomas: insights into thyroid function and Cowden disease pathogenesis. Cancer Res 2007;67:959–66.
134. Dahia PLM, Marsh DJ, Zheng Z, et al. Somatic deletions and mutations in the cowden disease gene, PTEN, in sporadic thyroid tumors. Cancer Res 1997;57:4710–3.
135. Halachmi N, Halachmi S, Evron E, et al. Somatic mutations of the PTEN tumor suppressor gene in sporadic follicular thyroid tumors. Genes Chromosomes Cancer 1998;23:239–43.
136. Samuels Y, Wang Z, Bardelli A, et al. High frequency of mutations of the PIK3CA gene in human cancers. Science 2004;304:554.
137. Hou P, Liu D, Shan Y, et al. Genetic alterations and their relationship in the phosphatidylinositol 3-kinase/Akt pathway in thyroid cancer. Clin Cancer Res 2007;13:1161–70.
138. García-Rostán G, Costa AM, Pereira-Castro I, et al. Mutation of the PIK3CA gene in anaplastic thyroid cancer. Cancer Res 2005;65:10199–207.
139. Santarpia L, El-Naggar AK, Cote GJ, et al. Phosphatidylinositol 3-kinase/akt and ras/raf-mitogen-activated protein kinase pathway mutations in anaplastic thyroid cancer. J Clin Endocrinol Metab 2008;93:278–84.
140. Burke JE, Perisic O, Masson GR, et al. Oncogenic mutations mimic and enhance dynamic events in the natural activation of phosphoinositide 3-kinase p110α (PIK3CA). Proc Natl Acad Sci U S A 2012;109:15259–64.
141. Ricarte-Filho JC, Ryder M, Chitale DA, et al. Mutational profile of advanced primary and metastatic radioactive iodine-refractory thyroid cancers reveals distinct pathogenetic roles for BRAF, PIK3CA, and AKT1. Cancer Res 2009;69:4885–93.
142. Laplante M, Sabatini DM. mTOR signaling in growth control and disease. Cell 2012;149:274–93.
143. Ringel MD, Hayre N, Saito J, et al. Overexpression and overactivation of Akt in thyroid carcinoma. Cancer Res 2001;61:6105–11.

144. Vasko V, Saji M, Hardy E, et al. Akt activation and localisation correlate with tumour invasion and oncogene expression in thyroid cancer. J Med Genet 2004;41:161–70.
145. Chen ML, Xu PZ, Peng XD, et al. The deficiency of Akt1 is sufficient to suppress tumor development in Pten+/− mice. Genes Dev 2006;20:1569–74.
146. Xu P-Z, Chen ML, Jeon SM, et al. The effect Akt2 deletion on tumor development in Pten(+/-) mice. Oncogene 2012;31:518–26.
147. Beroukhim R, Mermel CH, Porter D, et al. The landscape of somatic copy-number alteration across human cancers. Nature 2010;463:899–905.
148. Tang YC, Amon A. Gene copy-number alterations: a cost-benefit analysis. Cell 2013;152:394–405.
149. Knouse KA, Davoli T, Elledge SJ, et al. Aneuploidy in cancer: seq-ing answers to old questions. Annu Rev Cancer Biol 2017;1:335–54.
150. Wang Y, Hou P, Yu H, et al. High prevalence and mutual exclusivity of genetic alterations in the phosphatidylinositol-3-kinase/akt pathway in thyroid tumors. J Clin Endocrinol Metab 2007;92:2387–90.
151. Garcia-Rendueles ME, Ricarte-Filho JC, Untch BR, et al. NF2 loss promotes oncogenic RAS-induced thyroid cancers via YAP-dependent transactivation of RAS proteins and sensitizes them to MEK inhibition. Cancer Discov 2015;5:1178–93.
152. Duquette M, Sadow PM, Husain A, et al. Metastasis-associated MCL1 and P16 copy number alterations dictate resistance to vemurafenib in a BRAF V600E patient-derived papillary thyroid carcinoma preclinical model. Oncotarget 2015;6:42445–67.
153. Anders L, Ke N, Hydbring P, et al. A systematic screen for CDK4/6 substrates links FOXM1 phosphorylation to senescence suppression in cancer cells. Cancer Cell 2011;20:620–34.
154. Antonello ZA, Hsu N, Bhasin M, et al. Vemurafenib-resistance via de novo RBM genes mutations and chromosome 5 aberrations is overcome by combined therapy with palbociclib in thyroid carcinoma with BRAF^{V600E}. Oncotarget 2017;8:84743–60.
155. Liu Y, Cope L, Sun W, et al. DNA copy number variations characterize benign and malignant thyroid tumors. J Clin Endocrinol Metab 2013;98:E558–66.
156. Karin M. Nuclear factor-kappaB in cancer development and progression. Nature 2006;441:431–6.
157. Visconti R, Cerutti J, Battista S, et al. Expression of the neoplastic phenotype by human thyroid carcinoma cell lines requires NFkappaB p65 protein expression. Oncogene 1997;15:1987–94.
158. Starenki D, Namba H, Saenko V, et al. Inhibition of nuclear factor-kappaB cascade potentiates the effect of a combination treatment of anaplastic thyroid cancer cells. J Clin Endocrinol Metab 2004;89:410–8.
159. Pacifico F, Mauro C, Barone C, et al. Oncogenic and anti-apoptotic activity of NF-kappa B in human thyroid carcinomas. J Biol Chem 2004;279:54610–9.
160. Bommarito A, Richiusa P, Carissimi E, et al. BRAFV600E mutation, TIMP-1 upregulation, and NF-κB activation: closing the loop on the papillary thyroid cancer trilogy. Endocr Relat Cancer 2011;18:669–85.
161. Neely RJ, Brose MS, Gray CM, et al. The RET/PTC3 oncogene activates classical NF-κB by stabilizing NIK. Oncogene 2011;30:87–96.
162. Kato Y, Ying H, Zhao L, et al. PPARgamma insufficiency promotes follicular thyroid carcinogenesis via activation of the nuclear factor-kappaB signaling pathway. Oncogene 2006;25:2736–47.

163. Guigon CJ, Zhao L, Willingham MC, et al. PTEN deficiency accelerates tumour progression in a mouse model of thyroid cancer. Oncogene 2009;28:509–17.
164. Bauerle KT, Schweppe RE, Lund G, et al. Nuclear factor κB-dependent regulation of angiogenesis, and metastasis in an in vivo model of thyroid cancer is associated with secreted interleukin-8. J Clin Endocrinol Metab 2014;99: E1436–44.
165. Pozdeyev N, Berlinberg A, Zhou Q, et al. Targeting the NF-κB pathway as a combination therapy for advanced thyroid cancer. PLoS One 2015;10: e0134901.
166. Davies KJ, Ermak G, Rothermel BA, et al. Renaming the DSCR1/Adapt78 gene family as RCAN: regulators of calcineurin. FASEB J 2007;21:3023–8.
167. Martínez-Martínez S, Genescà L, Rodríguez A, et al. The RCAN carboxyl end mediates calcineurin docking-dependent inhibition via a site that dictates binding to substrates and regulators. Proc Natl Acad Sci U S A 2009;106:6117–22.
168. Hogan PG, Chen L, Nardone J, et al. Transcriptional regulation by calcium, calcineurin, and NFAT. Genes Dev 2003;17:2205–32.
169. Baek KH, Zaslavsky A, Lynch RC, et al. Down's syndrome suppression of tumour growth and the role of the calcineurin inhibitor DSCR1. Nature 2009; 459:1126–30.
170. Hesser BA, Liang XH, Camenisch G, et al. Down syndrome critical region protein 1 (DSCR1), a novel VEGF target gene that regulates expression of inflammatory markers on activated endothelial cells. Blood 2004;104:149–58.
171. Iizuka M, Abe M, Shiiba K, et al. Down syndrome candidate region 1,a downstream target of VEGF, participates in endothelial cell migration and angiogenesis. J Vasc Res 2004;41:334–44.
172. Minami T, Horiuchi K, Miura M, et al. Vascular endothelial growth factor- and thrombin-induced termination factor, Down syndrome critical region-1, attenuates endothelial cell proliferation and angiogenesis. J Biol Chem 2004;279: 50537–54.
173. Stathatos N, Bourdeau I, Espinosa AV, et al. KiSS-1/G protein-coupled receptor 54 metastasis suppressor pathway increases myocyte-enriched calcineurin interacting protein 1 expression and chronically inhibits calcineurin activity. J Clin Endocrinol Metab 2005;90:5432–40.
174. Espinosa AV, Shinohara M, Porchia LM, et al. Regulator of calcineurin 1 modulates cancer cell migration in vitro. Clin Exp Metastasis 2009;26:517–26.
175. Wang C, Saji M, Justiniano SE, et al. RCAN1-4 is a thyroid cancer growth and metastasis suppressor. JCI Insight 2017;2:e90651.
176. Kimura ET, Nikiforova MN, Zhu Z, et al. High prevalence of BRAF mutations in thyroid cancer: genetic evidence for constitutive activation of the RET/PTC-RAS-BRAF signaling pathway in papillary thyroid carcinoma. Cancer Res 2003;63:1454–7.
177. Henderson YC, Shellenberger TD, Williams MD, et al. High rate of BRAF and RET/PTC dual mutations associated with recurrent papillary thyroid carcinoma. Clin Cancer Res 2009;15:485–91.
178. Smallridge RC, Ain KB, Asa SL, et al. American Thyroid Association guidelines for management of patients with anaplastic thyroid cancer. Thyroid 2012;22: 1104–39.
179. Kaneshige M, Kaneshige K, Zhu X, et al. Mice with a targeted mutation in the thyroid hormone beta receptor gene exhibit impaired growth and resistance to thyroid hormone. Proc Natl Acad Sci U S A 2000;97(24):13209–14.

180. Suzuki H, Willingham MC, Cheng SY. Mice with a mutation in the thyroid hormone receptor beta gene spontaneously develop thyroid carcinoma: a mouse model of thyroid carcinogenesis. Thyroid 2002;12:963–9.
181. Ying H, Suzuki H, Zhao L, et al. Mutant thyroid hormone receptor beta represses the expression and transcriptional activity of peroxisome proliferator-activated receptor gamma during thyroid carcinogenesis. Cancer Res 2003;63:5274–80.
182. Araki O, Ying H, Furuya F, et al. Thyroid hormone receptor beta mutants: dominant negative regulators of peroxisome proliferator-activated receptor gamma action. Proc Natl Acad Sci U S A 2005;102:16251–6.
183. Furuya F, Hanover JA, Cheng S. Activation of phosphatidylinositol 3-kinase signaling by a mutant thyroid hormone beta receptor. Proc Natl Acad Sci U S A 2006;103:1780–5.
184. Guigon CJ, Zhao L, Lu C, et al. Regulation of beta-catenin by a novel nongenomic action of thyroid hormone beta receptor. Mol Cell Biol 2008;28:4598–608.
185. Guigon CJ, Kim DW, Zhu X, et al. Tumor suppressor action of liganded thyroid hormone receptor beta by direct repression of beta-catenin gene expression. Endocrinology 2010;151:5528–36.
186. Kim WG, Park JW, Willingham MC, et al. Diet-induced obesity increases tumor growth and promotes anaplastic change in thyroid cancer in a mouse model. Endocrinology 2013;154:2936–47.
187. Park JW, Han CR, Zhao L, et al. Inhibition of STAT3 activity delays obesity-induced thyroid carcinogenesis in a mouse model. Endocr Relat Cancer 2016;23:53–63.
188. Park J, Kim WG, Zhao L, et al. Metformin blocks progression of obesity-activated thyroid cancer in a mouse model. Oncotarget 2016;7:34832–44.
189. Zhu X, Zhao L, Park JW, et al. Synergistic signaling of KRAS and thyroid hormone receptor β mutants promotes undifferentiated thyroid cancer through MYC up-regulation. Neoplasia N Y N 2014;16:757–69.
190. Zhu X, Enomoto K, Zhao L, et al. Bromodomain and extraterminal protein inhibitor JQ1 suppresses thyroid tumor growth in a mouse model. Clin Cancer Res 2017;23:430–40.
191. Park S, Willingham M, Qi J, et al. Metformin and JQ1 synergistically inhibit obesity-activated thyroid cancer. Endocr Relat Cancer 2018. https://doi.org/10.1530/ERC-18-0071.

第4章
甲状腺结节临床诊断的评估

Carolyn Maxwell, Jennifer A.Sipos

关键词

- 甲状腺 ● 甲状腺结节 ● 超声 ● 淋巴结 ● 细针穿刺活检

要点

- 甲状腺结节的评估应包括颈部超声检查。
- 应根据患者临床表现、血清促甲状腺激素和超声报告确定甲状腺结节是否需要细针穿刺活检。
- 颈部淋巴结的超声检查是评估甲状腺结节的重要组成部分。

引言

甲状腺结节是一种常见的临床疾病,在 70 岁以上的中发病率高达 70%[1]。这些病变大多是良性,只有 5%~15% 的结节为恶性肿瘤[2,3]。庆幸的是,甲状腺癌有较高的可治疗性,大多数患者有良好的长期生存率。事实上,通过对较小的低风险的甲状腺癌的观察性研究表明,在没有手术干预的情况下,经过中位数为 6 年的随访,只有不到 10% 的患者病情出现恶化[4]。然而,并不是所有的甲状腺恶性肿瘤预后都如此良好;高达 20% 的患者在初次诊断时,其肿瘤可能已经处于更高的分期[5,6]。因此,临床医生有责任建立一个准确、有效的系统,从而可以对大量的甲状腺结节进行筛选,以便在患者尚未处于较高风险的情况下,对罕见且潜在致命的肿瘤进行甄别与切除。

流行病学

甲状腺结节的患病率取决于检测方法。约 5%~10% 的患者通过触诊检查出甲状腺结节[1]。然而,超声等敏感成像技术的应用检测出了高达 34.2% 的甲状腺结节性疾病[7]。甲状腺结节的发病率随年龄呈线性增加,30 岁以下的患者占 12.9%,然而,70 岁以上患者中 50%~70% 有 1 个或多个结节[7-9]。患病风险还受到性别的影响,女性患甲状腺结节的可能性是男性的 3~4 倍[7,10]。造成这种差异的原因尚不清楚。转诊偏倚[11]、代谢参数[12]和雌激素效应[13,14]是已公认的潜在因素。

危险因素

碘摄入不足或摄入过量都会增加甲状腺结节的患病风险[15]。另一个重要的危险因素是儿童时期暴露于电离辐射[16,17]。在一项针对儿童霍奇金病患者的大型回顾性研究中,甲状腺受到辐射的患者患结节的可能性是其对照组同胞的 27 倍[18]。在最近一项针对 119 名儿童癌症幸存者的研究中,暴露于电离辐射和接受化疗的患者(n=60)患甲状腺结节的可能性是仅接受化疗患者(18.6%,P=0.03)的 2 倍(36.7%)[19]。成人接受治疗性辐射对甲状腺结节发展的额外风险的定量仍然难以确定。

症状

病史及体格检查

虽然仅凭病史和体格检查不能准确鉴别结节的性质,但某些临床症状可能会提高其为甲状腺恶性肿瘤的可能性[20]。由于这些症状提高了甲状腺癌的可能性,因此,询问个人辐射史和甲状腺癌家族史或甲状腺癌综合征(多发性内分泌瘤、Cowden 综合征、家族性增生,或者加德纳综合征)和评估快速增长的颈部包块(如果患者确认)显得十分重要。此外,确定有固定结节、局部肿大的淋巴结或声带麻痹的存在,可将恶性的风险提高到 70% 以上[20]。

也应咨询有甲状腺结节的患者是否存在局部受压症状。明确地说,临床医生应确定患者是否有吞咽固体食物困难、发声困难或颈部发紧等症状。这些症状的存在不一定与结节的良恶性相关,但可能是确定手术的原因[21]。

诊断检查和影像实验室评估

所有怀疑有甲状腺结节的患者均应检验血清促甲状腺激素(thyroid-stimulating hormone,TSH)[21]。低 TSH 提示有亚临床或明显的甲状腺功能亢进,需要进一步的实验室检查、超声检查和可能的显像检查来评估"热"结节(见甲状腺显像检查)[22]。另外,TSH 正常或升高则不太可能是自主结节,此时显像检查的价值有限,应该进一步行超声诊断评估。

促甲状腺素是已知的甲状腺滤泡细胞生长因子,血清 TSH 的抑制与晚期甲状腺癌患者生存的改善有关[23]。进一步说,TSH 升高会增加甲状腺结节恶性的概率[24]。一项前瞻性研究表明,与 TSH 水平较低的患者相比,血清 TSH ≥ 2.26mU/ml 的患者患甲状腺癌的风险要高出 3 倍[25]。此外,术前伴有较高 TSH 水平的患者,也预示着其肿瘤具有更高的分期,伴有腺外侵犯和淋巴结转移[26,27]。

尽管血清降钙素是甲状腺髓样癌(medullary thyroid cancer,MTC)的一种标志物,但是是否应该对所有甲状腺结节患者行降钙素检测仍然具有一定争议[21]。一项针对超过 10 000 名甲状腺结节患者的大型前瞻性研究发现,与单用细针穿刺活检(fine-needle aspiration,FNA)相比,常规血清降钙素检测可提高诊断的敏感性和特异性。与行常规降钙素检测前被诊断的患者相比,这些经过筛查更早被诊断为 MTC 的患者,其痊愈的可能性更高[28]。这项研究和其他研究均表明,通过五肽胃泌素刺激试验对基础值升高的患者行常规降钙素检测确诊 MTC 是有益的。不过,美国目前还没有广泛应用这种刺激试验。基础降钙素值为 50~100pg/ml 的特异性仅为 25%;假阳性可见于肾衰竭、吸烟、慢性自身免疫性甲状腺炎和其他神经内分泌肿瘤等[29]。因此,缺乏确证性的试验会给许多患者带来严重过度治疗的风险。鉴于缺乏支持或反对筛查作用的明确数据,目前,美国甲状腺协会(American Thyroid Association,ATA)指南不推荐也不反对常规进行降钙素检测[21]。

血清甲状腺球蛋白对确定甲状腺结节的良恶性没有很大作用[21]。虽然甲状腺癌患者的甲状腺球蛋白通常很高,但良性多结节性甲状腺肿患者的甲状腺球蛋白也会显著升高[30]。

甲状腺显像

放射性核素显像提供了有关结节功能状态的信息。碘同位素(通常为

^{123}I)或锝 -99m(^{99m}Tc)高锝酸盐通过带针孔准直器的伽马照相机进行平面成像。这些扫描分辨率较差,限制了其对 1cm 以上结节的探测应用。对于有多个甲状腺结节的患者,二维成像可能会混淆重叠结节功能状态的准确特征。

相比正常甲状腺组织,恶性结节通常对放射性同位素的富集程度较低,会表现为"冷"或无功能状态。但是大多数良性结节也没有功能,降低了这一发现的特异性。因此,超声特征决定了对冷结节行进一步细胞学评估的必要性。核素显像的临床价值在于鉴别出比邻近甲状腺组织更能集碘的结节。这些自主性(或"热")结节很少有恶性的,因此不需要进行 FNA[22]。

超声

所有怀疑有甲状腺结节的患者均应行超声检查[21]。高达 63% 的患者有超声学改变[31]。在针对 114 例临床发现甲状腺结节的患者的回顾性研究中,16% 患者的超声检查没有显示出结节[31]。此外,超声在 23% 的患者中发现了甲状腺其他部位的隐匿性病变[31]。在对甲状腺结节患者进行初步评估时,对侧颈部超声评估有助于确定甲状腺癌确诊后的手术范围。除此之外,一些研究还发现,在术前颈部超声检查之后,40% 以上患者的手术方式发生了改变[32,33]。

门诊超声的优势

超声检查为临床医生和患者提供了许多好处。作为体格检查的补充,实时超声检查允许临床医生将探头直接放置在重点关注部位,以确定治疗方案。许多灰阶超声图在实时观察中比静止图像更容易识别,特别是将高回声病灶描述为胶质或微钙化时(两者具有相反的临床意义)[34]。

如何行颈部超声检查

患者在行颈部超声检查时最好呈仰卧位,可以在肩膀之间放一个枕头或卷毛巾使颈部完全伸展。使用高频探头(5~13MHz)可实现高分辨率成像。

为了确保检查的全面性,操作者用一个标准化的区域清单来检查。甲状腺本身分三个部分:峡部、左侧腺叶和右侧腺叶,在横视图和矢状视图中都可以看到(图 4.1)。腺叶的大小记录在三维以及腺体的整体特征中(表 4.1)。

甲状腺结节的记录应实现标准化(表 4.1),以改进研究时的决策,并提高监测检查的敏感性。

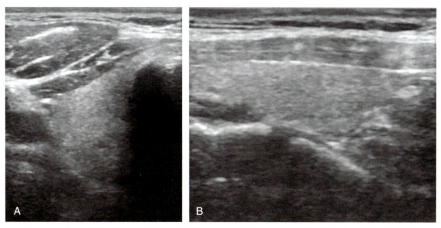

图 4.1 （A）横切面上正常的右甲状腺叶和峡部。（B）正常甲状腺矢状面（纵向）

表 4.1
超声检查报告的特点

甲状腺特征	结节特征	淋巴结特征
每个腺叶大小	大小	大小
回声反射	位置	形状
结构（平滑/异质性）	回声反射	钙化/囊性改变
血流情况	成分	位置
气管偏离	回声灶	血流分布
峡部厚度	边缘	回声反射
	血流分布	

中央区（甲状腺后方）和侧颈区域的详细检查是颈部全面超声检查的关键组成部分；发现异常颈部淋巴结有助于危险分层，并为手术计划提供信息。中央区，又称作第Ⅵ区，包含气管旁淋巴结，从舌骨上部延伸到胸骨切口下部。在甲状腺完整的情况下，中央区检查的灵敏度比较有限[35]。

侧颈也应该进行系统的检查，从第Ⅳ区到第Ⅱ区，在锁骨下方和颈动脉鞘内侧接壤，胸锁乳突肌后边缘的侧面，下颌骨的上部。胸锁乳突肌外侧的Ⅴ区包括颈部后室的结节，通过环状软骨分为上（ⅤA）和下（ⅤB）两区。

超声危险分层

一直以来，甲状腺结节的一些超声特征与乳头状甲状腺癌（papillary

thyroid cancer,PTC)增长的危险性相关,一些多变量分析已经证实,当这些特征在单个结节中都观察到时,危险性将增加[36,37]。结节声像图的评估由六个基本组成部分,以确定恶性的可能性:成分、回声、形状、边缘、回声病灶和结节内血流。

成分

结节分为全实性、全囊性或混合囊性和实性。大多数甲状腺癌是实性的;一项针对360个恶性结节的回顾性研究发现,88%的甲状腺癌或为完全实性,或只有不到5%的为囊性[38]。然而,实性结节的成分并不特殊,因为大多数实性结节是良性的。全囊性或无回声结节,也基本都是良性的[39],且无细胞,这些结节的取样通常得不出诊断结果。囊性和实性成分混合的结节比全实性结节恶性的概率低[38,40],但在出现可疑的超声特征时,则可能需要进一步分析。例如,海绵状图像(图4.2A),其中远超过50%的结节是由微囊性改变构成,恶性风险非常低[36,39,41,42]。在其他混合实性和囊性结节中,当实性成分与结节壁成锐角接触、形状偏离或含有微钙化时,结节恶性风险则会增加[38,40,43](图4.2B)。

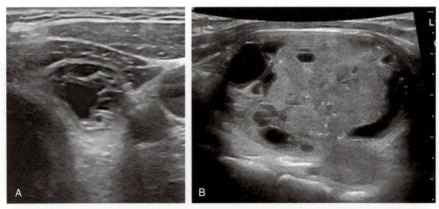

图4.2 (A)海绵状结节。(B)超声表现为可疑的混合性结节(边缘不规则,微钙化)

回声

相对于正常甲状腺组织来说,结节的回声可分为两类:高/等回声和低回声。高/等回声结节(比正常甲状腺组织的回声强或具有相同的回声)通常是良性的,而结节一旦为恶性则可能预示着滤泡型肿瘤[44,45](图4.3A)。低回声比正常甲状腺组织回声暗,此时结节有更高恶性的风险,由于超过一半的低回声结节是良性的,所以这又不算一个特殊发现(图 4.3B)。有的结节明显低回声,与周围的肌肉组织一样或更暗,此时,结节有更高恶性的风险[37,41](图 4.3C)。

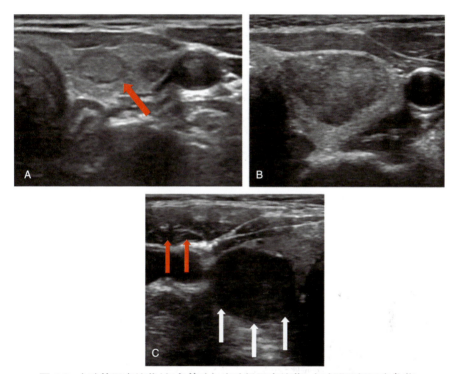

图 4.3 (A)等回声结节(红色箭头)。(B)低回声结节。(C)明显低回声结节,注意结节回声(白色箭头)比前带肌(红色箭头)暗

形状

当患者仰卧时,良性甲状腺结节在水平面上自然生长(图 4.4A)。与该平面反方向生长,或高>宽时,则暗示结节有更强的侵袭性并且可能为恶性[46](图 4.4B)。一些研究报道,在横向或纵向成像中,纵向>横向会增加恶性的风险[47,48],但仅见于 12% 的甲状腺结节[36]。据报道,这一发现的特异性高达 94%[48]。这一发现的效用可能限于结节的大小,因为一项研究发现,与较大结节相比,1cm 以下的病灶的形状特异性更高[46]。

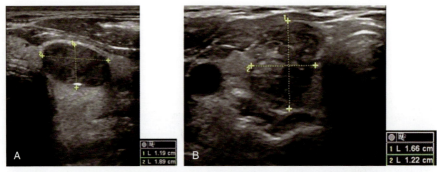

图 4.4 （A）椭圆形结节（水平生长面）。（B）高＞宽的形状

边缘

甲状腺结节边缘不规则（浸润性、毛刺状或微分叶）会增加其恶性的风险，尽管这一特点缺乏敏感性，33%~93% 的恶性结节可能有平滑或规则的边界[49]（图 4.5A）。但重要的是在结节的边界与周围的甲状腺分辨不清时，区分不规则的边界和边界不清的边缘。边界不清常见于良性等回声或轻度低回声结节，不会增加恶性风险（图 4.5B）[41]。晕环，即围绕结节的无回声（超声透明）边缘（图 4.5C），以前被认为与良性结节有关。最近的超声分层系统没有将这一特征纳入风险评估，因为它难以区分或定义，可能存在于不规则边缘的情况下，并且还在某些癌症中可见[37,49]。当结节通过甲状腺包膜扩散到邻近的肌肉或血管系统时，则高度怀疑为恶性肿瘤[37,50,51]。

回声灶

结节内的回声区有助于风险分层，但准确分类至关重要，因为某些形式（而不是所有形式）的钙化提高了肿瘤恶性的风险。巨大钙化指超过 1mm 的粗大高回声包涵体，伴有后部声学阴影[36]（图 4.6A）。一些研究[52,53]报道，结节内巨大钙化使癌症的可能性增加，但一些分析发现，如没有其他可疑特征，孤立的巨型钙化并不是恶性肿瘤的可靠预测因子[36,54,55]。外周线性钙化，也称为边缘或蛋壳钙化（图 4.6B），一些数据也表明其与结节为恶性的风险相冲突。然而，受软组织挤压断裂的边缘则具有很高的恶性可能[56]。

小于 1mm 的小点状回声病灶可能是胶质体或微钙化，代表着风险谱的两端，准确区分这些全然不同的特点十分重要，但又极具挑战性。胶质体的标志性特征是后方混响伪影，通常也称为彗尾征或 V 形伪影（图 4.6C）。实时超声比在静态图像上更容易识别这些特点。缺少彗尾征的点状病灶（图 4.6D）更可能代表着微钙化,这通常与甲状腺乳头状癌密切相关[36,41]。最后,位于微囊性区域后方的线性高回声包涵体,如在海绵状结节所见,是混合结节固体成分内的后方声增强伪影,不会增加恶性的风险(图 4.6E)。

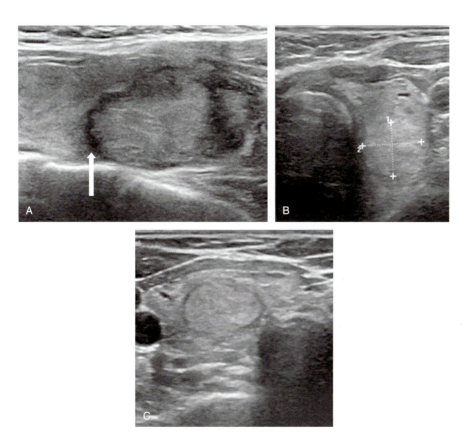

图 4.5 (A)白色箭头表示浸润性/分叶边缘。(B)边界不清,结节和甲状腺的回声非常相似,使结节的定义极具挑战性。(C)等回声结节周围的晕环——超声透光圈

结节内血流

结节内血流增加以前被认为是恶性的危险因素[57,58],但最近已被证明没有预测能力[59,60]。一项对近 700 个甲状腺肿瘤的研究发现,超过一半的恶性结节,达到 63%,在术前超声图像上无结节内血管[60]。实际上,ATA[21]和美国放射学会(Thyroid Imaging Reporting and Data System,TIRADS)[37]最新的风险分层指南没有将血流状态纳入其超声分层系统。然而,应该注意的是,结节内血流可能与一些肿瘤和传统 PTC 以外的其他恶性肿瘤的恶性风险相

关,包括具有乳头状特征的非侵袭性滤泡性甲状腺肿瘤(noninvasive follicular thyroid neoplasm with papillary-like nuclear feature,NIFTP),滤泡型乳头状甲状腺癌(follicular variant of papillary thyroid carcinoma,FVPTC),滤泡型甲状腺癌(follicular thyroid carcinoma,FTC)和 MTC [39,60-62]。

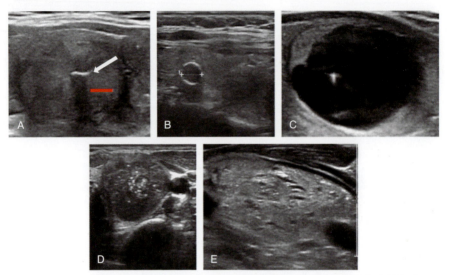

图 4.6 (A)巨大钙化(白色箭头)伴后声影(红色箭头)。(B)不间断的蛋壳样钙化。(C)彗尾征。(D)微钙化。(E)囊性内容物后面的明亮线性反射

非乳头状甲状腺癌

经典的可疑声像图特征,如纵横比>1、微钙化和低回声,是较准确预测 PTC 的指标,但很少与其他形式的甲状腺癌相关。FTC 和 FVPTC 在超声上更不确定:等回声,缺乏微钙化,并且为椭圆形(而不是高)[44,45,63]。由于这个原因,没有这些可疑特征的结节仍然要观察和穿刺[21]。然而,由于 2cm 以下的滤泡癌转移率非常低,所以,这些超声难以判断性质的结节,其行 FNA 的阈值更大[64]。

很少有研究探讨 MTC 的具体声像图特征。现有数据表明,MTC 与 PTC 都具有某些可疑的特征,如明显的低回声和粗糙的钙化,但更有可能是圆形(不高不宽),其边界规则,结节内血流特征比 PTC 更明显[62,65-67]。一项研究报告,亚厘米级 MTC 的超声特征与 PTC 相仿,具有高>宽和毛刺边缘的特点;然而,较大(>1cm)的髓样癌往往具有较少可疑的元素,如圆形规则的边界[68]。

假结节

甲状腺实质内的某些声像图特征可能会给出结节或"假结节"的假象。这种情况最常发生在自身免疫性甲状腺炎患者中,慢性炎症使甲状腺实质出现异质性,大量淋巴细胞沉积为低回声斑块,可能被误认为结节。这一发现,通常被称为"长颈鹿"型(图 4.7A 和 B)或"瑞士奶酪"型(图 4.7C),这只代表淋巴细胞浸润,此时不应立即于低回声区采样。此外,慢性炎症导致的纤维化表现为高回声线形条带,这可能给人以甲状腺结节在其边界内的错误印象(图 4.7D)。这些区域通常可以通过它们在横断面和矢状面的成像中缺乏明显的结节外观,并且不随探针的移动而示踪证明,从而与真正的结节区分开来。

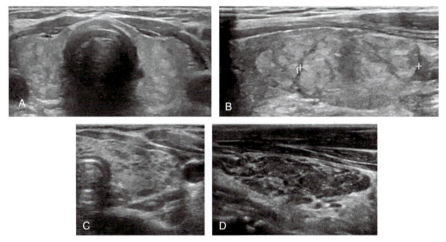

图 4.7 (A)自身免疫性甲状腺炎的"长颈鹿"型,横断面。(B)自身免疫性甲状腺炎的"长颈鹿"型,矢状面。(C)早期桥本甲状腺炎的微囊性改变("瑞士奶酪"型)。(D)自身免疫性甲状腺炎的纤维带

淋巴结评估

因为对颈部中央区和侧区的超声检查可识别触及不到的可疑淋巴结,并影响到恶性风险的评估,进而改变大约 1/3 患者的手术计划,所以这是颈部超声全面检查的关键因素[32,33],良性淋巴结具有特征性的超声表现——扁平或卵圆形-高回声的淋巴门、纯囊性病变和引流至淋巴管[69](图 4.8A)。30%~80% 的正常淋巴结可见淋巴门[70-73]。在良性和癌变的结节中都可以看

到门的缺失,但它的存在基本上排除了恶性过程[74]。

　　淋巴结肿大,通常定义为最短轴长>8~10mm,此时提示为恶性,但非特异性,因为淋巴结肿大是感染或炎症的正常反应。若结节从椭圆形转变为圆形,则提示为恶性(图4.8B)。客观来说,圆形的定义为短长轴比为0.5或更大,尽管这种转变也可以发生在良性反应过程中[75],但重要的是检查横断面和矢状面上的每个淋巴结。基于探头的位置,在一个节点上看起来可能是圆形的,但是在不同的平面上可能会显示节点的延伸。

　　几个更明确的超声特征与甲状腺癌转移至淋巴结的存在有关。在淋巴结内出现的高回声组织(外观与甲状腺组织相似),无论是最初的小沉积,还是最终整个淋巴结的替代,都是由恶性滤泡细胞和胶质浸润所致[71,76]。结节内的血流供应也有助于区分良性或恶性过程。良性或反应性淋巴结通常显示淋巴门(图4.8C)或无血流,而在转移性结节(图4.8D)可观察到无组织或周围血管[71,77]。囊性变也具有高度的恶变预测能力,可表现为淋巴结内散在的小囊性区域或整个淋巴结被囊性液替代[70,71,76](图4.8E)。在PTC的转移性淋巴结中,46%~69%可见结节内钙化,而在甲状腺髓样癌中少见。它们通常位于淋巴结周围,呈点状(图4.8F)。放疗或化疗后淋巴结内也可见钙化[78]。

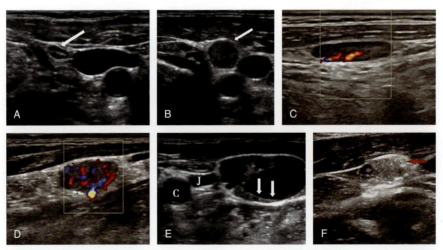

图4.8　(A)良性侧区的淋巴门,梭形(卵圆形)。白色箭头表示淋巴门。(B)左侧颈动脉前圆形恶性结节(白色箭头)。(C)良性淋巴结,门部多普勒血流正常。(D)恶性结节伴周围血流。(E)恶性结节伴有内囊性变性和小的外周固体成分(白色箭头)。C,颈动脉,J,颈静脉。(F)恶性结节伴有微钙化(红色箭头)

风险分层系统

基于上述甲状腺结节的超声特征,多个风险分层系统得以建立[21,37,79-84],致力于创建一种共同的方法来描述和分类发病率最高的结节,同时避免对良性结节进行不必要的活检。早期的系统建议对具有单一可疑特征的结节进行活检[79,80],而最近的分类方案使用了模式识别或采用定量方法[21,37,81,82]。虽然结节恶性的可能性随着可疑征象的增加而增加,但其对任何单个超声元素的敏感性都很低。不同的超声医师也并不是常常可以达成一致,即使有经验的超声医师在检查单独的超声特征时也是如此[87]。然而,基于模式分类系统的使用却能显著改善观察者之间的协议[88,89]。

甲状腺成像、报告和数据系统

TIRADS 首字母缩写最早是由 Horvath 及其同事[82]提出的,它是根据美国放射学会(American College of Radiology,ACR)广泛使用的乳腺影像报告数据系统(Breast Imaging Reporting and Data System,BIRADS)改编而来。随后公布了名为 TIRADS 的多个甲状腺风险分层系统[90],使用 5~10 个风险等级。由 Horvath 及其同事[82]首先提出的 10 层系统已经在一项单独的研究中得到验证,据报道,对于高风险模式中的恶性肿瘤,其敏感度为 99.6%,特异度为 74.4%[91]。

由美国放射学会(ACR-TIRADS)[37]认可的 TIRADS 系统包括一针对个人特征指定的积分系统,如高>宽、不规则的边缘等,然后进一步分为 5 个 TIRADS 级别(表 4.2 和表 4.3)。ACR-TIRADS 已在一项大型多机构研究[86]中得到验证,该研究评估了 3422 个结节,并将相应的 TIRADS 分级进行评分(0~10 分),结果发现,随着评分的增加,恶性肿瘤的风险也相应增加了,从 1 分的 0.3% 增加到 10 分或以上的 68.4%。肿瘤的恶性风险与 TIRADS 的分类相关联:TR1 0.3%,TR2 1.5%,TR3 4.8%,TR4 为 9.1%,TR5 为 35%。

ATA[21]、美国内分泌学会(American College of Endocrinology,ACE)[84]和韩国甲状腺放射学会(Korean Society for Thyroid Radiology,K-IRADS)[81]提出的其他分类系统包括没有定量点系统的基于模式的分类。K-TIRADS 包括 4 种基于灰阶超声图的模式:良性、低度、中度、高度可疑。该系统在 902 个结节的前瞻性研究中得到验证,其报告的恶性肿瘤风险分别为 0%、7.8%、25.4% 和 79.3%[85]。

表 4.2
ACR-TIRADS 结节特征和每个特征的相关点

成分		回声		形状		边缘		回声灶	
囊性	0	无回声	0	宽大于高	0	光滑	0	无	0
海绵状	0	超/等回声	1	高大于宽	3	不确定	0	彗尾征	0
混合性	1	低回声	2			分叶状/不规则	2	巨大钙化	1
实性	2	明显低回声	3			腺外扩散	3	周边/边缘	2
								点状	3

Tessler FN, Middleton WD, Grant EG, et al. ACR thyroid imaging, reporting and data system (TI-RADS): white paper of the ACR TI-RADS Committee. J Am Coll Radiol 2017; 14(5): 589.

表 4.3
ACR-TIRADS 评分

分数	0	2	3	4~6	7
TIRADS 分级	TR1	TR2	TR3	TR4	TR 5
临床描述	良性	不可疑	轻度可疑	中度可疑	高度可疑

Tessler FN, Middleton WD, Grant EG, et al. ACR thyroid imaging, reporting and data system (TI-RADS): white paper of the ACR TI-RADS Committee. JAm Coll Radiol 2017; 14(5): 589.

ATA 危险分层系统包括 5 个类别，基于灰阶超声图的各种组合：良性、极低恶性、低度恶性、中度恶性、高度恶性，相应恶性风险的估计分别为：不超过 1%、不超过 3%、5%~10%、10%~20% 和 70%~90%[21]。这些对结节恶性风险的评估在一项 206 个结节的前瞻性研究中得到验证，报告的极低恶性率为 2%、低度恶性率为 8%、中度恶性率为 11%，超声模式报告的高度可疑恶性率为 100%[92]。其他研究发现，在 ATA 分类中属于高度恶性结节，其恶性程度低至 55%~58%[93,94]。ATA 系统的一个缺陷是，有的结节有一个可疑的特征，如微钙化，不是低回声，不能归类，因此恶性的风险无法量化。在验证性研究中，不属于 ATA 归类的结节数量从 0% 至 14% 不等[86,92,94]，一项研究发现，这些无法归类的结节有 18% 是恶性的[94]。

很少有比较各种分层系统性能的研究。Middleton 及其同事[86]用他们 3422 个结节的数据集来比较 ACR-TIRADS 与 ATA 和 K-TIRADS，得出的结论是，依靠 ACR-TIRADS 活检的良性结节均低于其他两种系统。意大利一项对 987 个结节的研究发现，将 5 级 ATA 系统分别与 ACE[84]和英国甲状腺协会推荐的 3 级和 4 级系统相比较，其准确性不相上下[93]（表 4.4）。

表 4.4
ATA 分层体系中管理建议的比较

分类	描述	FNA 阈值大小	细胞学检查为良性的监测时间间隔
ATA			
良性	无回声囊肿	不推荐	不推荐
非常低度	混合性；海绵状	≥2cm	≥24 个月或临床监测
低度	混合性或实行高/等回声	≥1.5cm	12~24 个月
中度	实性低回声	≥1cm	12~24 个月
高度	有可疑特征的低回声	≥1cm	在第 12 个月进行重复的 FNA 或超声复查
ACR-TIRADS			
0 良性	0 分(图 4.2)	不推荐	
2 不怀疑	2 分(图 4.2)	不推荐	
3 轻度怀疑	3 分(图 4.2)	FNA≥2.5cm 随访≥1.5cm	第 1,3,5 年
4 中度怀疑	4~6 分(图 4.2)	FNA≥1.5cm 随访≥1.0cm	第 1,2,3,5 年
5 高度怀疑	≥7 分(图 4.2)	FNA≥1.0cm 随访≥0.5cm	每 5 年
K-TIRADS			
2 良性	囊状,海绵状,混合性与胶体包裹物	≥2cm	未说明
3 低度可疑	混合性或实性高/等回声	≥1.5cm	12~24 个月
4 中度可疑	无可疑特征的实性低回声或有可疑特征的高/等回声	≥1cm	12~24 个月
5 高可疑	伴可疑特征的实性低回声	≥0.5~1cm	在 6~12 个月内 FNA 和超声复查
ACE			
低度	囊状,海绵状,有胶体包裹物的混合性	≥2cm 且大小一直增加或其他临床危险因素	≥12 个月或临床监测
中度	实性或混合性,无可疑特征	≥2cm	≥12 个月或临床监测
高度	明显低回声或其他可疑特征	≥0.5~1cm	再次行 FNA

数据引自文献[21,37,81,84]

管理

细针穿刺活检的适应证

风险分层系统提供了关于甲状腺结节管理的两个基本问题：应该对哪些结节进行活检？应该多久对那些没有活检的结节进行一次监测扫描？大小是决定活检最常用的因素，但需要注意的是，这种趋势是基于其对在临床上有意义的恶性肿瘤的预测价值，而不是仅针对恶性肿瘤的存在[95]。事实上，几项对经活检证实的较小（<1cm）的癌症的观察研究显示，甲状腺乳头状癌很少生长或转移到甲状腺以外，当这种情况发生时，推迟手术时间并不影响总体生存[96]。这些数据，加上手术并发症的风险，促使大多数甲状腺结节管理指南仅推荐对最大尺寸≥1cm的结节取样[21]。虽然之前推荐使用不加区分的1cm阈值来决定所有实性结节的活检，但最近的指南将超声表现纳入了活检的大小标准。具体的大小阈值根据分层系统而异（表4.4）。但一般情况下，>1cm的可疑特征的实性结节和>2~2.5cm的具有较可靠模式或囊性占优的结节建议采用FNA，当中度至低度怀疑特征的结节为恶性时，更有可能是FTC而不是PTC[90]。基于此类型结节更大的纳入阈值，说明<2cm的滤泡癌与远处转移或死亡率无关[21,64]。

可能影响临床决策的个体化因素包括头颈部照射史、甲状腺癌家族史或与甲状腺癌相关的综合征的个人病史，如多发性内分泌瘤、Cowden综合征、家族性腺瘤性息肉病或卡尼综合征。在[^{18}F]-氟代脱氧葡萄糖（^{18}F-FDG）正电子发射体层成像（PET）中，偶然发现的结节有35%的病例中被证明是恶性的[97]；然而，推荐这些结节活检的阈值仍然≥1cm[21]。此外，还应考虑患者的年龄、医学合并症和预期寿命。事实上，最近对1 129名70岁以上甲状腺结节患者的一项回顾性研究发现，14.4%的队列在平均4年的随访期中死亡。队列中只有0.9%（n=10）死于甲状腺癌；所有患者术前均经影像学和/或细胞学确诊为有临床意义的甲状腺癌。在评估结节时，与没有相同诊断的患者相比，患独立的非甲状腺恶性肿瘤或冠状动脉疾病患者的死亡率增加了2倍以上，证实了在甲状腺结节检查过程中，对同时共存其他医学问题的老年患者应采取明智的方法[98]。

如何行细针穿刺活检

甲状腺活检是一种安全、准确、快速评估甲状腺结节恶性风险的方式。在从甲状腺结节获得细胞学样本时，有许多变量需要考虑，包括影像引导的使用、针头大小、麻醉剂的使用和取样技术。

在门诊超声检查广泛应用之前,大多数活检都是在触诊下引导的。这种方法的局限性是在敏感区域缺乏直接的可视化探针。对于大的实性结节,触诊引导的活检在大多数情况下提供了足够的样本。然而,具有囊性成分但不易触诊的结节,若之前未行 FNA 或位于后方,最好在超声引导下穿刺取样[21]。

大多数临床医生更喜欢使用小口径针头(23~27 号)作为甲状腺取样的初始方法,这被称为 FNA。相反,一些人使用大针头(21 号或更大)为组织病理学分析提供甲状腺的核心组织,或者在先前未行诊断性 FNA 的情况下提供更多的细胞样本[99]。然而,这种大针活检在大多数情况下是不必要的,并且使患者面临出血和明显不适的风险增加。

虽然麻醉剂不是必需的,但有些人更喜欢使用注射利多卡因或局部使用利多卡因。有人争辩说,使用细针(25 号或 27 号)时,仅引起极小的不适,而注射利多卡因则是不必要的额外疼痛的来源。或者说,局部使用利多卡因可以避免额外的针扎,但在等待麻醉效果的同时,会增加手术时间。

有两种方法来引导超声针进入结节:平行和垂直。医生的偏好决定了大多数情况下使用的方法,但每种方法都有明显的优势。平行技术是将针放置在平行于超声波平面的探针外侧边缘,从而使针沿着其到结节的整个路径可视化。这种方法需要更精确地操纵指针来找到超声波束的平面。另一种方法,垂直于超声探头的中心,是进入结节更快和更直接的途径。使用这种方法,当针尖穿过超声束平面时,仅针尖可视化。

一旦用针刺穿结节,获得细胞材料的方法包括使用注射器抽吸(吸入)或在没有注射器的情况下的毛吸管技术。这两种技术在获得适当样本方面表现出相似的效果[100]。

细胞学结果和管理

2008 年,Bethesda 系统的引入为甲状腺细胞病理学报告[101]带来了一种及时、标准化的方法,以风险分层的方式报告细胞病理学发现,为临床医生提供了实践标准。Bethesda 系统自发布以来被广泛采用,并在 2017 年[102]进行了修订,以反映新的发展,如 NIFTP 分类的引入,以及在细胞学上不确定的结节中使用分子标志物。

2017 年,Bethesda 系统[102]保留了原始的 6 个细胞学分类,如表 4.5 所示。

第 I 类,不能诊断(nondiagnostic,ND)或不满意,指的是仅含血液或滤泡细胞数量不足的抽吸物,要求至少 6 组,每组至少 10 个滤泡细胞。有一个例外是滤泡细胞数量不足,但胶质丰富,也可归类为良性。很难准确评估Ⅰ类结节的恶性风险,因为许多结节在重复活检时被重新分类,而那些被切除的结节的恶化率可能是由于选择偏差而高估了所有ND结节的恶性程度。当收到ND结果时,超声特征有助于决定是密切监测结节(大多数囊性结节的超声检查结果令人安心)还是重复活检[103]。

表 4.5
Bethesda 系统在甲状腺结节细胞学诊断中的应用

类型	类型名称	细胞学特征	恶性风险 /%
Ⅰ	不能诊断或不满意(ND)	细胞不足,血液模糊	5~10
Ⅱ	良性	外观正常的卵泡细胞呈片状或大卵泡排列,胶质丰富	0~3
Ⅲ	意义不明的非典型性/意义不明的滤泡性病变(AUS/FUS)	细胞稀疏,微小滤泡,轻微核改变	10~30
Ⅳ	滤泡病变/可疑滤泡病变(FN/SFN)	细胞富集,拥挤,微小滤泡,胶体缺乏	25~40
Ⅴ	可疑恶性病变(SFM)	一些提示但不确定为恶性的特征	50~75
Ⅵ	恶性病变	乳头状结构,明确的核改变	97~99

Cibas ES, Ali SZ.The 2017 Bethesda System for Reporting Thyroid Cytopathology.Thyroid 2017;27(11):1341-6.

第Ⅱ类,良性最为常见(60%~70%)[101],表示<3%的恶性风险。Ⅱ类结节有超细胞,拥挤,微滤泡,缺乏胶体。第Ⅱ类还包括以淋巴细胞性甲状腺炎和肉芽肿性(亚急性)甲状腺炎为特征的抽吸物。

第Ⅲ类[意义不明的非典型性/意义不明的滤泡性病变(atypia of undetermined significance,AUS/follicular lesion of undetermined significance,FUS)]和第Ⅳ类[滤泡性肿瘤或可疑性滤泡性肿瘤(follicular neoplasm or suspicious for follicular neoplasm,FN/SFN)]的异常细胞学特征增加了结节恶性的风险,但并不确定就是恶性。往往正是在这一区域,管理方式存在细微差别,人们才探索进一步对调查结果进行风险分层。在 AUS/FLUS 类别中,微滤泡中排列着稀疏的细胞样本,这些细胞有轻微的核改变,或者有大量的 Hürthle 细胞。

AUS/FLUS 分类的恶性风险范围很大,在 5%~48%[102~105],但是比例会根据具体的细胞学发现、病理学家的解释和社区人口而变化。由于许多 NIFTP 肿瘤最初在 FNA 上被归类为 AUS,因此,NIFTP 分类的引入进一步增加了恶性风险评估的复杂性。如果 NIFTP 不被认为是一种癌症,那么总体恶性肿瘤的比例将下降。一项分析报告显示,如果 NIFTP 不是癌症,那么恶性肿瘤的风险为 6%~18%,如果 NIFTP 被认为是癌症,则为 10%~30%[103,106]。虽然理论上 NIFTP 并不是一种癌症,但它确实需要手术切除,所以当涉及手术计划时,较高的估计值可能更有意义[103]。

第Ⅳ类,FN/SFN,由超细胞的细胞学结果组成,呈微滤泡或小梁状排列。可见聚集,胶体常稀少。当这些结节被发现为恶性时(10%~40%),典型的就是滤泡性癌或滤泡性乳头状癌,这两种类型都是根据包膜受侵犯定义的,因此不能通过 FNA 诊断。同样,当 NIFTP 被重新归类为非恶性时(10%~40% vs. 25%~40%),恶性率同样会降低[103]。

为了进一步对不确定性结节进行危险分层而进行分子检测已经成为常见的方法,并将在本书中进行阐述。最近的数据表明,超声特征也可能有助于不确定结节的危险分层和随后的决策[107]。

最后两类,Ⅴ类[可疑恶性(SFN)]和Ⅵ类(恶性),恶性率极高(分别为 60%~75% 和 97%~99%),几乎都建议切除。甲状腺乳头状癌的细胞学改变包括典型的核和结构特征:大细胞、核仁突出、核沟和包涵体、砂粒体和呈乳头状排列的细胞[101]。

监测

应根据超声特征对细胞学为良性的结节进行适当监测,对于具有多个可疑声像图特征但细胞学检查为良性的结节,由于担心其细胞学结果为假阴性,大多数指南建议在 6~12 个月内再次行 FNA[21,81,84](表 4.4),几项研究已确定细胞学假阴性率与结节的超声形态有关。细胞学为良性且有相对可靠的超声表现的结节,其恶性风险<2%,而当超声表现可疑时,其恶性风险为 17%~20%[108,109]。FNA 为良性的结节超声表现稳定,建议随访时间为 12~24 个月。ATA 进一步建议,超声评估为低风险且细胞学良性的结节可能不需要任何后续影像检查[21]。对超声较稳定的结节的长期监测间隔时长应适当延长,但理想的监测间隔时长尚不明确,由于循证指导有限,5 年以上评估的需要尚不明确。

对于稳定结节的定义,主要的关注点在肿瘤的大小。定义为:至少在结节的两个平面上出现 20% 的尺寸增加（至少增加 2mm）或体积增长超过 50%[21]。最近，可疑超声特征的出现使那些未被认知的恶性肿瘤得到了更多关注。几项研究证实，许多良性结节都在增长，但其变为恶性的可能性并不随着（FNA 之后）结节的增大而增加[108~110]。然而，最近的一项研究比较了细胞学良性结节和 1cm 以上没有立即切除的恶性结节的生长速度，发现恶性结节更易生长，生长速度超过 2mm/年则预示着恶性。此外，更高的生长率与更高侵袭性的亚型癌症紧密相关[111]。因此，将超声特征和明显的增长纳入 FNA 复检的决定非常合理。

一个两次活检结果均为良性的结节，其恶性的可能性几乎为零，则不再需要超声监测[21,108]。从实用的观点来看，这对单个结节很有帮助，但是对于多结节的甲状腺，通常需要持续监测。此外，如果未行超声学检查，由于较大的或位置偏中间的良性结节有可能在其生长过程中引起压迫性症状，最终可能需要切除或消融手术，此时，长期的临床随访显得非常重要。

未行活检的结节通常需要持续的超声检查，建议的间隔时间为 6~24 个月，同样根据超声特征（表 4.4），ATA 建议低风险类型的亚厘米级结节不需要行后续的超声随访[21]。

（殷德涛）

参考文献

1. Mazzaferri EL. Management of a solitary thyroid nodule. N Engl J Med 1993; 328(8):553–9.
2. Yang J, Schnadig V, Logrono R, et al. Fine-needle aspiration of thyroid nodules: a study of 4703 patients with histologic and clinical correlations. Cancer 2007; 111(5):306–15.
3. Yassa L, Cibas ES, Benson CB, et al. Long-term assessment of a multidisciplinary approach to thyroid nodule diagnostic evaluation. Cancer 2007;111(6): 508–16.
4. Ito Y, Miyauchi A, Kihara M, et al. Patient age is significantly related to the progression of papillary microcarcinoma of the thyroid under observation. Thyroid 2014;24(1):27–34.
5. SEER database. Available at: https://seer.cancer.gov/statfacts/html/thyro.html. Accessed March 20, 2018.
6. Hundahl SA, Fleming ID, Fremgen AM, et al. A national cancer data base report on 53,856 cases of thyroid carcinoma treated in the U.S., 1985-1995 [see commetns]. Cancer 1998;83(12):2638–48.

7. Moon JH, Hyun MK, Lee JY, et al. Prevalence of thyroid nodules and their associated clinical parameters: a large-scale, multicenter-based health checkup study. Korean J Intern Med 2018;33(4):753–62.
8. Acar T, Ozbek SS, Acar S. Incidentally discovered thyroid nodules: frequency in an adult population during Doppler ultrasonographic evaluation of cervical vessels. Endocrine 2014;45(1):73–8.
9. Liu Y, Lin Z, Sheng C, et al. The prevalence of thyroid nodules in northwest China and its correlation with metabolic parameters and uric acid. Oncotarget 2017;8(25):41555–62.
10. Libutti SK. Understanding the role of gender in the incidence of thyroid cancer. Cancer J 2005;11(2):104–5.
11. Germano A, Schmitt W, Almeida P, et al. Ultrasound requested by general practitioners or for symptoms unrelated to the thyroid gland may explain higher prevalence of thyroid nodules in females. Clin Imaging 2018;50:289–93.
12. Ding X, Xu Y, Wang Y, et al. Gender disparity in the relationship between prevalence of thyroid nodules and metabolic syndrome components: the SHDC-CDPC community-based study. Mediators Inflamm 2017;2017:8481049.
13. Manole D, Schildknecht B, Gosnell B, et al. Estrogen promotes growth of human thyroid tumor cells by different molecular mechanisms. J Clin Endocrinol Metab 2001;86(3):1072–7.
14. Xu S, Chen G, Peng W, et al. Oestrogen action on thyroid progenitor cells: relevant for the pathogenesis of thyroid nodules? J Endocrinol 2013;218(1):125–33.
15. Zhao W, Han C, Shi X, et al. Prevalence of goiter and thyroid nodules before and after implementation of the universal salt iodization program in mainland China from 1985 to 2014: a systematic review and meta-analysis. PLoS One 2014;9(10):e109549.
16. Ron E, Brenner A. Non-malignant thyroid diseases after a wide range of radiation exposures. Radiat Res 2010;174(6):877–88.
17. Schneider AB, Ron E, Lubin J, et al. Dose-response relationships for radiation-induced thyroid cancer and thyroid nodules: evidence for the prolonged effects of radiation on the thyroid. J Clin Endocrinol Metab 1993;77(2):362–9.
18. Sklar C, Whitton J, Mertens A, et al. Abnormalities of the thyroid in survivors of Hodgkin's disease: data from the Childhood Cancer Survivor Study. J Clin Endocrinol Metab 2000;85(9):3227–32.
19. Agrawal C, Guthrie L, Sturm MS, et al. Comparison of thyroid nodule prevalence by ultrasound in childhood cancer survivors with and without thyroid radiation exposure. J Pediatr Hematol Oncol 2016;38(1):43–8.
20. Hamming JF, Goslings BM, van Steenis GJ, et al. The value of fine-needle aspiration biopsy in patients with nodular thyroid disease divided into groups of suspicion of malignant neoplasms on clinical grounds. Arch Intern Med 1990;150(1):113–6.
21. Haugen BR, Alexander EK, Bible KC, et al. 2015 American Thyroid Association Management guidelines for adult patients with thyroid nodules and differentiated thyroid cancer: the American Thyroid Association guidelines task force on thyroid nodules and differentiated thyroid cancer. Thyroid 2016;26(1):1–133.
22. Ross DS, Burch HB, Cooper DS, et al. 2016 American Thyroid Association guidelines for diagnosis and management of hyperthyroidism and other causes of thyrotoxicosis. Thyroid 2016;26(10):1343–421.
23. Jonklaas J, Sarlis NJ, Litofsky D, et al. Outcomes of patients with differentiated thyroid carcinoma following initial therapy. Thyroid 2006;16(12):1229–42.

24. Boelaert K, Horacek J, Holder RL, et al. Serum thyrotropin concentration as a novel predictor of malignancy in thyroid nodules investigated by fine-needle aspiration. J Clin Endocrinol Metab 2006;91(11):4295–301.
25. Golbert L, de Cristo AP, Faccin CS, et al. Serum TSH levels as a predictor of malignancy in thyroid nodules: a prospective study. PLoS One 2017;12(11): e0188123.
26. Haymart MR, Repplinger DJ, Leverson GE, et al. Higher serum thyroid stimulating hormone level in thyroid nodule patients is associated with greater risks of differentiated thyroid cancer and advanced tumor stage. J Clin Endocrinol Metab 2008;93(3):809–14.
27. McLeod DS, Cooper DS, Ladenson PW, et al. Prognosis of differentiated thyroid cancer in relation to serum thyrotropin and thyroglobulin antibody status at time of diagnosis. Thyroid 2014;24(1):35–42.
28. Elisei R, Bottici V, Luchetti F, et al. Impact of routine measurement of serum calcitonin on the diagnosis and outcome of medullary thyroid cancer: experience in 10,864 patients with nodular thyroid disorders. J Clin Endocrinol Metab 2004; 89(1):163–8.
29. Daniels GH. Screening for medullary thyroid carcinoma with serum calcitonin measurements in patients with thyroid nodules in the United States and Canada. Thyroid 2011;21(11):1199–207.
30. Suh I, Vriens MR, Guerrero MA, et al. Serum thyroglobulin is a poor diagnostic biomarker of malignancy in follicular and Hurthle-cell neoplasms of the thyroid. Am J Surg 2010;200(1):41–6.
31. Marqusee E, Benson CB, Frates MC, et al. Usefulness of ultrasonography in the management of nodular thyroid disease. Ann Intern Med 2000;133(9):696–700.
32. Kouvaraki MA, Shapiro SE, Fornage BD, et al. Role of preoperative ultrasonography in the surgical management of patients with thyroid cancer. Surgery 2003; 134(6):946–54 [discussion: 954–5].
33. Stulak JM, Grant CS, Farley DR, et al. Value of preoperative ultrasonography in the surgical management of initial and reoperative papillary thyroid cancer. Arch Surg 2006;141(5):489–94 [discussion: 494–6].
34. Moon HJ, Kim EK, Yoon JH, et al. Differences in the diagnostic performances of staging US for thyroid malignancy according to experience. Ultrasound Med Biol 2012;38(4):568–73.
35. Shimamoto K, Satake H, Sawaki A, et al. Preoperative staging of thyroid papillary carcinoma with ultrasonography. Eur J Radiol 1998;29(1):4–10.
36. Kwak JY, Han KH, Yoon JH, et al. Thyroid imaging reporting and data system for US features of nodules: a step in establishing better stratification of cancer risk. Radiology 2011;260(3):892–9.
37. Tessler FN, Middleton WD, Grant EG, et al. ACR thyroid imaging, reporting and data system (TI-RADS): white paper of the ACR TI-RADS committee. J Am Coll Radiol 2017;14(5):587–95.
38. Henrichsen TL, Reading CC, Charboneau JW, et al. Cystic change in thyroid carcinoma: prevalence and estimated volume in 360 carcinomas. J Clin Ultrasound 2010;38(7):361–6.
39. Brito JP, Gionfriddo MR, Al Nofal A, et al. The accuracy of thyroid nodule ultrasound to predict thyroid cancer: systematic review and meta-analysis. J Clin Endocrinol Metab 2014;99(4):1253–63.
40. Li W, Zhu Q, Jiang Y, et al. Partially cystic thyroid nodules in ultrasound-guided fine needle aspiration: prevalence of thyroid carcinoma and ultrasound features. Medicine 2017;96(46):e8689.

41. Moon WJ, Jung SL, Lee JH, et al. Benign and malignant thyroid nodules: US differentiation–multicenter retrospective study. Radiology 2008;247(3):762–70.
42. Bonavita JA, Mayo J, Babb J, et al. Pattern recognition of benign nodules at ultrasound of the thyroid: which nodules can be left alone? AJR Am J Roentgenol 2009;193(1):207–13.
43. Kim DW, Lee EJ, In HS, et al. Sonographic differentiation of partially cystic thyroid nodules: a prospective study. AJNR Am J Neuroradiol 2010;31(10):1961–6.
44. Jeh SK, Jung SL, Kim BS, et al. Evaluating the degree of conformity of papillary carcinoma and follicular carcinoma to the reported ultrasonographic findings of malignant thyroid tumor. Korean J Radiol 2007;8(3):192–7.
45. Kim DS, Kim JH, Na DG, et al. Sonographic features of follicular variant papillary thyroid carcinomas in comparison with conventional papillary thyroid carcinomas. J Ultrasound Med 2009;28(12):1685–92.
46. Ren J, Liu B, Zhang LL, et al. A taller-than-wide shape is a good predictor of papillary thyroid carcinoma in small solid nodules. J Ultrasound Med 2015;34(1):19–26.
47. Chen SP, Hu YP, Chen B. Taller-than-wide sign for predicting thyroid microcarcinoma: comparison and combination of two ultrasonographic planes. Ultrasound Med Biol 2014;40(9):2004–11.
48. Moon HJ, Kwak JY, Kim EK, et al. A taller-than-wide shape in thyroid nodules in transverse and longitudinal ultrasonographic planes and the prediction of malignancy. Thyroid 2011;21(11):1249–53.
49. Grant EG, Tessler FN, Hoang JK, et al. Thyroid ultrasound reporting lexicon: white paper of the ACR thyroid imaging, reporting and data system (TIRADS) committee. J Am Coll Radiol 2015;12(12 Pt A):1272–9.
50. Kuo EJ, Thi WJ, Zheng F, et al. Individualizing surgery in papillary thyroid carcinoma based on a detailed sonographic assessment of extrathyroidal extension. Thyroid 2017;27(12):1544–9.
51. Lee CY, Kim SJ, Ko KR, et al. Predictive factors for extrathyroidal extension of papillary thyroid carcinoma based on preoperative sonography. J Ultrasound Med 2014;33(2):231–8.
52. Taki S, Terahata S, Yamashita R, et al. Thyroid calcifications: sonographic patterns and incidence of cancer. Clin Imaging 2004;28(5):368–71.
53. Arpaci D, Ozdemir D, Cuhaci N, et al. Evaluation of cytopathological findings in thyroid nodules with macrocalcification: macrocalcification is not innocent as it seems. Arq Bras Endocrinol Metabol 2014;58(9):939–45.
54. Kim MJ, Kim EK, Kwak JY, et al. Differentiation of thyroid nodules with macrocalcifications: role of suspicious sonographic findings. J Ultrasound Med 2008;27(8):1179–84.
55. Lee J, Lee SY, Cha SH, et al. Fine-needle aspiration of thyroid nodules with macrocalcification. Thyroid 2013;23(9):1106–12.
56. Park YJ, Kim JA, Son EJ, et al. Thyroid nodules with macrocalcification: sonographic findings predictive of malignancy. Yonsei Med J 2014;55(2):339–44.
57. American Thyroid Association (ATA) Guidelines Taskforce on Thyroid Nodules and Differentiated Thyroid Cancer, Cooper DS, Doherty GM, et al. Revised American Thyroid Association management guidelines for patients with thyroid nodules and differentiated thyroid cancer. Thyroid 2009;19(11):1167–214.
58. Papini E, Guglielmi R, Bianchini A, et al. Risk of malignancy in nonpalpable thyroid nodules: predictive value of ultrasound and color-Doppler features. J Clin Endocrinol Metab 2002;87(5):1941–6.

59. Moon HJ, Kwak JY, Kim MJ, et al. Can vascularity at power Doppler US help predict thyroid malignancy? Radiology 2010;255(1):260–9.
60. Yang GCH, Fried KO. Most thyroid cancers detected by sonography lack intranodular vascularity on color Doppler imaging: review of the literature and sonographic-pathologic correlations for 698 thyroid neoplasms. J Ultrasound Med 2017;36(1):89–94.
61. Cappelli C, Castellano M, Pirola I, et al. The predictive value of ultrasound findings in the management of thyroid nodules. QJM 2007;100(1):29–35.
62. Lai X, Liu M, Xia Y, et al. Hypervascularity is more frequent in medullary thyroid carcinoma: compared with papillary thyroid carcinoma. Medicine 2016;95(49): e5502.
63. Hong MJ, Na DG, Baek JH, et al. Impact of nodule size on malignancy risk differs according to the ultrasonography pattern of thyroid nodules. Korean J Radiol 2018;19(3):534–41.
64. Machens A, Holzhausen HJ, Dralle H. The prognostic value of primary tumor size in papillary and follicular thyroid carcinoma. Cancer 2005;103(11):2269–73.
65. Lee S, Shin JH, Han BK, et al. Medullary thyroid carcinoma: comparison with papillary thyroid carcinoma and application of current sonographic criteria. AJR Am J Roentgenol 2010;194(4):1090–4.
66. Kim SH, Kim BS, Jung SL, et al. Ultrasonographic findings of medullary thyroid carcinoma: a comparison with papillary thyroid carcinoma. Korean J Radiol 2009;10(2):101–5.
67. Liu MJ, Liu ZF, Hou YY, et al. Ultrasonographic characteristics of medullary thyroid carcinoma: a comparison with papillary thyroid carcinoma. Oncotarget 2017;8(16):27520–8.
68. Zhou L, Chen B, Zhao M, et al. Sonographic features of medullary thyroid carcinomas according to tumor size: comparison with papillary thyroid carcinomas. J Ultrasound Med 2015;34(6):1003–9.
69. Langer JE, Mandel SJ. Sonographic imaging of cervical lymph nodes in patients with thyroid cancer. Neuroimaging Clin N Am 2008;18(3):479–89, vii-viii.
70. Kuna SK, Bracic I, Tesic V, et al. Ultrasonographic differentiation of benign from malignant neck lymphadenopathy in thyroid cancer. J Ultrasound Med 2006; 25(12):1531–7 [quiz: 1538–40].
71. Leboulleux S, Girard E, Rose M, et al. Ultrasound criteria of malignancy for cervical lymph nodes in patients followed up for differentiated thyroid cancer. J Clin Endocrinol Metab 2007;92(9):3590–4.
72. Sohn YM, Kwak JY, Kim EK, et al. Diagnostic approach for evaluation of lymph node metastasis from thyroid cancer using ultrasound and fine-needle aspiration biopsy. AJR Am J Roentgenol 2010;194(1):38–43.
73. Park JS, Son KR, Na DG, et al. Performance of preoperative sonographic staging of papillary thyroid carcinoma based on the sixth edition of the AJCC/UICC TNM classification system. AJR Am J Roentgenol 2009;192(1):66–72.
74. Leenhardt L, Erdogan MF, Hegedus L, et al. 2013 European thyroid association guidelines for cervical ultrasound scan and ultrasound-guided techniques in the postoperative management of patients with thyroid cancer. Eur Thyroid J 2013; 2(3):147–59.
75. Solbiati L, Osti V, Cova L, et al. Ultrasound of thyroid, parathyroid glands and neck lymph nodes. Eur Radiol 2001;11(12):2411–24.
76. Rosario PW, de Faria S, Bicalho L, et al. Ultrasonographic differentiation between metastatic and benign lymph nodes in patients with papillary thyroid carcinoma. J Ultrasound Med 2005;24(10):1385–9.

77. Ahuja AT, Ying M, Ho SS, et al. Distribution of intranodal vessels in differentiating benign from metastatic neck nodes. Clin Radiol 2001;56(3):197–201.
78. Ahuja A, Ying M. Sonography of neck lymph nodes. Part II: abnormal lymph nodes. Clin Radiol 2003;58(5):359–66.
79. Kim EK, Park CS, Chung WY, et al. New sonographic criteria for recommending fine-needle aspiration biopsy of nonpalpable solid nodules of the thyroid. AJR Am J Roentgenol 2002;178(3):687–91.
80. Frates MC, Benson CB, Charboneau JW, et al. Management of thyroid nodules detected at US: Society of Radiologists in Ultrasound consensus conference statement. Radiology 2005;237(3):794–800.
81. Shin JH, Baek JH, Chung J, et al. Ultrasonography diagnosis and imaging-based management of thyroid nodules: revised Korean Society of Thyroid Radiology consensus statement and recommendations. Korean J Radiol 2016;17(3):370–95.
82. Horvath E, Majlis S, Rossi R, et al. An ultrasonogram reporting system for thyroid nodules stratifying cancer risk for clinical management. J Clin Endocrinol Metab 2009;94(5):1748–51.
83. Park JY, Lee HJ, Jang HW, et al. A proposal for a thyroid imaging reporting and data system for ultrasound features of thyroid carcinoma. Thyroid 2009;19(11):1257–64.
84. Gharib H, Papini E, Garber JR, et al. American Association of Clinical Endocrinologists, American College of Endocrinology, and Associazione Medici Endocrinologi Medical guidelines for clinical practice for the diagnosis and management of thyroid nodules–2016 update. Endocr Pract 2016;22(5):622–39.
85. Na DG, Baek JH, Sung JY, et al. Thyroid imaging reporting and data system risk stratification of thyroid nodules: categorization based on solidity and echogenicity. Thyroid 2016;26(4):562–72.
86. Middleton WD, Teefey SA, Reading CC, et al. Multiinstitutional analysis of thyroid nodule risk stratification using the American College of Radiology thyroid imaging reporting and data system. AJR Am J Roentgenol 2017;208(6):1331–41.
87. Park CS, Kim SH, Jung SL, et al. Observer variability in the sonographic evaluation of thyroid nodules. J Clin Ultrasound 2010;38(6):287–93.
88. Russ G, Royer B, Bigorgne C, et al. Prospective evaluation of thyroid imaging reporting and data system on 4550 nodules with and without elastography. Eur J Endocrinol 2013;168(5):649–55.
89. Grani G, Lamartina L, Cantisani V, et al. Interobserver agreement of various thyroid imaging reporting and data systems. Endocr Connect 2018;7(1):1–7.
90. Ha EJ, Baek JH, Na DG. Risk stratification of thyroid nodules on ultrasonography: current status and perspectives. Thyroid 2017;27(12):1463–8.
91. Horvath E, Silva CF, Majlis S, et al. Prospective validation of the ultrasound based TIRADS (thyroid imaging reporting and data system) classification: results in surgically resected thyroid nodules. Eur Radiol 2017;27(6):2619–28.
92. Tang AL, Falciglia M, Yang H, et al. Validation of American Thyroid Association ultrasound risk assessment of thyroid nodules selected for ultrasound fine-needle aspiration. Thyroid 2017;27(8):1077–82.
93. Persichetti A, Di Stasio E, Guglielmi R, et al. Predictive value of malignancy of thyroid nodule ultrasound classification systems: a prospective study. J Clin Endocrinol Metab 2018;103(4):1359–68.
94. Yoon JH, Lee HS, Kim EK, et al. Malignancy risk stratification of thyroid nodules: comparison between the thyroid imaging reporting and data system and the

2014 American Thyroid Association management guidelines. Radiology 2016; 278(3):917–24.
95. Frates MC, Benson CB, Doubilet PM, et al. Prevalence and distribution of carcinoma in patients with solitary and multiple thyroid nodules on sonography. J Clin Endocrinol Metab 2006;91(9):3411–7.
96. Ito Y, Miyauchi A, Inoue H, et al. An observational trial for papillary thyroid microcarcinoma in Japanese patients. World J Surg 2010;34(1):28–35.
97. Soelberg KK, Bonnema SJ, Brix TH, et al. Risk of malignancy in thyroid incidentalomas detected by 18F-fluorodeoxyglucose positron emission tomography: a systematic review. Thyroid 2012;22(9):918–25.
98. Wang Z, Vyas CM, Van Benschoten O, et al. Quantitative analysis of the benefits and risk of thyroid nodule evaluation in patients >/=70 years old. Thyroid 2018; 28(4):465–71.
99. Carpi A, Nicolini A, Sagripanti A, et al. Large-needle aspiration biopsy for the preoperative selection of palpable thyroid nodules diagnosed by fine-needle aspiration as a microfollicular nodule or suspected cancer. Am J Clin Pathol 2000;113(6):872–7.
100. Tublin ME, Martin JA, Rollin LJ, et al. Ultrasound-guided fine-needle aspiration versus fine-needle capillary sampling biopsy of thyroid nodules: does technique matter? J Ultrasound Med 2007;26(12):1697–701.
101. Baloch ZW, Cibas ES, Clark DP, et al. The National Cancer Institute Thyroid fine needle aspiration state of the science conference: a summation. Cytojournal 2008;5:6.
102. Pusztaszeri M, Rossi ED, Auger M, et al. The Bethesda system for reporting thyroid cytopathology: proposed modifications and updates for the second edition from an international panel. Acta Cytol 2016;60(5):399–405.
103. Cibas ES, Ali SZ. The 2017 Bethesda system for reporting thyroid cytopathology. Thyroid 2017;27(11):1341–6.
104. Wang CC, Friedman L, Kennedy GC, et al. A large multicenter correlation study of thyroid nodule cytopathology and histopathology. Thyroid 2011;21(3):243–51.
105. Olson MT, Clark DP, Erozan YS, et al. Spectrum of risk of malignancy in subcategories of 'atypia of undetermined significance. Acta Cytol 2011;55(6):518–25.
106. Faquin WC, Wong LQ, Afrogheh AH, et al. Impact of reclassifying noninvasive follicular variant of papillary thyroid carcinoma on the risk of malignancy in The Bethesda system for reporting thyroid cytopathology. Cancer Cytopathol 2016;124(3):181–7.
107. Valderrabano P, McGettigan MJ, Lam CA, et al. Thyroid nodules with indeterminate cytology: utility of the American Thyroid Association sonographic patterns for cancer risk stratification. Thyroid 2018;28(8):1004–12.
108. Kwak JY, Koo H, Youk JH, et al. Value of US correlation of a thyroid nodule with initially benign cytologic results. Radiology 2010;254(1):292–300.
109. Rosario PW, Purisch S. Ultrasonographic characteristics as a criterion for repeat cytology in benign thyroid nodules. Arq Bras Endocrinol Metabol 2010;54(1): 52–5.
110. Durante C, Costante G, Lucisano G, et al. The natural history of benign thyroid nodules. JAMA 2015;313(9):926–35.
111. Angell TE, Vyas CM, Medici M, et al. Differential growth rates of benign vs. malignant thyroid nodules. J Clin Endocrinol Metab 2017;102(12):4642–7.

第5章
甲状腺结节的分子诊断

Sarah E. Mayson, Bryan R. Haugen

关键词

- 甲状腺结节 • 细胞学不确定 • 分子检测 • ThyroSeq • Afirma

要点

- 灵敏度和特异度是评价一种检测方法固有的指标,而阳性预测值和阴性预测值则取决于检测人群的患病率。
- 灵敏度和阴性预测值高的分子诊断检测可以用于甲状腺癌的排除诊断,而特异度和阳性预测值高者可以用于确定诊断。
- 二代测序分子检测、Afirma GSC RNA 测序试剂盒和 ThyroSeq v3 112-基因试剂盒,灵敏度高且特异度也较好,可以作为排除和确定诊断的有效方法。
- 好的分子诊断方法应该经过分析验证、临床验证以及临床实践应用,并应该由临床实验室改进修正案批准的实验室来完成。

引言

对细胞学不确定的甲状腺结节,以往的处理方法通常是诊断性腺叶切除或全切除。这种方法的缺点是,很多术后被证明为良性结节的患者,也要承受手术的风险、术后并发症、医疗花费和误工,等等。在过去的 10 年中,分子诊断检测被用来指导细胞学不确定结节的治疗,最终减少了出于诊断性目的的甲状腺手术的数量。

讨论

Bethesda 细胞学分级/细针穿刺不确定诊断

甲状腺结节患者的临床评估，包括 Bethesda 甲状腺细胞学报告系统（the Bethesda System for Reporting Thyroid Cytopathology，TBSRTC），在本书的其他章节中已有阐述。TBSRTC 最早在 2007 年被提出，并在最近进行了更新，纳入了近期的研究，以及"具有乳头状核特征的非侵袭性滤泡性肿瘤（noninvasice follicular thyroid neoplasm，NIFTP）"这一术后病理诊断[1-3]。TBSRTC 作为甲状腺细胞学的标准报告系统被广泛接受，不论 NIFTP 被归为术后病理良性还是恶性，应用 TBSRTC 进行良恶性分类都能得到较高的正确率；TBSRTC 分类为良性的结节恶性风险为 0%~3%，分类为恶性的结节恶性风险为 94%~99%[1]。

意义不明的细胞非典型性病变或滤泡性病变（atypia of undetermined significance/follicular lesion of undetermined significance，AUS/FLUS；Bethesda Ⅲ）和滤泡性肿瘤或可疑滤泡性肿瘤（follicular neoplasm/suspicious for follicular neoplasm，FN/SFN；Bethesda Ⅳ）的恶性风险，没有高到需要对所有患者都进行手术，也没有低到可以对所有患者都进行观察。Cibas 和 Ali1 在 2017 版 TBSRTC 中指出，如果将 NIFTP 算作良性，AUS/FLUS 的恶性风险为 6%~18%；如果 NIFTP 算为恶性，恶性风险为 10%~30%。同样，如果将 NIFTP 算作良性，FN/SFN 的恶性风险为 10%~40%；如果 NIFTP 算为恶性，恶性风险为 25%~40%。这说明，对于任意一个细胞学不确定的患者，恶性风险可能受病例选择、部分验证和发表偏倚等因素影响，其真实的恶性风险可能被高估，也可能被低估[2]。

以往对细胞学不确定患者的处理，特别是在 TBSRTC 应用以前，多为诊断性甲状腺腺叶切除或全切除。这种处理方式导致 60%~94% 的不确定结节患者接受了不必要的手术。2015 年版美国甲状腺学会（American Thyroid Association，ATA）甲状腺结节和分化型甲状腺癌指南针对 AUS/FLUS 和 FN/SFN 给出了几种选择[4]，对 AUS/FLUS 患者首选的处理方法是重复细针穿刺活检（fine needle aspiration，FNA）或分子检测，而 FN/SFN 患者建议行诊断性腺叶切除或分子检测。这两类患者的处理都应该结合临床和超声特征，以及患者的意愿来作出决定。ATA 指南还建议可以考虑病理会诊，特别是对于 AUS/FLUS 患者。2017 年版 TBSRTC 建议对 AUS/FLUS 患者行重复 FNA、分子检测或诊断性腺叶切除,对 FN/SFN 患者进行分子诊断或诊断性腺叶切除。因此,分子检测是很多细胞学 Bethesda Ⅲ类和Ⅳ类患者的核心诊断工具。图 5.1 解释了分子诊断检测在细胞学不确定的甲状腺结节处理中所起的作用。

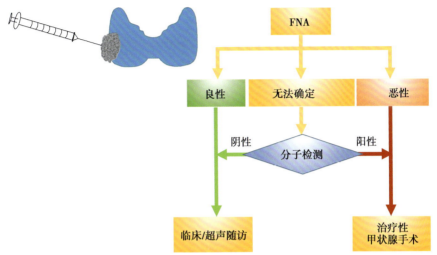

图 5.1　分子诊断检测在细胞学不确定的甲状腺结节处理中的建议流程
FNA:细针穿刺活检

分子诊断评估甲状腺结节的原则

对患者的甲状腺结节应用分子诊断检测进行评估时需要注意三个重要的概念:分析验证、临床验证和临床价值。我们将详细论述分析验证和临床验证。临床价值是指检测带来的心理学、社会学和经济学结果,以及其对患者个人、家庭和社会所带来的影响。

分析验证

分析验证是指一种检测方法能对有限的输入样本进行检测的能力,包括分辨可能混入的非肿瘤细胞或血液污染,以及在相同技术条件下和不同操作者之间的可重复性[5]。112 基因测序试剂盒(ThyroSeq v3)在 238 例手术标本和 175 例 FNA 标本中完成了分析验证[6]。质控过程首先是查找非肿瘤标本,然后是非甲状腺标本,然后对通过测试的标本进行二代测序。这种检测可以准确检测出低至 2.5ng 输入标本的基因变异,准确区分出混合 12% 肿瘤细胞和 88% 正常甲状腺细胞的 10 个样本,并且能对被血液稀释至 12% 的 3 个样本检验正确。该方法还对 12 个标本用同样方法重复了 3 次（精确性），由不同操作者重复 3 次（可重复性），均得到同样的结果。穿刺得到的样本可以在室温下 2 小时内，转移到 –20℃或 4℃环境长达 72 小时内保持稳定。基因组测序分类器（genomic sequencing classifier，GSC）也进行过分析验证，结果已经投稿但尚未发表（Kennedy GC，个人交流）。167 基因表达分类器（Afirma gene expression classifier，Afirma GEC）使用标准的 FNA 标本进行分析验证，包括保存、分析前、分析中和可重复性研究[7]。这种检测可以对低至 10ng 的 RNA 标本准确区分出良性或可疑恶性，虽然它的输入标准定为 15ng。它还可以准确分辨混在正常组织内的 20%FNA 内容物，和混在血液中的 17%FNA 内容物。该方法还可达到 94% 的精确度（自身测试）和 100% 的可重复性（实验室间）。穿刺标本可以在室温下保持稳定长达 6 天。

1988 年，美国国会通过了临床实验室改进修正案，提出了实验室检测的质量标准。为了保证实验室检测质量，所有分子检测都应在临床实验室改进修正案批准的实验室进行。

临床验证

临床验证检验的是一种诊断方法对疾病排除诊断[灵敏度，阴性预测值（negative predictive value，NPV）]和确定诊断[特异度，阳性预测值（positive predictive value，PPV）]的能力。灵敏度和特异度评价的是诊断方法的固有特性，不受人群患病率的影响，而 NPV 和 PPV 则取决于人群患病率。灵敏度和特异度可以在对不同人群的研究之间直接比较，而 NPV 和 PPV 不能直接比较（图 5.2）。如果想对某一种分子检测的 NPV 和 PPV 进行充分评估，我们需要知道在这一机构或地区内，最好是近 3~5 年时间中，每种 Bethesda 细胞学分类结节的恶性比例[8]。对一种甲状腺结节分子标记物最切的临床验证研究设计，是对一系列连续患者进行检测，并对所有患者实施手术以得到病理验证的前瞻性、双盲研究[9,11]。另一项对 7 基因突变试剂盒的大样本研究是前瞻性，但没有双盲[12]。这一 7 基因突变试剂盒的灵敏度和特异度经过多个其他独立研究的验证[13-15]，也是另外一种形式的临床验证。最近发布的，也是应用最普遍的这两种分子检测方法还没有经过独立研究的验证[10,11]。

分子诊断检测的种类

关于细胞学不确定的甲状腺结节的第一代、第二代和下一代分子检测方法总结见表 5.1。

表 5.1
分子诊断检测的灵敏度、特异度、阴性预测值（NPV）和阳性预测值（PPV）比较

代数	检测名称	结节数量	Bethesda 分级	灵敏度/%	特异度/%	恶性比例/%	NPV/%	PPV/%
第一代	Afirma-GEC	265	Ⅲ～Ⅴ	92	52	32	93	47
	167 RNA GEC							
	7-基因试剂盒	513	Ⅲ～Ⅴ	61	98	24	89	90
第二代	ThyroSeq v2	95	Ⅲ	91	92	23	97	77
	19 基因试剂盒	143	Ⅳ	90	93	27	96	83
	ThyGenX/ThyraMIR	109	Ⅲ～Ⅳ	89	85	32	94	74
	8 基因试剂盒/microRNA GEC							
第三代	Afirma-GSC	191	Ⅲ～Ⅳ	91	68	24	96	47
	RNAseq 试剂盒							
	ThyroSeq v3	286	Ⅲ～Ⅳ	94	82	28*	97	66
	112 基因试剂盒							

*癌/具有乳头状核特征的非侵袭性滤泡性肿瘤（NIFTP）合计比例，NIFTP 的比例在其他研究中未标明

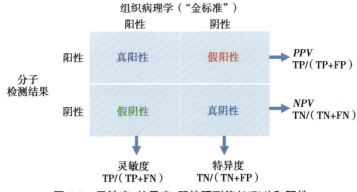

图 5.2 灵敏度、特异度、阴性预测值(NPV)和阳性预测值(PPV)的统计学定义
FN:假阴性,FP:假阳性,TN:真阴性,TP:真阳性

第一代分子检测

2011 年,Afirma GEC(Veracyte,South San Francisco,CA)作为细胞学不确定的甲状腺结节的诊断工具开始在临床应用。这种基于基因芯片技术的检测方法,使用一种专利算法来分析信使 RNA 表达模式,以鉴别良恶性。GEC 根据不同表达模式的恶性可能性不同,将甲状腺结节分为"良性"(检测阴性)和"可疑恶性"(检测阳性)[16]。为了保证标本足够,厂家建议做 FNA 时专门穿刺 2 针收集在核酸保存液中。

一项前瞻性、双盲、多中心的研究对该方法进行了临床验证,纳入 4 812 例 FNA 标本,577 例(12%)为细胞学不确定,对其中 265 例样本进行分析。对所有细胞学不确定的甲状腺结节(Bethesda Ⅲ/Ⅳ/Ⅴ)的灵敏度和特异度分别为 92% 和 52%。对 AUS/FLUS(Bethesda Ⅲ)的灵敏度和特异度分别为 90% 和 53%,对 FN/SFN(Bethesda Ⅳ)分别为 90% 和 49%。该研究中 Bethesda Ⅲ 和 Bethesda Ⅳ 结节的恶性比例分别为 24% 和 25%,对这两类结节的 NPV 和 PPV 分别为 95% 和 38%,94% 和 37%[9]。最近的一个 meta 分析总结了 18 项验证后研究(4 项前瞻性和 14 项回顾性),计算 GEC 在手术切除的不确定结节中的诊断特性。确认了灵敏度约为 90%,与临床验证研究基本一致。但是,特异度偏低,仅 27%(vs. 52%)[9,17]。Veracyte 同时提供 *BRAFV600E* 突变检测,但由于 Bethesda Ⅲ/Ⅳ 结节 *BRAFV600E* 突变率低,对检测结果改善得并不明显[18]。

此前验证研究中的 346 个经 GEC 检测的甲状腺不确定结节患者,在纳入 5 个中心的多中心随访研究中,51% 的结节为 GEC 检测良性,44% 为可疑恶性,其中一半患者的检测结果对临床决策产生了影响[19]。这项研究和其他研究一样,发现各个单位之间 GEC 分类为可疑恶性的结节中,良性比例(27%~53%)和恶性比例(15.6%~70.0%)存在较大差异[19-26]。这与各个单位之间 Bethesda Ⅲ 和 Bethesda Ⅳ 结节的恶性比例差异相一致[27]。

新版 AUS/FLUS(Bethesda Ⅲ)区分为结构非典型性和细胞非典型性,分别会对 GEC 可疑恶性结节的术后良性和恶性比例产生不同的影响。Baca 及其同事[28]对 227 个结节进行 AUS 细胞学和 GEC 检测,指出 GEC 对 AUS 结构非典型良性判断的准确率(65%)高于细胞非典型(59%)和两者兼有的结节(38%)。对 GEC 可疑恶性结节手术切除的恶性比例在结构非典型中是 19%,细胞非典型中为 45%,两者兼有中为 57%。重要的是,GEC 在 Hürthle 细胞肿瘤中的特异性非常低(大约 12%),因此,即使检测结果为阳性,最后病理为恶性的可能性也不会显著提高[29]。

当检测样本的恶性比例近似或低于验证研究的恶性比例时,灵敏度高这一特点使 GEC 可以用在 Bethesda Ⅲ/Ⅳ 结节中,作为排除甲状腺癌的检测方法。它的 NPV 较高,检测阴性者可以密切观察,而不需要立即行诊断性手术。但 GEC 的特异度和 PPV 较低,这意味着当检测结果为阳性时,不足以判断结节为恶性,下一步制订临床决策还应结合细胞学结果、超声所见和临床患病风险等综合评估。该检测在 Bethesda Ⅴ 结节中临床应用较少,因为此类结节恶性风险相对较高,不建议使用 GEC 检测。除了在检测样本的恶性比例较低时(<10%),对其他所有人群常规应用这种检测方法性价比并不高[30]。

对 GEC 检测为良性结节的远期随访研究结果还是令人放心的。很多研究认为,GEC 检测良性的结节需要外科切除的比例很低[8,31-34]。Angell 及其同事[32]发现 90 例 GEC 诊断良性的不确定结节中只有 5 例(5.5%)最终手术切除,其中仅 1 例是恶性的。在中位随访 13 个月时发现,GEC 诊断良性的结节与细胞学良性的结节生长速度相似。Deaver 及其同事[8]观察的 73 例 GEC 良性结节中有 5 例(6.8%)接受手术,只有 1 例发现伴随着 FNA 目标结节以外的微小乳头状癌。对 Bethesda Ⅲ 结节中位随访 46 个月,对 Bethesda Ⅳ 结节中位随访 62 个月,其中多数(>70%)GEC 良性的结节的大小没有变化。

Afirma GEC 已经被 Afirma GSC 取代,后者将在下文讨论。

甲状腺癌经常发生丝裂原活化蛋白激酶和磷脂酰肌醇 3- 激酶信号通路上的基因突变[35-37]。miRinform Thyroid 检测(Asuragen,Austin,TX),更名为 ThyGenX 甲状腺癌基因试剂盒(Interpace Diagnostics,Parsippany,NJ),检测常见的 7 个基因变异(*BRAFV600E*,*NRAS* 61 号密码子,*HRAS* 61 号密码子,

KRAS 12/13 号密码子点突变，以及 *RET/PTC1*、*RET/PTC3* 和 *PAX8/PPAR* 重排），这些变异可见于约 70% 的甲状腺癌[12]。标本收集要求 FNA 时专门穿刺 1 针放在核酸保存液中。对液基薄片和晾干涂片标本的 DNA 水平突变检测也获得了成功[38,39]。

评价这一 7 基因试剂盒的样本量最大的是一项单中心、非盲的前瞻性研究，该研究纳入了 1 056 例不确定结节，513 例结节有术后病理并进行了分析。共有 247 个 Bethesda Ⅲ 结节，214 个 Bethesda Ⅳ 结节，52 个 Bethesda Ⅴ 结节，恶性比例分别为 14%、27% 和 54%。该试剂盒在所有病例中的灵敏度和特异度分别为 61% 和 98%，对 Bethesda Ⅲ 结节为 63% 和 99%，对 Bethesda Ⅳ 结节为 57% 和 97%，对 Bethesda Ⅴ 结节为 68% 和 96%[12]。恶性可能性主要受突变种类的影响，如 *BRAF V600E* 突变的恶性可能性为 100%，而 *RAS* 突变在良性和恶性结节中都会出现。

在 2015 年版 ATA 甲状腺结节和分化型甲状腺癌指南发布以前，7 基因试剂盒检测阳性的患者被建议行甲状腺全切而不是腺叶切除，以避免诊断性切除后术后病理为恶性者还需行第二次手术。与之前的指南不同，2015 年版 ATA 指南认为，对多数 <4cm 的甲状腺癌，腺叶切除或全切除都是合适的手术方式，因此，不再需要二次补充全切除[4]。因此，7 基因突变试剂盒由于灵敏度较低，在目前的临床实践中，对手术决策的指导作用被弱化了。

第二代检测

第一代分子检测用来评估不确定甲状腺结节时，或灵敏度高，或特异度高，但无法两者兼顾。此后开发的检测方法的主要目标是改进这一特性，使一种检测可以同时作为确定诊断和排除诊断。ThyroSeq 使用二代基因测序技术，在 7 个基因的基础上扩展了基因变异的检测范围，同时 ThyrGenX/ThyraMIR 将 7 基因突变试剂盒与小分子非编码 microRNA（miRNA）表达分析分类器相结合。另一种 miRNA 分类检测——RosettaGX Reveal（Rosetta Genomics，美国）的特色之处在于，可以在已经制作好的细胞学涂片上检测，但是目前在临床上已经不再使用[40]。

ThyroSeq 检测（CBL Path Inc，美国）是包含与甲状腺癌相关的 12 个基因 284 个突变热点的专门试剂盒。FNA 标本的第一针中取 1 或 2 滴，或专门穿刺 1 针可以满足样本要求。为了验证这种检测的效能，Nikiforova 及其同事[41] 对 228 例甲状腺肿瘤和良性非肿瘤性病变的 DNA 样本进行测序，包括冷冻、福尔马林固定标本和甲状腺 FNA 标本，检测到了 145 例甲状腺癌中的 110 例（76%）和 83 例良性标本中的 5 例（6%）存在突变。接下来的

ThyroSeq v2 试剂盒扩大了基因范围,加入了端粒逆转录酶(telomerase reverse transcriptase, TERT)基因启动子突变,38 种 RET 融合基因,8 个基因的表达分析,用来确定滤泡上皮细胞足量以及鉴别非甲状腺来源病变(如甲状旁腺)。在一项单中心研究中,143 例 Bethesda Ⅳ类连续病例的 FNA 标本接受 ThyroSeq v2 检测(91 例回顾性和 52 例前瞻性样本),并经术后病理验证,灵敏度为 90%,特异度为 93%[42]。另一项研究纳入 462 例 Bethesda Ⅲ结节,使用升级版 ThyroSeq v2(14 个基因突变和 42 个基因融合)检测,其中 95 例进行了手术,灵敏度 91%,特异度 92%[43]。评价 ThyroSeq v2 的样本量最大的独立验证后研究包含了 190 例连续的不确定结节(Bethesda Ⅲ/Ⅳ),根据 102 例结节的术后病理计算其检验效能,总体灵敏度 70%,特异度 77%,NPV 91%,PPV 42%,样本中恶性/NIFTP 比例为 20%。作者发现,该方法在 Bethesda Ⅳ结节中的表现要显著优于 Bethesda Ⅲ[44]。

  ThyGenX/ThyraMIR(Interpace Diagnostics)将多种技术融合,即 5 个基因突变的靶向测序和 3 个基因融合的转录产物,可将结节分类为低危和高危的特定的 10-miRNA GEC 检测。当 ThyGenX 未检测到基因突变或检测到恶性特异性很低的突变时,会自动启动 ThyraMIR 检测。厂家建议将专门的 1 针 FNA 标本收集在核酸保存液中,以保证足够检测。其临床验证研究为来自 12 个临床中心的纳入 109 例 Bethesda Ⅲ/Ⅳ甲状腺结节的横断面研究。在检测人群恶性比例为 32% 时,灵敏度为 89%,特异度 85%,NPV 94%,PPV 74%。ThyGenX 阴性者再加上 ThyraMIR 低危结果,恶性风险仅剩 6%[45]。目前,尚无 ThyGenX/ThyraMIR 的验证后研究。

第三代检测

  ThyroSeq v3 基因组分类器(Genomic Classifier, GC)和 Afirma GSC 是目前可以用来评估细胞学不确定甲状腺结节的最新的分子检测方法,与上一代检测相比,两者的灵敏度和特异度都有所提高。

  ThyroSeq v3 GC 使用二代测序技术,对 112 个甲状腺癌相关基因的点突变、基因融合、拷贝数变异和基因异常表达进行检测。检测到的每种基因变异都被赋予 0~2 之间的一个分数,计算总分。总分为 0 或 1 被定义为阴性,2 分及以上为阳性。除阳性/阴性的二元结果以外,ThyroSeq v3 也会报告检测到的突变和其他基因变异,以及其相关的恶性风险。

  最近的一项研究评价了 GC 的分析效果,该研究纳入了 238 例组织标本(205 例甲状腺标本)作为训练集,175 例已知术后病理结果(恶性比例 52.6%)的细胞学不确定 FNA 标本(Bethesda Ⅲ~Bethesda Ⅳ)作为验证集。嗜酸性病变被包括在训练集（n=68）和验证集中（n=14）。得到的灵敏度、特异度和正确率在训练集中分别为94%、89.4%和92.1%，在验证集中分别为98%、81.8%和90.9%。虽然在分析验证研究中只需要2.5ng核酸样本，厂家还是建议专门穿刺1针（对结节进行穿刺的第二针）以保证样本足量，对于较大的结节，每一针的洗脱液都应保存到同一容器中。

一项在10个临床中心开展的前瞻、双盲临床验证研究最近发表，使用ThyroSeq v3 GC检测286个不确定甲状腺结节（Bethesda Ⅲ~Bethesda Ⅳ）[10]。20例样本（7%）因核酸含量低在测序前一步失败，9例样本（3%）因甲状腺细胞标志物低表达造成样本量不足，其余257例样本得到分子分析信息。对Bethesda Ⅲ结节（154例）的灵敏度和特异度分别是91.4%和84.9%，对Bethesda Ⅳ结节（93例）分别是97%和75%。NPV和PPV对Bethesda Ⅲ（癌/NIFTP比例23%）是97.1%和64%，对Bethesda Ⅳ（癌/NIFTP比例35%）是98%和68%。研究样本中共有11例NIFTP（4%），均被算为阳性。此外，所有的10例Hürthle细胞癌都被正确分类，嗜酸性病变的阴性率为53%（相比之下，Bethesda Ⅲ/Ⅳ结节整体为61%）。下一步研究需要弄清楚，使用灵敏度非常高的二代测序技术，在样本中检测到非常低水平（<10%）的等位基因突变有什么样的临床意义。另外，携带有低危基因变异（GC评分为1分）的结节，目前临床判断为阴性，其远期结局还需要观察。所幸在这一研究中，257例样本中仅有21例（8.2%）的GC评分为1分。

Afirma GSC是一种以RNA测序为基础的检测方法，包含10 196个基因（1 115个核心基因）的12个分类器，再加上7个额外成分来鉴别甲状旁腺病变、MTC、BRAFV600E突变、RET/PTC1或RET/PTC3融合，以及Hürthle细胞病变。目前没有已发表的研究来评价GSC的诊断效果，但有一项双盲的临床验证研究在49个中心进行，它使用的是GEC的验证研究所用的同一组病例，包含191个不确定甲状腺结节（Bethesda Ⅲ/Ⅳ）。该研究样本中，恶性比例为24%（NIFTP比例不详），得到的灵敏度较高，为91%，特异度一般，为68%，NPV为96%，PPV为47%。对Bethesda Ⅲ（114个结节）灵敏度和特异度分别为92.9%和70.9%，对Bethesda Ⅳ（76个结节）分别为88.2%和64.4%。NPV和PPV分别为96.8%和51%（Bethesda Ⅲ），95%和41.7%（Bethesda Ⅳ）。为了弥补GEC在Hürthle细胞病变中特异度不佳，GSC设置了2个专门的Hürthle细胞分类器。对该研究中的26例Hürthle细胞肿瘤亚组进行分析得到的灵敏度和特异度分别为88.9%和58.8%（相比之下，GEC分别为88.9%和11.8%）[11]。虽然GSC被设计为可以将NIFTP识别为可疑恶性，但因为验证研究所用样本在 NIFTP 这一概念被提出之前就存在，故 GSC 在 NIFTP 中的诊断表现尚不明确。厂家建议 FNA 时专门穿刺 2 针，并将标本收集在核酸保存液中以保证足量。

我们的经验

在科罗拉多州大学医院，很多因素会影响我们决定是否会向不确定甲状腺结节患者推荐分子诊断检测。在我们的临床工作中，应用分子检测最常见的指征是需要通过细胞学结果为 Bethesda Ⅲ / Ⅳ 患者决策是否选择临床观察，而不是立即行诊断性手术。以此为目的，我们会选择灵敏度高（>90%）的检测方法，以在我们患者人群中获得较高的 NPV。最近我们对 2011—2015 年期间在我院行 FNA 的 2 019 例甲状腺结节进行总结发现，恶性比例在不同年度之间差别较大，Bethesda Ⅲ 结节范围在 8%~38%（3 年平均 21%~30%），Bethesda Ⅳ 结节在 0~42%（3 年平均 24%~34%）[8]。因为分子诊断方法的 NPV 和 PPV 依赖于检测人群中的恶性比例，为了帮助解读分子检测结果并指导临床决策，持续与病理科医生沟通非常重要。当检测前患者的恶性可能性就已经很大时，我们不会为了排除甲状腺癌而建议分子检测，比如临床甲状腺癌风险高的患者（如有头颈部射线暴露史）出现了不确定的细胞学结果，ATA 指南描述的高度可疑恶性的超声表现，或 Bethesda Ⅴ 结节。

因为我们中心可以进行实时细胞学评估，当穿刺活检时初步细胞学结果提示不确定可能性大时，我们经常可以有机会留取标本用作分子检测。我们在实践中，会另外穿刺 1 针用于分子检测，或者把细胞学涂片针道的洗脱液（通常 2~3 针）收集到核酸保存液中代替额外穿刺。我们通常将分子检测所需样本保存在冰箱中，等待病理结果。当分子检测完成后，我们将结果结合患者的临床恶性风险、超声所见和细胞学结果进行解读，并综合以上信息指导临床处理。据我们所知，还没有已经发表的研究来评价不同的超声表现对不同细胞学和分子检测结果恶性可能性产生的影响。这一领域需要在将来的研究中引起注意。

总结

对不确定甲状腺结节的分子诊断检测大约出现在 10 年前，此后经历了显著的改进，这归功于检测方法的进步和我们对甲状腺肿瘤发生机制了解的深入。最新一代分子检测（如 Afirma GSC 和 ThyroSeq v3）的灵敏度和特异度都取得了较大的改进。这些检测可能会对细胞学不确定的甲状腺结节目前的临床处理产生显著的影响。对分子检测阴性的患者远期结局的观察和对新一代分子检测的独立临床验证研究，将会指导我们在临床实践中如何应用这些检测。

（宋韫韬　张　彬）

参考文献

1. Cibas ES, Ali SZ. The 2017 Bethesda System for Reporting Thyroid Cytopathology. Thyroid 2017;27(11):1341–6.
2. Pusztaszeri M, Rossi ED, Auger M, et al. The Bethesda System for Reporting Thyroid Cytopathology: proposed modifications and updates for the second edition from an international panel. Acta Cytol 2016;60(5):399–405.
3. Ali SZ, Cibas ES, SpringerLink (Online service). The Bethesda System for Reporting Thyroid Cytopathology: definitions, criteria, and explanatory notes. New York: Springer; 2010.
4. Haugen BR, Alexander EK, Bible KC, et al. 2015 American Thyroid Association management guidelines for adult patients with thyroid nodules and differentiated thyroid cancer: the American Thyroid Association guidelines task force on thyroid nodules and differentiated thyroid cancer. Thyroid 2016;26(1):1–133.
5. Pankratz DG, Hu Z, Kim SY, et al. Analytical performance of a gene expression classifier for medullary thyroid carcinoma. Thyroid 2016;26(11):1573–80.
6. Nikiforova MN, Mercurio S, Wald AI, et al. Analytical performance of the ThyroSeq v3 genomic classifier for cancer diagnosis in thyroid nodules. Cancer 2018; 124(8):1682–90.
7. Walsh PS, Wilde JI, Tom EY, et al. Analytical performance verification of a molecular diagnostic for cytology-indeterminate thyroid nodules. J Clin Endocrinol Metab 2012;97(12):E2297–306.
8. Deaver KE, Haugen BR, Pozdeyev N, et al. Outcomes of Bethesda categories III and IV thyroid nodules over 5 years and performance of the Afirma gene expression classifier: a single-institution study. Clin Endocrinol (Oxf) 2018. [Epub ahead of print].
9. Alexander EK, Kennedy GC, Baloch ZW, et al. Preoperative diagnosis of benign thyroid nodules with indeterminate cytology. N Engl J Med 2012;367(8):705–15.
10. Steward DL, Carty SE, Sippel RS, et al. Performance of a multigene genomic classifier in thyroid nodules with indeterminate cytology: a prospective blinded multicenter study. JAMA Oncol 2018. [Epub ahead of print].
11. Patel KN, Angell TE, Babiarz J, et al. Performance of a genomic sequencing classifier for the preoperative diagnosis of cytologically indeterminate thyroid nodules. JAMA Surg 2018;153(9):817–24.
12. Nikiforov YE, Ohori NP, Hodak SP, et al. Impact of mutational testing on the diagnosis and management of patients with cytologically indeterminate thyroid nodules: a prospective analysis of 1056 FNA samples. J Clin Endocrinol Metab

2011;96(11):3390-7.
13. Nikiforov YE, Steward DL, Robinson-Smith TM, et al. Molecular testing for mutations in improving the fine-needle aspiration diagnosis of thyroid nodules. J Clin Endocrinol Metab 2009;94(6):2092-8.
14. Cantara S, Capezzone M, Marchisotta S, et al. Impact of proto-oncogene mutation detection in cytological specimens from thyroid nodules improves the diagnostic accuracy of cytology. J Clin Endocrinol Metab 2010;95(3):1365-9.
15. Moses W, Weng J, Sansano I, et al. Molecular testing for somatic mutations improves the accuracy of thyroid fine-needle aspiration biopsy. World J Surg 2010;34(11):2589-94.
16. Chudova D, Wilde JI, Wang ET, et al. Molecular classification of thyroid nodules using high-dimensionality genomic data. J Clin Endocrinol Metab 2010;95(12):5296-304.
17. Vargas-Salas S, Martinez JR, Urra S, et al. Genetic testing for indeterminate thyroid cytology: review and meta-analysis. Endocr Relat Cancer 2018;25(3):R163-77.
18. Kloos RT, Reynolds JD, Walsh PS, et al. Does addition of BRAF V600E mutation testing modify sensitivity or specificity of the Afirma Gene Expression Classifier in cytologically indeterminate thyroid nodules? J Clin Endocrinol Metab 2013;98(4):E761-8.
19. Alexander EK, Schorr M, Klopper J, et al. Multicenter clinical experience with the Afirma gene expression classifier. J Clin Endocrinol Metab 2014;99(1):119-25.
20. Harrell RM, Bimston DN. Surgical utility of Afirma: effects of high cancer prevalence and oncocytic cell types in patients with indeterminate thyroid cytology. Endocr Pract 2014;20(4):364-9.
21. McIver B, Castro MR, Morris JC, et al. An independent study of a gene expression classifier (Afirma) in the evaluation of cytologically indeterminate thyroid nodules. J Clin Endocrinol Metab 2014;99(11):4069-77.
22. Harrison G, Sosa JA, Jiang X. Evaluation of the Afirma gene expression classifier in repeat indeterminate thyroid nodules. Arch Pathol Lab Med 2017;141(7):985-9.
23. Al-Qurayshi Z, Deniwar A, Thethi T, et al. Association of malignancy prevalence with test properties and performance of the gene expression classifier in indeterminate thyroid nodules. JAMA Otolaryngol Head Neck Surg 2017;143(4):403-8.
24. Jug R, Jiang X. Noninvasive follicular thyroid neoplasm with papillary-like nuclear features: an evidence-based nomenclature change. Patholog Res Int 2017;2017:1057252.
25. Lastra RR, Pramick MR, Crammer CJ, et al. Implications of a suspicious Afirma test result in thyroid fine-needle aspiration cytology: an institutional experience. Cancer Cytopathol 2014;122(10):737-44.
26. Sacks WL, Bose S, Zumsteg ZS, et al. Impact of Afirma gene expression classifier on cytopathology diagnosis and rate of thyroidectomy. Cancer Cytopathol 2016;124(10):722-8.
27. Bongiovanni M, Spitale A, Faquin WC, et al. The Bethesda System for Reporting Thyroid Cytopathology: a meta-analysis. Acta Cytol 2012;56(4):333-9.
28. Baca SC, Wong KS, Strickland KC, et al. Qualifiers of atypia in the cytologic diagnosis of thyroid nodules are associated with different Afirma gene expression classifier results and clinical outcomes. Cancer Cytopathol 2017;125(5):313-22.
29. Brauner E, Holmes BJ, Krane JF, et al. Performance of the Afirma gene expres-

sion classifier in Hurthle cell thyroid nodules differs from other indeterminate thyroid nodules. Thyroid 2015;25(7):789–96.
30. Wu JX, Lam R, Levin M, et al. Effect of malignancy rates on cost-effectiveness of routine gene expression classifier testing for indeterminate thyroid nodules. Surgery 2016;159(1):118–26.
31. Duick DS, Klopper JP, Diggans JC, et al. The impact of benign gene expression classifier test results on the endocrinologist-patient decision to operate on patients with thyroid nodules with indeterminate fine-needle aspiration cytopathology. Thyroid 2012;22(10):996–1001.
32. Angell TE, Frates MC, Medici M, et al. Afirma benign thyroid nodules show similar growth to cytologically benign nodules during follow-up. J Clin Endocrinol Metab 2015;100(11):E1477–83.
33. Sipos JA, Blevins TC, Shea HC, et al. Long-term nonoperative rate of thyroid nodules with benign results on the Afirma gene expression classifier. Endocr Pract 2016;22(6):666–72.
34. Witt RL. Outcome of thyroid gene expression classifier testing in clinical practice. Laryngoscope 2016;126(2):524–7.
35. Cancer Genome Atlas Research Network. Integrated genomic characterization of papillary thyroid carcinoma. Cell 2014;159(3):676–90.
36. Landa I, Ibrahimpasic T, Boucai L, et al. Genomic and transcriptomic hallmarks of poorly differentiated and anaplastic thyroid cancers. J Clin Invest 2016;126(3):1052–66.
37. Pozdeyev N, Gay LM, Sokol ES, et al. Genetic analysis of 779 advanced differentiated and anaplastic thyroid cancers. Clin Cancer Res 2018;24(13):3059–68.
38. Eszlinger M, Krogdahl A, Munz S, et al. Impact of molecular screening for point mutations and rearrangements in routine air-dried fine-needle aspiration samples of thyroid nodules. Thyroid 2014;24(2):305–13.
39. Krane JF, Cibas ES, Alexander EK, et al. Molecular analysis of residual ThinPrep material from thyroid FNAs increases diagnostic sensitivity. Cancer Cytopathol 2015;123(6):356–61.
40. Lithwick-Yanai G, Dromi N, Shtabsky A, et al. Multicentre validation of a microRNA-based assay for diagnosing indeterminate thyroid nodules utilising fine needle aspirate smears. J Clin Pathol 2017;70(6):500–7.
41. Nikiforova MN, Wald AI, Roy S, et al. Targeted next-generation sequencing panel (ThyroSeq) for detection of mutations in thyroid cancer. J Clin Endocrinol Metab 2013;98(11):E1852–60.
42. Nikiforov YE, Carty SE, Chiosea SI, et al. Highly accurate diagnosis of cancer in thyroid nodules with follicular neoplasm/suspicious for a follicular neoplasm cytology by ThyroSeq v2 next-generation sequencing assay. Cancer 2014;120(23):3627–34.
43. Nikiforov YE, Carty SE, Chiosea SI, et al. Impact of the multi-gene ThyroSeq next-generation sequencing assay on cancer diagnosis in thyroid nodules with atypia of undetermined significance/follicular lesion of undetermined significance cytology. Thyroid 2015;25(11):1217–23.
44. Valderrabano P, Khazai L, Leon ME, et al. Evaluation of ThyroSeq v2 performance in thyroid nodules with indeterminate cytology. Endocr Relat Cancer 2017;24(3):127–36.
45. Labourier E, Shifrin A, Busseniers AE, et al. Molecular testing for miRNA, mRNA, and DNA on fine-needle aspiration improves the preoperative diagnosis of thyroid nodules with indeterminate cytology. J Clin Endocrinol Metab 2015;100(7):2743–50.

第6章
分化型甲状腺癌的临床评估和风险分层

Fernanda Vaisman, R. Michael Tuttle

关键词

- 风险分层 • 甲状腺癌 • 死亡率 • 复发率 • 治疗反应

要点

- 初始风险分层为肿瘤分期、治疗以及随访提供了重要信息。
- 动态风险分层进一步调整初始风险分层,有助于制订更准确的后续管理策略。
- 第 8 版 AJCC/TNM 分期系统将大量患者降至较低分期,并改进了对疾病结局的预测。

引言

在过去的数十年中,分化型甲状腺癌的分期和管理经历了从标准化到个体化评估和治疗的模式转变。这得益于风险分层的发展,使得在疾病随访的早期便能够预测出诸如疾病特异性死亡率、持续或复发风险,以及治疗失败的可能性。

2009 年修订的 ATA 指南是引导其进行模式转变的一个里程碑。指南强烈推荐将肿瘤复发和疾病持续风险同包括病死率在内的预后结局列入风险分层,这对甲状腺癌的管理具有重要意义,因为甲状腺癌的疾病特异性死亡率通常较低[1]。指南还强调了其他因素,如初次手术的组织病理和质量,术后甲状腺球蛋白(thyroglobulin,Tg)的评估和制订放射性碘(radioactive iodine,RAI)

辅助治疗决策的重要性[2]。

虽然初次治疗后的再评估可以更好预测远期预后和制订随访方案,但是 Tuttle 等人[3]在 2010 年提出的基于治疗反应的动态风险分层方法已成为个体化管理分化型甲状腺癌(differentiated thyroid cancer,DTC)的基石。

10 年后的今天,随着风险评估方式的不断改进,其中一些细节的改变使得我们可以从预后良好的患者中区分出可能具有不良结局的群体。本章旨在回顾这些风险评估方式并简述人们近年来为改善预后而作出的改进。

讨论

评估死亡风险

死亡率往往是患者初次走进诊室最为关切的问题。因此,术后第一次随访时,给出精确肿瘤分期至关重要,因为其能帮助预测肿瘤特异性死亡率。同其他实体肿瘤一样,美国癌症联合会(the American Joint Committee on Cancer,AJCC)提出的 TNM(肿瘤、淋巴结、远处转移)分期系统也广泛应用于甲状腺癌中。它将肿瘤大小、原发肿瘤局部浸润情况、有无淋巴结转移和远处转移按照年龄分组。和其他肿瘤分期系统相比,AJCC/TNM 分期系统的制定更佳,已成为全世界范围内最常使用的分期体系。第 7 版的诊断年龄截点是 45 岁[4]。

最近发表的第 8 版 AJCC/TNM 分期系统进一步强调了疾病特异性死亡率预测的准确性[5,6]。

第一,将诊断时用于分期的截点年龄从 45 岁提高到 55 岁。一项纳入了近 10 000 名患者的国际多中心研究认为:提高年龄截点可以更好地把Ⅲ期患者从过去标准下的Ⅳ期患者群体中区别出来。这项研究表示,使用 45 岁年龄截点时,Ⅰ~Ⅳ期患者的 10 年疾病特异性生存率(disease specific survival,DSS)分别为 99.7%、97.3%、96.6% 和 76.3%。使用 55 岁年龄截点时,Ⅰ~Ⅳ期患者的 10 年疾病 DSS 分别为 99.5%、94.7%、94.1% 和 67.6%。这一改变最终使得大量患者在获得疾病降期的同时保留了肿瘤分期的区分度[7]。Kim 等人在 2018 年提出另一项从基因角度支持 55 岁作为年龄截点的研究[8],他们的研究结果显示,确诊时年龄>55 岁的患者群体相比<55 岁的群体,有 103 个与高度恶性相关通路(如 TGF-β)的基因出现异常表达。

第二,重新评估了微小腺外浸润(minor extrathyroidal extension,mETE)对于结局的预测意义。mETE 被定义为:只能在组织学切片中才能发现的亚临床甲状腺周围组织浸润(查体和影像学检查阴性)。在第 7 版中,任何伴有

mETE 的肿瘤都被定为 T_3 期,有分析指出,显微镜下的微小腺外浸润并不会对无瘤生存期、疾病特异性生存期、局部转移和远处转移产生影响。Tam 等人近期的研究[9]提示,肿瘤大小才是上述不良结局的独立预测因子。综上,AJCC 将 T_3 分期重新定义为 T_{3a}:肿瘤直径>4cm 且局限在甲状腺内;T_{3b}:无论肿瘤大小,肉眼见肿瘤腺外侵犯带状肌。

第三,淋巴结分区的变更(主要针对Ⅶ区淋巴结)。原先的 N_{1a} 专指Ⅵ区(如:中央区气管前、气管旁、喉前等)发现转移淋巴结。现在第 8 版将纵膈淋巴结转移也归为 N_{1a},同时 N_{1b} 专指颈侧区淋巴结转移(Ⅱ~Ⅴ区)[5,10]。

第四,TNM 分期的变更。N_1 期病变不再把高龄患者升级为Ⅲ期或Ⅳ期。虽然淋巴结转移对高龄患者的疾病特异性死亡率确实有显著影响,但是这一影响对年轻人和高龄患者中具有更高死亡风险的Ⅲ/Ⅳ期患者而言并不重要[6]。因此,N_1 期患者在确诊年龄<55 岁的患者群中被归为Ⅰ期,而在确诊年龄>55 岁的群体中被分为Ⅱ期。

多篇文献报道,相较第 7 版分期体系而言,第 8 版分期体系确实将大量低风险患者降至较低分期,并提供了更好的分期区分度[6,10-13]。

确诊年龄<55 岁的患者群体只能被归为Ⅰ期(无远处转移)或Ⅱ期(有远处转移)。而确诊年龄>55 岁的患者若有远处转移会被分类为Ⅳb 期。如果没有远处转移或远处转移不明确时(M_0/M_x),有无肉眼可见的腺外侵犯就是下一个重大判定点。当没有肉眼可见腺外侵犯时,≤4cm 的肿瘤且局限在甲状腺内(N_0/N_x)者属于Ⅰ期;肿瘤>4cm 或有颈部淋巴结转移的属于Ⅱ期。相反,当出现肉眼可见腺外侵犯时,患者会因周围不同组织结构受侵而被归为Ⅱ、Ⅲ、Ⅳa 期。需要强调的是,初次手术后 4 个月内获得的任何信息都应该用于 AJCC 分期,这包括任何后续结构/功能影像学检查或查体发现的新发转移灶。

评估复发/疾病持续性风险

前文提到,2009 年 ATA 甲状腺结节及甲状腺癌指南提出了新的评价体系,即基于复发及疾病持续性进行风险评估,取代了以往仅关注死亡率的评估方式。这种评价体系的恰当性在于,低病死率和高复发/疾病持续率之间的矛盾性,尤其是在年轻患者群体中。Mazzaferri 等人在 2001 年的研究显示,虽然疾病特异性病死率随年龄增长,但是复发率和年龄却呈 U 形关系,即在高龄和低龄两端的复发风险最高[14]。针对这个问题,2009 年,ATA 推出了一个依靠病理学特征、淋巴结转移情况、远处转移情况以及一些术后评估指标(例如,甲状腺球蛋白测值、碘扫描情况和横断面影像学等参数信息)的风险分层方法。

在 2010 年，Tuttle 等人[3]提出的这一新的风险分层体系相比 AJCC 系统而言，能够更加精确地预测复发和疾病持续性风险，因为它可以解释 34% 的变异。同时也优于其他常用的分期系统，如 MACIS 系统和以前的 MSKCC 系统[4,15,16]。

2015 年，更新后的 ATA 指南将新的数据引入这一风险预测体系，包括转移淋巴结的大小和数目、血管侵犯、特殊病理类型、细胞学特征分析等，这些变量均有助于改善风险预测。淋巴结转移对预后的影响仍然有争议[17,18]。大多数研究都显示，出现淋巴结转移对总体生存率只有很小的影响，而对高龄患者群的复发或疾病持续率以及全年龄组生活质量影响更大[4,5]。

过去，淋巴结转移与否以及转移部位是仅有的淋巴结病变分层指标[6]。现在，受累淋巴结数目、大小和部位以及出现淋巴结外侵犯（extranodal extension，ENE）等参数对淋巴结病变复发/疾病持续性预测具有重要意义[7]。2015 版 ATA 推荐把低风险疾病分层定义为：无淋巴结转移临床证据（cN_0）或出现不超过 5 枚淋巴结微转移（<2mm）；中风险疾病分层定义为：出现有临床证据的淋巴结转移（cN_1）和/或多于 5 枚淋巴结转移（受累淋巴结<3cm）；高风险疾病分层定义为：转移淋巴结>3cm。ENE 并非独立预测因子，出现 3 处转移淋巴结伴 ENE 方被认为具有高风险特征，具有 40% 复发/疾病持续性风险[18]。血管侵犯程度是甲状腺滤泡状癌风险分层中一项重要参考变量（>4 处局灶血管浸润被认为具有更高风险）。此外，虽然并非必备条件，但基因突变也可用于风险分层。

新版风险分层体系的临床意义对放射性碘（RAI）辅助治疗同样有意义，例如：微小淋巴结转移者可以不用 RAI 治疗[3]，所以微小浸润性 FTC 可以归为低风险组，这使得初始治疗可以个体化。

Ghaznavi 等人最近提议[13]融合 AJCC/TNM 第 8 版分期系统和 ATA 风险分层体系以促进个体化风险评估的完善。他们基于 AJCC 分期系统、ATA 风险分层体系和年龄这三个维度开展了 6 个队列研究，并展示了随访 6 年后的疾病特异性生存率（disease-free survival，DSS）数据：

Ⅰ 期/ATA 低风险，低龄加高龄，100%DSS[2]

Ⅰ 期/ATA 中风险，低龄加高龄，98%DSS[3]

Ⅰ 期/ATA 高风险，低龄，95%DSS[4]

Ⅰ 期/ATA 高风险，高龄，89%DSS[5]

Ⅱ 期/ATA 高风险，低龄，78%DSS[6]

Ⅱ 期/ATA 高风险，高龄，61%DSS

这一评估体系在高风险组内有巨大差异，未来需要对其更加个体化[13]。

与死亡风险不同,分析疾病复发/持续风险时,年龄一般不纳入考虑。但年龄因素在某些特殊组内却很重要。Shah 和 Boucai 等人的研究结果[19]展示了在 ATA 高风险组中,<55 岁的患者对治疗反应良好的概率是那些>55 岁的患者的 2 倍。由此,作者提出:在甲状腺癌 ATA 高风险组内,年龄可作为疾病特异性生存率和治疗反应的关键预测因子。

评估远期复发/疾病持续性风险并制订长期随访策略

临床医生早就认识到,虽然初始风险分层能够为其提供重要的预后参考信息以制订个体化管理策略,但是风险预测需要及时调整,因为初次治疗后的功能性应答和疾病生物学行为会随之改变。2010 年,MSKCC 甲状腺癌工作组提出了一个新的命名法和一个基于随访数据可用于修改初始风险预测的动态风险分层体系[3]。这个体系包括反应良好、反应不确定、反应不全(生化性和结构性)三个组,患者会被不断地再次评估而被重新划分到这些组内。定义如下:

反应良好组:无临床、生化或结构性疾病证据;

生化性反应不全:在无可定位的局灶性病变前提下,出现异常升高的血清甲状腺球蛋白(Tg)或具有升高趋势的抗甲状腺球蛋白抗体(antithyroglobulin antibody,TgAb);

结构性反应不全:具有持续存在的或新发局灶性病变或出现远处转移,伴或不伴随异常 Tg 或 TgAb;

反应不确定性:不典型的生化或结构性改变,既不能确定分类为良性也不能确定为恶性病变(表 6.1)[3]。

表 6.1
治疗反应——甲状腺全切 +^{131}I 治疗(初次治疗 6~24 个月后)

反应良好	反应不确定性	生化反应不全	结构性反应不全
满足以下所有:	满意以下任意一条:	在未发现明确结构性病变的前提下,满意以下任意一条:	满足以下任意一条,不论 Tg 为何值:
• 抑制性 Tg<0.2ng/ml 且刺激性 Tg<1ng/ml	• 抑制性 Tg<1ng/ml 同时刺激性 Tg>1ng/ml 且<10ng/ml	• 抑制性 Tg>1ng/ml	• 持续存在或新发横断面影像和/或核医学影像结果阳性
• 颈部彩超未见疾病证据	• 非特异性影像学检查结果,无确切疾病证据	• 刺激性 Tg>10ng/ml	
• 横断面影像和/或核医学影像结果阴性(若有)		• 逐步升高的 Tg 值	
		• 逐步升高的 TgAb	

正如预期,不论首次风险预测如何,对治疗反应良好的患者群相比反应不全的患者,在术后 2 年内的复发 / 疾病持续风险大大降低(复发 / 疾病持续率:反应良好组<3%~5% vs. 结构性反应不全组>85%)。以上数据由世界范围内多个队列研究证实[20-22]。Vaisman 等人[23]在巴西的研究显示了相似的结果:在 10 年随访期内无疾病证据的患者中,对治疗反应良好的患者组中有 99%,在对治疗反应不确定的患者组中有 81%,在生化性反应不全的患者组有 56%,在结构性反应不全的患者组内只有 10% 的患者在最初 2 年内病灶持续存在,但在 10 年随访期结束时无疾病证据。

在接下来的几年里,治疗反应分层体系已经被应用于指导长期随访策略。2015 版 ATA 指南推荐,一旦患者对治疗具有良好反应,应该早期降低随访强度和频率,并降低促甲状腺激素(thyroid-stimulating hormone,TSH)抑制力度,因为此时的复发概率处于低值(1%~4%)。大部分生化反应不全患者表现出稳定或降低趋势的血清 Tg 值时,应该继续 TSH 抑制和随访观察。发现持续升高的 Tg 或 TgAb 时,鼓励增加额外检查甚至开始进行治疗;对治疗反应不确定性患者应该持续观察随访,并针对非特异性病损进行影像学检查,监测血清 Tg 水平。随访中发现可疑的非特异性改变应该进一步行影像学检查或活检,结构性反应不全患者需要根据多项临床病理学因素综合判断,最终可能进行额外治疗或进行性观察,需要参考的因素有:病灶大小,位置,增长率,RAI 亲和性,[^{18}F]- 氟代脱氧葡萄糖(^{18}F-FDG)亲和性,以及结构性病变的病理学指标[18]。值得指出的是,对结构性反应不全患者群体即使给予额外治疗也很可能只有不到 15% 的概率最终达到无病生存,换言之,此时大多数治疗的意义在于姑息减瘤。因此,在这种情况下若提议治疗,慎重评估风险和获益显得尤为关键。

另一方面,ATA 指南对低、中风险患者还提议了一些比较缓和的初次处置方式。虽然这些治疗反应分组定义是为接受甲状腺全切加 RAI 治疗的患者量身订制的,但以下治疗方式并不适用于每一位患者。比如,低风险患者不需要常规行 RAI 治疗,如果肿瘤小,且局限在甲状腺腺体内,也可以考虑腺叶切除。正因如此,需要进一步扩展对治疗的不同反应产生的四组分类的定义,因为初始治疗方案有所不同。为阐述这一问题,Momesso 等人[24]发表了一篇文章,验证了初次手术范围少于甲状腺全切且未行 RAI 的治疗反应分类表现。不出所料,基于 ATA 风险分层,反应良好组大幅降低了结构性复发 / 疾病持续风险,低风险组和中风险组分别从 2.5% 和 9.5% 降低至 0。相似地,反应不确定性组未行 RAI 治疗者也基于 ATA 风险预测相应降低了复发风险(表 6.2)。

表 6.2
治疗应答——甲状腺全切未行 ^{131}I 治疗和腺叶切除（初次治疗 6~24 个月后）

良好应答	不确定性应答	生化不完全性应答	结构性不完全应答
甲状腺全切 满足以下全部：	甲状腺全切 满意以下任意一条：	甲状腺全切 在未发现明确结构性病变的前提下满足以下任意一条：	甲状腺全切 满足以下任意一条不论 Tg 为何值：
• 非刺激性 Tg<0.2ng/ml 且刺激性 Tg<1ng/ml	• 非刺激性 Tg 0.2~5ng/ml 同时刺激性 Tg>2ng/ml 且<10ng/ml	• 非刺激性 Tg>5ng/ml	• 持续存在或新发横断面影像和/或核医学影像结果阳性
• 颈部彩超未见疾病证据	• 非特异性影像学检查结果，无确切疾病证据	• 刺激性 Tg>10ng/ml	腺叶切除
腺叶切除 满足以下全部：	腺叶切除	• 逐步升高的 Tg 值	• 持续存在或新发横断面影像和/或核医学影像结果阳性
• 非刺激性 Tg<30ng/ml 且刺激性 Tg<1ng/ml	• 非特异性影像学检查结果，无确切疾病证据	• 逐步升高的 TgAb	
• 颈部彩超未见疾病证据		腺叶切除	
		• 非刺激性 Tg≥30ng/ml	
		• Tg 逐步升高伴相似 TSH 水平	
		• 逐步升高的 TgAb	

预测治疗失败的风险

当考虑风险分层方案时，明确预测何种预后结局是十分关键的。临床医生习惯上会把复发、转移和疾病死亡风险看作主要感兴趣的结局事件。但是，从临床实用角度考虑，真正需要预测的是首次治疗失败的风险。需要强调，高龄伴有肉眼腺外浸润和放射性碘抵抗的转移灶[^{18}F-FDG 正电子放射体层成像（positron emission tomography，PET）阳性]的患者病死率高，是由于肿瘤生物学恶性度本身和对首次治疗无反应合力为之。少数高风险高龄且对初次治疗（肿瘤彻底切除甚至连带部分颈部结构一并切除，转移灶 RAI 亲和性良好）反应良好的患者，相比那些治疗反应不良的持续性病灶者而言，具有更好的预后。

从这种意义上讲，为了更加了解肿瘤有多大可能对治疗产生反应以及对每个患者的个性化治疗，提议通过更多额外检查综合评估。

指南建议，初次治疗后横断面影像学结果阴性，但仍然保持高血清 Tg 水平或具有持续升高趋势 Tg 的患者，行 FDG-PET/CT 检查[18]。虽然这种检查敏感性（85%~100%）很高，但是 PET/CT 的特异性仍然较低（约 75%），而且依赖肿瘤负荷量[25]。

最近，FDG-PET/CT 被用作一种预后评估工具。Wang 等人[26]的研究展示：FDG-PET/CT 显像阳性的病灶对高剂量 RAI 不敏感。同样的研究队列提示，具有 FDG-PET/CT 阳性转移灶患者，相比阴性群体而言，具有更差的预后，不管其对 RAI 的亲和力如何[27]。

所谓的"人字拖"现象，描述了一种情形，当肿瘤不再有摄碘能力或摄碘率低时，FDG 摄取率反而升高，是因为此时肿瘤具有更高的葡萄糖摄取率和代谢水平。相比 FDG-PET/CT 阴性肿瘤而言，阳性肿瘤往往体积更大，且侵犯范围更广[28]，更加具有侵袭性[29]，以及有更多基因突变[30]。现如今，FDG-PET/CT 已被用作一种有效预测肿瘤产生碘抵抗的工具。

为了深化个体化诊治，甲状腺癌风险分层已经深入基因水平，在不远的将来，基因突变很可能会融合到更完善、准确性更高的综合临床评估中来。比如，多个研究均提示：相比 *BRAF+TERT* 基因突变的人群而言[32-35]，携带 *RAS* 基因位点突变的肿瘤更可能具有 RAI 亲和性[31]。

总结

综上所述，风险分层体系经历了一个逐步发展的过程。由 AJCC 和 ATA 指南分别提出的疾病特异性死亡风险分层和疾病复发/持续风险分层，有助于临床医生制订初始治疗决策。而持续的治疗反应评估和动态风险分层对于调整患者的管理具有长期意义。这种不断迭代优化的过程，正在引领我们抵达新的目标——维持患者最大利益和最小风险的平衡——才是个体化的肿瘤管理方式。

（张　琨　李志辉）

参考文献

1. Cooper DS, Doherty GM, Haugen BR, et al. Revised American Thyroid Association management guidelines for patients with thyroid nodules and differentiated thyroid cancer. Thyroid 2009;19:1167–214.
2. Rondeau G, Tuttle RM. Similarities and differences in follicular cell-derived thyroid cancer management guidelines used in Europe and the United States. Semin Nucl Med 2011;41(2):89–95.
3. Tuttle RM, Tala H, Shah J, et al. Estimating risk of recurrence in differentiated thyroid cancer after total thyroidectomy and radioactive iodine remnant ablation: using response to therapy variables to modify the initial risk estimates predicted by the new American Thyroid Association staging system. Thyroid 2010;20(12): 1341–9.
4. Brierley JD, Panzarella T, Tsang RW, et al. A comparison of different staging systems predictability of patient outcome. Thyroid carcinoma as an example. Cancer 1997;79(12):2414–23.
5. Perrier ND, Brierley JD, Tuttle RM. Differentiated and anaplastic thyroid carcinoma: major changes in the American Joint Committee on Cancer eighth edition cancer staging manual. CA Cancer J Clin 2018;68(1):55–63.
6. Tuttle RM, Haugen B, Perrier ND. Updated American Joint Committee on Cancer/tumor-node-metastasis staging system for differentiated and anaplastic thyroid cancer (eighth edition): what changed and why? Thyroid 2017;27(6):751–6.
7. Nixon IJ, Wang LY, Migliacci JC, et al. An international multi-institutional validation of age 55 years as a cutoff for risk stratification in the AJCC/UICC staging system for well-differentiated thyroid cancer. Thyroid 2016;26(3):373–80.
8. Kim K, Kim JH, Park IS, et al. The updated AJCC/TNM staging system for papillary thyroid cancer (8th Edition): from the perspective of genomic analysis. World J Surg 2018. [Epub ahead of print].
9. Tam S, Boonsripitayanon M, Amit M, et al. Survival in differentiated thyroid cancer: comparing the AJCC cancer staging 7th and 8th editions. Thyroid 2018; 28(10):1301–10.
10. van Velsen EFS, Stegenga MT, van Kemenade FJ, et al. Comparing the prognostic value of the eighth edition of the American Joint Committee on Cancer/tumor node metastasis staging system between papillary and follicular thyroid cancer thyroid cancer. Thyroid 2018;28(8):976–81.
11. Kim TH, Kim YN, Kim HI, et al. Prognostic value of the eighth edition AJCC TNM classification for differentiated thyroid carcinoma. Oral Oncol 2017;71:81–6.
12. Pontius LN, Oyekunle TO, Thomas SM, et al. Projecting survival in papillary thyroid cancer: a comparison of the seventh and eighth editions of the American Joint Commission on Cancer/Union for International Cancer Control Staging Systems in two contemporary national patient cohorts. Thyroid 2017;27(11):1408–16.
13. Ghaznavi SA, Ganly I, Shaha AR, et al. Using the ATA risk stratification system to refine and individualize the AJCC 8th edition disease specific survival estimates in differentiated thyroid cancer. Thyroid 2018;28(10):1293–300.
14. Mazzaferri EL, Kloos RT. Clinical review 128: current approaches to primary therapy for papillary and follicular thyroid cancer. J Clin Endocrinol Metab 2001;86(4): 1447–63.

15. Sherman SI, Brierley JD, Sperling M, et al. 3rd Prospective multicenter study of thyroid carcinoma treatment: initial analysis of staging and outcome. National Thyroid Cancer Treatment Cooperative Study Registry Group. Cancer 1998;83: 1012–21.
16. Verburg FA, Mader U, Kruitwagen CL, et al. A comparison of prognostic classification systems for differentiated thyroid carcinoma. Clin Endocrinol (Oxf) 2010; 72:830–8.
17. Randolph GW, Duh Q, Heller KS, et al. The prognostic significance of nodal metastasis from papillary thyroid carcinoma can be stratified based on the size and number of metastatic lymph nodes, as well as the presence of extranodal extension. Thyroid 2012;22(11):1144–52.
18. Haugen BR, Alexander EK, Bible KC, et al. 2015 American Thyroid Association management guidelines for adult patients with thyroid nodules and differentiated thyroid cancer: the American Thyroid Association Guidelines Task Force on Thyroid Nodules and Differentiated Thyroid Cancer. Thyroid 2016;26(1):1–133.
19. Shah S, Boucai L. Effect of age on response to therapy and mortality in patients with thyroid cancer at high risk of recurrence. J Clin Endocrinol Metab 2018; 103(2):689–97.
20. Vaisman F, Tala H, Grewal R, et al. In differentiated thyroid cancer and incomplete structural response to therapy is associated with significantly worse clinical outcomes than only an incomplete thyroglobulin response. Thyroid 2011;21: 1317–22.
21. Castagna MG, Maino F, Cipri C, et al. Delayed risk stratification, to include the response to initial therapy (surgery and radioiodine ablation), has better outcome predictivity in differentiated thyroid cancer patients. Eur J Endocrinol 2011;165: 441–6.
22. Pitoia F, Bueno F, Urciuoli C, et al. Outcome of patients with differentiated thyroid cancer risk stratified according to the American thyroid association and Latin-American thyroid society risk of recurrence classification systems. Thyroid 2013;23:1401–7.
23. Vaisman F, Momesso D, Bulzico DA, et al. Spontaneous remission in thyroid cancer patients after biochemical incomplete response to initial therapy. Clin Endocrinol 2012;77:132–8.
24. Momesso DP, Vaisman F, Yang SP, et al. Dynamic risk stratification in patients with differentiated thyroid cancer treated without radioactive iodine. J Clin Endocrinol Metab 2016;101(7):2692–700.
25. Leboulleux S, Schroeder PR, Schlumberger M, et al. The role of PET in follow-up of patients treated for differentiated epithelial thyroid cancers. Thyroid 2001; 11(12):1169–75.
26. Wang W, Larson SM, Tuttle RM, et al. Resistance of [18f]-fluorodeoxyglucose-avid metastatic thyroid cancer lesions to treatment with high-dose radioactive iodine. Thyroid 2001;11(12):1169–75.
27. Richard RJ, Wan Q, Grewal RK, et al. Larson real- time prognosis for metastatic thyroid carcinoma based on 2-[18F]Fluoro-2-Deoxy-D-glucose positron emission tomography scanning. J Clin Endocrinol Metab 2006;91(2):498–505.
28. Esteva D, Muros MA, Llamas-Elvira JM, et al. Clinical and pathological factors related to 18F-FDG-PET positivity in the diagnosis of recurrence and/or metastasis in patients with differentiated thyroid cancer. Ann Surg Oncol 2009;16(7): 2006–13.

29. Rivera M, Ghossein RA, Schoder H, et al. Histopathologic characterization of radioactive iodine-refractory fluorodeoxyglucose-positron emission tomography-positive thyroid carcinoma. Cancer 2008;113(1):48–56.
30. Ricarte-Filho JC, Ryder M, Chitale DA, et al. Mutational profile of advanced primary and metastatic radioactive iodine-refractory thyroid cancers reveals distinct pathogenetic roles for BRAF, PIK3CA, and AKT1. Cancer Res 2009;69(11): 4885–93.
31. Sabra MM, Dominguez JM, Grewal RK, et al. Clinical outcomes and molecular profile of differentiated thyroid cancers with radioiodine-avid distant metastases. J Clin Endocrinol Metab 2013;98(5):E829–36.
32. Yang X, Li J, Li X, et al. TERT Promoter mutation predicts radioiodine-refractory character in distant metastatic differentiated thyroid cancer. J Nucl Med 2017; 58(2):258–65.
33. Penna GC, Pestana A, Cameselle JM, et al. TERTp mutation is associated with a shorter progression free survival in patients with aggressive histology subtypes of follicular-cell derived thyroid carcinoma. Endocrine 2018;61(3):489–98.
34. Liu R, Bishop J, Zhu G, et al. Mortality risk stratification by combining BRAF V600E and TERT promoter mutations in papillary thyroid cancer: genetic duet of BRAF and TERT promoter mutations in thyroid cancer mortality. JAMA Oncol 2017;3(2):202–8.
35. Xing M, Liu R, Liu X, et al. BRAF V600E and TERT promoter mutations cooperatively identify the most aggressive papillary thyroid cancer with highest recurrence. J Clin Oncol 2014;32(25):2718–26.

第 7 章
基因检测指导甲状腺癌风险评估与诊治决策

邢明照（Mingzhao Xing）

关键词

- 甲状腺癌 ● 遗传分子标志 ● *BRAF V600E* 突变 ● *TERT* 启动子突变
- *RAS* 突变 ● 风险分层 ● 预后

要点

- 因为基于临床特征评估甲状腺癌预后往往不确定，所以关于如何精准诊治甲状腺癌尚存争议。
- 以 *BRAF V600E* 和 *TERT* 启动子突变为例的甲状腺癌预后分子标记，可以很好地指导风险分层，并受到广泛认可。
- 联合检测 *BRAF V600E/RAS* 和 *TERT* 启动子突变，是评估分化型甲状腺癌不良预后的最有效方法。
- 预后相关的分子标志物的阴性预测值较高，同样很有意义。
- 通过分子遗传指导临床风险分层和个体化诊治，才能实现分子标记物在甲状腺癌预后评估中的最大价值。

引言

甲状腺癌是常见的内分泌恶性肿瘤，组织学包括滤泡上皮细胞来源的甲状腺癌和滤泡旁 C 细胞来源的甲状腺髓样癌（medullary thyroid cancer, MTC）[1]。前者包括甲状腺乳头状癌（papillary thyroid cancer, PTC），甲状腺滤泡癌（follicular thyroid cancer,FTC)和甲状腺未分化癌(anaplastic thyroid cancer,ATC)。PTC 和 FTC 是最常见的甲状腺癌,分别占所有甲状腺癌的 80%~90% 和 5%~10%。ATC 和 MTC 较少见,分别占甲状腺癌的 2%~3%。PTC 又进一步分为若干亚型,包括最常见的经典型 PTC(conventional PTC,CPTC),其次是滤泡亚型 PTC(follicular-variant PTC,FVPTC),高细胞型 PTC(tall-cell PTC,TCPTC),以及其他一些罕见亚型[1-3]。

PTC 和 FTC 属于分化型甲状腺癌(differentiated thyroid cancer,DTC),总死亡率低,临床多数表现为惰性,但目前诊疗下同时存在复发率较高的现状。甲状腺癌复发与患者发病和死亡风险增加相关。ATC 可由 DTC 失分化发展而来,也可能发病时即为 ATC。尽管 ATC 不常见,但因其短期使患者致死,成为侵袭性最强的甲状腺癌。低分化甲状腺癌(poorly differentiated thyroid cancer,PDTC),也可从 DTC 发展而来,临床侵袭性中等,介于 DTC 和 ATC 之间。PTC 癌灶直径 ≤ 1.0cm 时定义为甲状腺微小乳头状癌(papillary thyroid microcarcinoma,PTMC)[4],总体临床预后良好,但也有部分患者预后较差甚至死亡。甲状腺癌临床治疗的主要目的是预防疾病复发,在降低患者发病率和死亡率的同时,最大限度地减少治疗相关的并发症。在治疗获益和并发症之间取得最佳平衡,取决于准确的甲状腺癌风险分层。近年来,基于临床病理特征评估指导诊治策略,已提高了其准确性[5]。然而关键问题在于,经典的基于临床病理的甲状腺癌风险评估,通常不准确。举个例子,临床表现明显低风险的甲状腺癌,可能发展为高侵袭性、预后较差,这给临床诊断和治疗决策带来了挑战,导致持续低风险的甲状腺癌过度治疗,而潜在侵袭性的甲状腺癌治疗不足,都较常见。鉴于近几十年来甲状腺癌发病率迅速增加,以及目前巨大的甲状腺癌患者量[2,6],更好地进行风险分层,以便更准确地治疗甲状腺癌,已比以往任何时候都更为重要。

近年来,应用基于分子标志物的风险分层指导甲状腺癌精确分期,备受青睐[7]。鉴于 DTC 的高发病率[2,6]和众所周知的预后分子标志物[1,7-14],以上在 DTC 临床中特别重要且很有前景,作为本章讨论的重点。

甲状腺癌主要的致癌基因改变

在甲状腺癌众多的遗传改变中评估预后最佳的是癌基因突变,最突出的是 *BRAF V600E* 和 *TERT* 启动子突变以及其他一些突变[1,7-14]。这些突变的发生与原发性 DTC 和相应的转移之间有着极好的一致性,与其在甲状腺癌进展中的作用相契合[15]。

甲状腺癌 BRAF V600E 突变

人们最初在 2003 年发现 BRAF V600E 突变存在于甲状腺癌[16-21]，发生率在 PTC 中约 45%~50%，在 ATC 中约为 25%~30%，而 FTC 和甲状腺良性肿瘤中则不存在此突变[13]。这是 BRAF 基因中最常见的激活突变位点，导致 BRAF 蛋白内缬氨酸变为谷氨酸，BRAF 蛋白激酶激活，从而激活微管相关蛋白（microtubule-associated protein，MAP）激酶通路[22]。过去 15 年，大量研究致力于揭示这一突变的预后价值[1,7,9,10,12-14,23]。2005 年，Johns Hopkins 的一项研究首次证明了 BRAF V600E 与 PTC 的不良临床转归相关，包括增加疾病复发，复发性肿瘤放射性碘（radioactive iodine，RAI）耐受，以及侵袭性的病理学行为：甲状腺外侵犯、淋巴结转移[24]。尽管也有结果不一致的报道，但随后的研究广泛证实了这些发现[14,25]。一项 2 099 例 PTC 的多中心研究表明，BRAF V600E 对 PTC 的复发具有独立的预后价值[26]。另一项 1 849 例 PTC 患者的多中心研究表明，BRAF V600E 与 PTC 特异性死亡率之间存在显著相关性[27]。综上，这些及其他研究提示，BRAF V600E 在 PTC 的进展和侵袭性方面发挥着重要的癌基因作用。

甲状腺癌端粒酶逆转录酶启动子突变

20 世纪 80 年代初，端粒酶逆转录酶（telomerase reverse transcriptase，TERT）最初被证实，并被定义其基本功能是通过在染色体末端添加端粒来维持其完整性[28,29]。现在众所周知，TERT 还可以促进多种具有癌症特征的细胞和分子活性[30]。TERT 的这些功能可驱动细胞永生和致癌。在黑色素瘤[31,32]和其他癌症（包括甲状腺癌）[33]中，发现了 TERT 基因启动子的两个体细胞突变，分别是 chr5：1,295,228C> T 和 chr5：1,295,250C> T（下文分别称为 C228T 和 C250T）。两种 TERT 启动子突变都可进一步产生 ETS 转录因子的共有结合位点，增加 TERT 启动子转录活性[31,32]。ETS 转录因子 GABPA 选择性结合 TERT 基因的突变启动子，促进 TERT 表达[34]。另外也发现 TERT 启动子突变与信使 RNA 表达、TERT 蛋白以及端粒长度的增加有关[35]。甲状腺癌中，TERT C228T 比 TERT C250T 更普遍，这两种突变共同发生在 10%~15% 的 DTC，40%~45% 的 PDTC 和 ATC 中，而在良性甲状腺肿瘤中几乎不存在[8,11]。已经广泛证实 TERT 启动子突变与甲状腺癌侵袭性行为和不良临床转归相关；在侵袭性 DTC、PDTC 和 ATC 中特别常见，并且与 DTC 的复发和死亡率增加相关[15,33,36-45]。

这些研究表明，TERT 启动子突变在甲状腺癌侵袭性发展中发挥着强大的致癌作用。

甲状腺癌中的 BRAF V600E 与端粒酶逆转录酶启动子突变共存

2013 年，研究者首次报告了甲状腺癌 TERT 启动子突变，同时报告了在 PTC 中 BRAF V600E 与 TERT 启动子突变之间的有趣的相关性[33]。这一现象在许多其他包括 PTC 原发灶和转移灶的研究中得到广泛证实[8,11,15]。在 PTC 原发灶，BRAF V600E 和 TERT 启动子突变共存的平均发生率为 7.7%（145/1 892）[11]。一些研究也报道了黑色素瘤中 TERT 启动子突变与 BRAF V600E 突变共存[31,46]，表明这是人类癌症中的普遍现象。考虑到 BRAF V600E 和 TERT 启动子突变各自在甲状腺癌中已知的致癌作用，可推测并证明，双突变共存是导致 PTC 最严重侵袭性的强大遗传背景，因此也预示临床转归最差[45]。该项队列研究分为四组：无突变、BRAF V600E 突变、TERT 启动子突变和双突变共存，每个突变单独存在均表现出对 PTC 的临床病理转归的中等影响，而双突变共存影响明显，包括甲状腺外侵犯、淋巴结转移、远处转移和甲状腺癌复发（图 7.1）[45]。BRAF V600E 和 TERT 启动子双突变共存还与 PTC 所致死亡存在相关[44]，一项 1 051 例 PTC 的大样本研究也显示，双突变共存协同作用对 PTC 相关生存不良影响显著；突变阴性时死亡率几乎为 0，单突变时死亡率略有升高，而双突变共存时明显上升（图 7.2）[39]。随后的许多研究也表明，BRAF V600E 和 TERT 启动子突变共存对甲状腺癌的临床病理转归具有强大的协同不良作用[15,37,42,47,48]。近期报道的一种新的分子机制很好地解释了双突变共存的这一不凡的临床发现[49]：BRAF V600E 组成性激活 MAP 激酶通路，导致 FOS 磷酸化和激活，而 FOS 作为 GABPB 基因新的转录因子，结合并激活 GABPB 的启动子并上调其表达。上调的 GABPB 驱动 GABPA/GABPB 复合物的形成，选择性结合并激活突变型 TERT 启动子，明显促进 TERT 表达，使 TERT 表现出强大的致癌性。这揭示了 BRAF V600E 和 TERT 启动子的突变协同作用，促进甲状腺癌侵袭性和不良临床转归的强大分子机制。

甲状腺癌中的 RAS 突变及其与端粒酶逆转录酶启动子突变共存

RAS 突变在甲状腺滤泡性肿瘤中常见，发生在大约 20%~25% 的甲状腺滤泡腺瘤、30%~45% 的 FVPTC、30%~45% 的 FTC、20%~40% 的 PDTC 和 ATC，很少在 CPTC 中发生，而在 TCPTC 中几乎不存在[1]。多项研究表明，特别是在 FTC 和 FVPTC 中，甲状腺癌 RAS 突变和 TERT 启动子突变存在明显相关[15,42,48]。RAS 和 TERT 启动子突变共存也显示与甲状腺癌的不良临床转归有关，包括明显增加疾病复发和患者的死亡[15,42,48]。之前也有研究表明，在 FTC[50] 和 PDTC[51,52] 中，RAS 突变与不良临床病理转归相关。RAS 突变的这种影响实际上可能是 RAS 和 TERT 启动子突变共存在起作用，因为 RAS 单突变常发生于良性滤泡腺瘤和低危 DTC。TERT 启动子突变在 FTC 中相当常见，在 PDTC 和 ATC 中也非常常见[8,11,15]。因此，RAS 和 TERT 启动子突变共存可能很常见，并构成了这些癌症侵袭性的重要遗传背景。实际上，已证明 RAS 和 TERT 启动子突变共存在 FTC 原发灶和转移灶高度一致，并与不良临床转归相关[15]。RAS 和 TERT 启动子突变在甲状腺癌侵袭性中的协同作用的分子机制尚待阐明，但可能也涉及 BRAF V600E 和 TERT 启动子双突变的 MAP 激酶/ROS/GABP/TERT 通路，因为 RAS 也可激活 MAP 激酶通路，尽管作用较弱。RAS 和 BRAF 突变相互排斥[1,13]，所以它们与 TERT 启动子突变的协同作用提示，RAS 和 BRAF 突变在驱动甲状腺癌侵袭性方面机制互补。

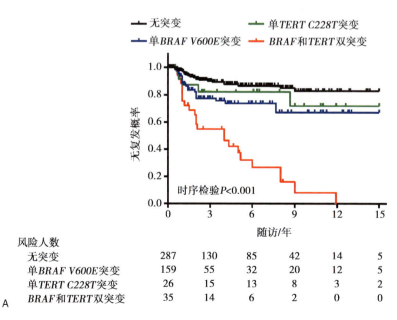

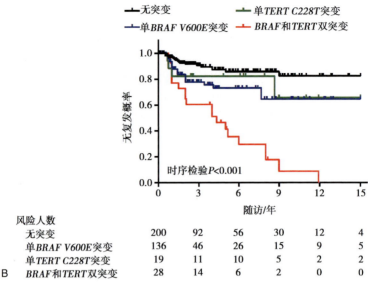

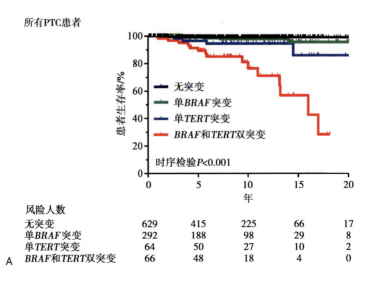

图7.1 单 BRAF V600E 突变、单 TERT 启动子突变、双突变共存对甲状腺乳头状癌(PTC)患者无病生存的影响。对 507 例 PTC 患者进行 Kaplan-Meier 分析。(A)显示所有 PTC 亚型患者分析结果。(B)只显示 PTC 经典亚型患者分析结果。两图的患者均分为四组,包括 BRAF V600E、TERT 启动子双突变阴性(黑线),TERT 启动子突变(绿线),BRAF V600E 突变(蓝线)和双突变共存(红线)的患者 Adapted from Xing M, Liu R, Liu X, et al. BRAF V600E and TERT promoter mutations cooperatively identify the most aggressive papillary thyroid cancer with highest recurrence. J Clin Oncol 2014;32(25):2718-26. Reprinted with permission.ª 2014 American Society of Clinical Oncology. All rights reserved.)

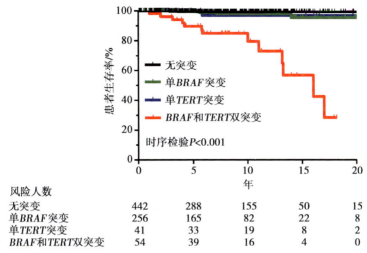

图 7.2 单 *BRAF V600E* 或 *TERT* 启动子突变及双突变共存对 PTC 患者疾病特异性生存率的影响。对 1 051 例 PTC 患者进行 Kaplan-Meier 分析。A,B 图分别为 PTC 所有亚型、经典亚型患者的分析结果。在每图中,将患者分为四个基因型组:*BRAF V600E*、*TERT* 启动子双突变阴性(黑线),*TERT* 启动子突变(蓝线),*BRAF V600E* 突变(绿线)和双突变共存(红线)

Adapted from Liu R, Bishop J, Zhu G, et al. Mortality risk stratification by combining BRAF V600E and TERT promoter mutations in papillary thyroid cancer: genetic duet of BRAF and TERT promoter mutations in thyroid cancer mortality. JAMA Oncol 2017;3(2):206; with permission.

甲状腺癌其他相关癌基因

还有其他一些致癌基因改变,促进甲状腺癌侵袭,并可能具有评估预后的价值。其中包括 *TP53*、*EIF1A* 和 *β-catenin* 突变,在 PDTC 和 ATC 中常见,但很少见于 DTC[53-60]。这样的分布差别提示,这些基因改变与甲状腺癌的侵袭性增强和复发有关,并且如果有的话,它们可能对 DTC 不良预后具有很强的评估效力。但是,DTC 中这些突变的罕见性表明,它们在 DTC 风险分层中的临床实用性比较局限。

近年来,基因组和大样本遗传研究揭示了甲状腺癌的最新发现。大样本甲状腺癌表观遗传研究也发现了的大量分子信息,如异常的 microRNA 和甲基化[54,59,60]。这些为发现新的甲状腺癌预后分子标志物带来了潜在的令人振奋的机会[23,54,61]。然而,人们对甲状腺癌中新的基因组/遗传/表观遗传分子变化的生物学功能尚知之甚少。与 *BRAF V600E* 和 *TERT* 启动子突变不同,这些新的分子标记大多数在评估甲状腺癌的临床预后方面潜力有限。一些常见的基因重排，如 *RET/PTC* 和 *PAX8/PPARg*，对甲状腺癌侵袭性强弱的影响不明显，预后评估价值有限[1,13]。

甲状腺癌遗传标志物的临床应用

鉴于 *BRAF V600E* 和 *TERT* 启动子突变等致癌遗传标记物在甲状腺癌内存在较高的突变率，并与甲状腺癌不良临床转归密切相关，应用它们评估预后具有强大的临床价值。然而，根据基因分型和临床特征，这些突变不一定总是预示甲状腺癌的不良预后。因此，应用基因评估预后不可一概而论，而应根据特定的临床特征进行个性化检测。在甲状腺癌治疗决策中，当医生基于常规临床病理无法准确进行风险评估时，合理应用预后遗传标记辅助诊断，无疑"雪中送炭"。此时，值得关注的是，这些甲状腺癌预后不良的基因标志物的高阴性预测值（negative predictive value，NPV），使检测为阴性时同样有价值。以下甲状腺癌特定的临床特征进一步说明了预后遗传标志物，特别是 *BRAF V600E* 和 *TERT* 启动子突变的临床应用价值。

高风险预测分子标志物临床应用的概览

从上述讨论我们可以得出，一些高风险的致病基因改变具有强大的致癌作用，并能导致甲状腺癌侵袭性增强，死亡率增高，这足以支持对合并基因突变的 DTC 给予更积极的治疗。其中包括 *BRAF V600E* 和 *TERT* 启动子突变共存，*RAS* 和 *TERT* 启动子突变共存，以及少见的 *TP53*、*EIF1A* 和 *β-catenin* 突变。有人甚至推荐对所有存在此类遗传标记的 DTC 患者，包括 PTMC，行全甲状腺切除术。治疗性和预防性颈淋巴清扫术以及 RAI 治疗也常被推荐。由于 PTC 中 *BRAF V600E* 和 *TERT* 启动子突变共存平均发生率只有 7.7%[11]，因而只有不足 10% 的 PTC 患者需要更加激进的治疗。由于 PTMC 中极少发生高风险基因改变，因此，只有少数 PTMC 患者根据基因检测会更加积极地治疗。直径大的肿瘤存在 *BRAF V600E* 突变时复发风险增加[62]，且高风险预测遗传标志与复发病灶对 RAI 耐受相关[1,24,63]，因此，初治彻底切除转移性淋巴结尤为重要，对直径 1.0~2.0cm 特别是直径>2.0cm 的 PTC，行预防性中央颈淋巴结清扫术也可能更加合理。FTC 患者存在高风险基因改变时，如 *TP53*、*EIF1A* 和 *β-catenin* 突变以及 *RAS* 和 *TERT* 启动子突变共存，也倾向于更加积极的治疗。

腺内单发甲状腺乳头状癌中 BRAF V600 突变的临床应用

对于临床上明显外浸/转移的甲状腺癌,采取更积极的治疗策略,如全甲状腺切除术,以及必要时行治疗性/预防性颈淋巴清扫术和放射性碘治疗,已被广泛接受。然而,如何治疗腺内 PTC,即无甲状腺外侵袭、淋巴结转移和远处转移的 PTC,尚未达成共识。现行的美国甲状腺协会指南对于直径 1~4cm 的腺内单发 PTC(solitary intrathyroidal PTC, SI-PTC),推荐腺叶切除术替代全甲状腺切除[5]。这种临床上看来低风险的甲状腺癌并不都是预后良好,在面对某个患者时,决定腺叶切除还是全甲状腺切除术并非易事,所以,该推荐尚存争议。最近的一项多中心研究解决了这一难题,即应用 BRAF V600E 突变作为预后遗传标记物,可以指导此类患者的更好的风险分层[62]。在这项研究中,BRAF V600E 突变的 SI-PTC 直径>1.0cm 的复发率,特别是>2.0cm 的肿瘤复发率为 20%~30%,而对应的 BRAF 突变阴性的 SI-PTC 的复发率仅为 2%~3%,其中,如果仅考虑结构性复发,则 BRAF V600E 预测复发的 NPV 为 97%~98% 或 100%。值得注意的是,即使在直径>4.0cm 的 SI-PTC 中也是如此。对于腺内 PTMC,BRAF V600E 突变阳性和阴性患者,结构复发率均较低,仅为 1%~2%。综上,如果将 BRAF 突变纳入评估预后条件,SI-PTC 决策可以更加精准:支持甲状腺叶切除术治疗任何大小(甚至包括直径>4.0cm)的 BRAF 突变阴性的 SI-PTC;直径>1.0cm 的 BRAF V600E 阳性的 SI-PTC,特别是>2.0cm 者,应治疗更加积极,行全甲状腺切除术和预防性颈淋巴清扫术,必要时行 RAI 治疗。BRAF 突变阳性 SI-PTC 中,直径 1.0~4.0cm 和 2.0~4.0cm 者分别占所有 SI-PTC 病例的 23.1% 和 8.3%。因此,只有极少数的 SI-PTC 需要更积极的治疗。由于复发率低,对于直径<2.0cm 的 SI-PTC,尤其是<1.0cm(即低危 PTMC)者,无论 BRAF 突变与否,都可行腺叶切除术。通过 BRAF 突变指导手术策略,多数 SI-PTC 患者仅行甲状腺叶切除,有效减少了手术并发症,并且保留了患者的部分甲状腺,可避免终身服用甲状腺激素替代。相对保守的动态随访那些 BRAF 突变阴性的直径<1.0cm 的 SI-PTC,可能成为合理的替代治疗方案(下文会进行进一步讨论)。

BRAF V600E 突变在临床诊断低危甲状腺微小乳头状癌中的临床应用

临床诊断的侵袭性 PTMC 的治疗方案应遵守 PTC 治疗原则,已得到共识。然而,关于临床诊断低风险的 PTMC,即无甲状腺外侵犯,无淋巴结转移,无远处转移,也不合并其他侵袭性特征的 PTMC,如何治疗存在争议。目前,多数医生倾向于将手术(通常是腺叶切除术)作为此类 PTMC 的首要治疗选择。近年来,部分医生对临床诊断低风险 PTMC 的治疗方案,已由动态随访替代手术。主要基于日本的几项前瞻性研究显示,动态随访 5~6 年,临床诊断低风险 PTMC 中多数患者保持惰性状态,并无严重的疾病进展[64-66]。然而众所周知,也有小部分的 PTMC 侵袭性明显,甚至导致患者死亡,并且所有 PTC 均由 PTMC 发展而来。最主要的挑战就是,没有任何临床特征,可以可靠地将相对少数的注定疾病进展的 PTMC 患者,从其他相对惰性的大量的 PTMC 患者中区分开。即使肿瘤大小可能相对保持不变,仍然可能发生严重的疾病进展如转移,所以,对所有临床上诊断低风险的 PTMC 不加选择地进行动态随访,尤其是长期随访(例如 10 年)是否合理,值得关注。

检测 BRAF 突变可能有助于简化此类 PTMC 的治疗决策。如上所述,BRAF 突变阴性的 PTC,无论肿瘤大小,一般死亡风险都非常低,而临床诊断低风险 PTMC 的死亡风险更低。临床诊断低风险的 BRAF 突变阴性的 PTC(包括 PTMC)的复发率也非常低[62]。因此,对临床诊断低风险 BRAF 突变阴性的 PTMC 进行动态随访是合理的,并且具有避免手术并发症和保持正常甲状腺功能的优势。由于缺乏具体的长期前瞻性数据,临床诊断低风险但 BRAF V600E 阳性的 PTMC,长期动态随访是否合理尚不清楚。近期研究显示,在 SI-PTC 中,BRAF V600E 对已行手术的临床诊断低危的 PTMC 的结构性复发无明显影响[62]。可能是由于在 PTMC 早期,即在 BRAF V600E 发挥促癌作用之前手术,因此严重的临床不良后果,甚至复发均未发生。BRAF V600E 突变阳性时,肿瘤大小增加会影响临床转归。在临床低风险的 SI-PTC 中,即使在全甲状腺切除术后,BRAF V600E 突变与>1.0cm 的肿瘤复发增加相关,特别在>2.0cm 的肿瘤中复发率显著增加[62]。理论上,如果时间足够长,BRAF V600E 突变可能会导致肿瘤进展,例如转移。目前,在动态随访期间,PTMC 大小超过多少建议行甲状腺手术,尚无共识。如果对 BRAF V600E 阳性但临床表现明显低风险的 PTMC,动态随访至大小>1.0cm,尤其是 2.0cm,则可能增加癌症进展的风险,如难治的 RAI 耐受转移灶,甚至死亡。相反,如果 BRAF 突变阴性,一些动态随访中的 PTMC 因肿瘤大小增加(如>3mm)而进行了手术[64-66],根据以上分析则不必担心。

BRAF V600E 突变促进 PTC 肿瘤侵袭性行为(如腺外侵袭、淋巴结转移和远处转移),但不影响 PTC 相关死亡率,已众所周知[27]。因此,对 BRAF V600E 阳性、临床低风险的 PTMC,在突变有足够的时间造成不良临床后果前,进行手术治疗而不是动态随访,似乎是合理的。但是,以上情况即当 *BRAF V600E* 尚未发挥不良作用时,在该早期阶段行甲状腺叶切除术可能是足够的。因为只有少数甲状腺癌属于 *BRAF V600E* 突变阳性,同时临床低风险的 PTMC,这条策略看起来可行[62]。如前所述,对临床低风险的 PTMC,如果发现合并高风险遗传变异(如 *BRAF V600E/RAS* 和 *TERT* 启动子突变共存,*TP53*、*EIF1A* 和 *β-catenin* 突变),采用更加积极的治疗方式(如全甲状腺切除术)是最佳策略。

甲状腺滤泡癌预后遗传标志物的临床应用

PTC 中 *BRAF V600E* 的预后价值已比较明朗。与 PTC 不同,FTC 的预后分子有待阐明。尽管如此,一些遗传标记有望用于评估 FTC 的预后。*RAS* 突变以前被报道与 FTC 的侵袭性行为有关[50]。*RAS* 和 *TERT* 启动子突变在 FTC 中都很常见,且它们之间存在显著相关性[11,15,42,48]。与 *BRAF V600E* 和 *TERT* 启动子突变共存在 PTC 强大的预后价值相似,*RAS* 和 *TERT* 启动子突变共存在 FTC 可能具有重要的预后价值。实际上,这在包括 FTC 在内的多项 DTC 研究中得到充分证明[15,42,48]。因此,*RAS* 和 *TERT* 启动子突变共存是 FTC 临床预后不良的重要遗传背景和预后遗传模式。因此,对 *RAS* 和 *TERT* 启动子突变共存的 FTC 积极治疗,包括全甲状腺切除和 RAI 消融治疗,是合理的。如果发现其他高危遗传改变,如 *TP53*、*EIF1A* 和 *β-catenin* 突变,则应视为 FTC 临床预后不良的重要遗传预测因素,应推荐更积极的治疗。

应用遗传标记评估甲状腺癌放射碘耐受

2005 年,人们首次报道了 *BRAF V600E* 与 PTC 复发、RAI 耐受以及因此导致的复发 PTC 疗效不佳相关[24],之后的许多研究也证实了这一发现,并证明了携带 *BRAF V600E* 突变的 PTC 中,甲状腺碘代谢基因表达减少甚至缺失,包括甲状腺刺激激素受体、钠/碘共转运体、甲状腺过氧化物酶、甲状腺球蛋白(Tg)、甲状腺转录因子 1 和 PAX8 转录因子的基因[1,7,13,14]。在正常甲状腺细胞中引入 *BRAF V600E* 表达会导致甲状腺碘代谢基因沉默,阻断 *BRAF V600E* 表达或抑制 BRAF/MAP 激酶通路可恢复甲状腺基因的表达,证明 *BRAF V600E* 与甲状腺碘代谢基因表达减少之间存在直接功能关系[67]。后续动物模型甚至临床试验也证实[68]:对 RAI 耐受的 PTC 患者应用 MAP 激酶通路拮抗剂,可以恢复肿瘤摄取 RAI 的能力[69]。最近的研究表明,*TERT* 启动子突变也可能与摄 RAI 功能受损或丧失有关,实际上,*BRAF V600E* 和 *TERT* 启动子突变共存与转移 PTC 的 RAI 耐受密切相关[63]。儿童 PTC 通常可通过 RAI 治疗达到高度治愈,这与其 *BRAF V600E* 突变率低[13]以及 *TERT* 启动子突变的罕见表达相符[70]。由于 BRAF V600E 与复发 PTC(多数为复发转移淋巴结)的 RAI 耐受风险增加相关,因此检测 *BRAF V600E* 突变阳性,尤其是 *BRAF V600E* 和 *TERT* 启动子突变共存,有利于通过彻底的颈淋巴结清扫对合适的病例进行预防性颈淋巴清扫术,可以最大限度地降低 RAI 耐受肿瘤的复发风险。如上文所述,*BRAF* 突变阳性、直径>2.0cm 的 PTC 推荐行预防性颈淋巴清扫。但是,因为摄 RAI 力通常只是部分丧失,所以当符合临床 RAI 治疗指征时,也应对 *BRAF V600E* 突变阳性的 PTC 进行 RAI 治疗。同样,由于突变阳性的癌症疾病复发甚至死亡风险增加,需要确保全甲状腺切除术后的随访是有效的。因此,可靠的特异性 Tg 检测尤为重要,可通过 RAI 清甲治疗实现。目前尚不清楚如果摄 RAI 功能受损,更高剂量的 RAI 是否对 *BRAF V600E* 突变阳性的 PTC 有益。

预后遗传标志物在临床高危分化型甲状腺癌中的应用

在合并腺外侵犯、淋巴结转移和远处转移的临床高侵袭性 DTC 中,检测侵袭性遗传标记也可指导预后评估。此类患者通常需要更积极的初始治疗,但当前治疗标准下疾病的转归也根据肿瘤 *BRAF* 和 *TERT* 突变有所不同。*BRAF V600E* 和 *TERT* 启动子突变阴性时,PTC 特别是 CPTC 和 FVPTC 的死亡率极低,而相比 *BRAF V600E* 和 *TERT* 启动子突变共存时,无论临床病理危险因素如何,死亡率都显著升高[39]。*RAS* 和 *TERT* 启动子突变共存具有同样预后效力[15,42,48]。同样,如上所述,这些突变与摄 RAI 功能丧失,以及进一步复发疾病治疗经常失败而显著相关。即使患者肿瘤侵袭性的最初临床表现相似,但是根据这些患者是否存在这些突变,疾病预后也有所不同。因此,这些遗传标志物仍有助于临床高侵袭性 DTC 预后评估。合并这些遗传标志物,意味着应用当前治疗方法,治疗失败风险增加,需要强调在初始治疗时彻底根治的重要性,以及动态随访疾病复发时保持密切关注的必要。

遗传标志物在甲状腺未分化癌和低分化甲状腺癌中潜在的预后价值

尽管 ATC 通常是一种极具侵袭性的癌症,但其侵袭性也因某些遗传模式而不同。例如,*TERT* 启动子突变阳性的 ATC 合并远处转移更常见[43],进一步导致死亡率快速升高。*BRAF V600E* 和 *TERT* 启动子突变共存可能代表了 ATC 更高侵袭性的遗传背景。也有报道称 *RAS* 突变与 PDTC 侵袭性增强相关[51,52]。如上所述,*RAS* 突变的这种影响可能源自 *RAS* 和 *TERT* 启动子突变共存。治疗上,近期研究证明,应用 BRAF V600E 和 MEK 拮抗剂联合治疗

BRAF V600E 突变阳性的 ATC，效果明显[71]，促进美国食品药品管理局加快批准将 BRAF V600E 拮抗剂达拉非尼和 MEK 拮抗剂曲美替尼联合治疗 *BRAF V600E* 阳性 ATC。因此，检测某些 ATC 遗传标记可能同时具有预后和疗效预测意义。对于 PTC 治疗，也可能成为现实。

几种临床情况下 *RAS* 突变的特殊考虑

由于甲状腺良性和恶性肿瘤均可发生 *RAS* 突变，因此其作为诊断和预后标志物的价值尚未确定[72]。近期研究表明，长期随访细胞学良性但 *RAS* 突变阳性的甲状腺结节，临床进展并不明显，DTC 中仅 *RAS* 突变时，通常与疾病低风险以及良好的临床转归相关[73]。如上所述，*RAS* 和 *TERT* 启动子突变共存与 DTC 的不良临床转归显著相关[15,42,48]。基于以上和其他研究，除非临床上有其他提示，当其他高危基因改变（如 *TERT* 启动子突变）阴性的甲状腺肿瘤仅存在 *RAS* 突变时，执行以下建议比较合理[72]：①细胞学良性但 *RAS* 突变阳性的甲状腺结节可长期随访，无须行手术；② *RAS* 突变阳性的甲状腺结节，伴有细胞学意义不明的非典型改变或滤泡性肿瘤，可进行小范围手术治疗（如腺叶切除术）；③临床上低风险但 *RAS* 突变阳性的 DTC 通常也可行小范围手术治疗（如腺叶切除术）。

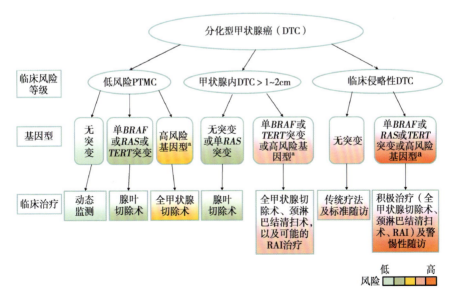

图 7.3　甲状腺癌主要预后遗传标志物推荐临床应对策略。表现各种临床特征、处于不同临床风险分层的甲状腺癌，在特定个体化基因型的指导下得以精准治疗。a 高风险基因型包括 *BRAF V600E/RAS* 和 *TERT* 启动子突变，*TP53*, *EIF1A*, *β-catenin* 突变等

总结

基于预后遗传标记进行甲状腺癌风险分层和精确诊治的价值已广为认可。有效分类和临床实用的预后遗传标记，首推 *BRAF V600E* 和 *TERT* 启动子突变。*BRAF V600E/RAS* 和 *TERT* 启动子突变共存对 DTC 不良临床转归具有很强的预后效力。这些预后遗传标志物的 NPV 在临床上同样重要。目前，遇到有争议的情况，如甲状腺叶切除与全甲状腺切除，预防性颈淋巴结清扫与不行颈淋巴结清扫，RAI 消融治疗与否，动态随访还是手术时，正确运用这些预后标志物可以显著提高甲状腺癌诊治的精准性。图 7.3 描绘了在 DTC 中，预后遗传标志物临床应用的推荐策略。通过这种方法，可在指导甲状腺癌治疗中发挥遗传标记物的最佳预后效用，可以实现临床风险分层和基因型个体化的诊疗模式。

（刘晓莉　孙　辉）

参考文献

1. Xing M. Molecular pathogenesis and mechanisms of thyroid cancer. Nat Rev Cancer 2013;13(3):184–99.
2. Mao Y, Xing M. Recent incidences and differential trends of thyroid cancer in the USA. Endocr Relat Cancer 2016;23(4):313–22.
3. Shi X, Liu R, Basolo F, et al. Differential clinicopathological risk and prognosis of major papillary thyroid cancer variants. J Clin Endocrinol Metab 2016;101(1): 264–74.
4. Lloyd RV, Osamura RY, Klöppel G, et al, editors. WHO classification of tumours of endocrine organs. 4th edition. Lyon (France): International Agency for Research on Cancer (IARC); 2017.
5. Haugen BR, Alexander EK, Bible KC, et al. 2015 American Thyroid Association Management Guidelines for adult patients with thyroid nodules and differentiated thyroid cancer: The American Thyroid Association Guidelines Task Force on thyroid nodules and differentiated thyroid cancer. Thyroid 2016;26(1):1–133.
6. Noone AM, Howlader N, Krapcho M, et al. SEER cancer statistics review, 1975-2015. Bethesda (MD): National Cancer Institute; 2018. Available at: https://seer.cancer.gov/csr/1975_2015/. based on November 2017 SEER data submission, posted to the SEER web site.
7. Xing M, Haugen BR, Schlumberger M. Progress in molecular-based management of differentiated thyroid cancer. Lancet 2013;381(9871):1058–69.
8. Alzahrani AS, Alsaadi R, Murugan AK, et al. TERT promoter mutations in thyroid cancer. Horm Cancer 2016;7(3):165–77.

9. D'Cruz AK, Vaish R, Vaidya A, et al. Molecular markers in well-differentiated thyroid cancer. Eur Arch Otorhinolaryngol 2018;275(6):1375–84.
10. Li F, Chen G, Sheng C, et al. BRAFV600E mutation in papillary thyroid microcarcinoma: a meta-analysis. Endocr Relat Cancer 2015;22(2):159–68.
11. Liu R, Xing M. TERT promoter mutations in thyroid cancer. Endocr Relat Cancer 2016;23(3):R143–55.
12. Tufano RP, Teixeira GV, Bishop J, et al. BRAF mutation in papillary thyroid cancer and its value in tailoring initial treatment: a systematic review and meta-analysis. Medicine (Baltimore) 2012;91(5):274–86.
13. Xing M. BRAF mutation in thyroid cancer. Endocr Relat Cancer 2005;12(2):245–62.
14. Xing M. BRAF mutation in papillary thyroid cancer: pathogenic role, molecular bases, and clinical implications. Endocr Rev 2007;28(7):742–62.
15. Sohn SY, Park WY, Shin HT, et al. Highly concordant key genetic alterations in primary tumors and matched distant metastases in differentiated thyroid cancer. Thyroid 2016;26(5):672–82.
16. Cohen Y, Xing M, Mambo E, et al. BRAF mutation in papillary thyroid carcinoma. J Natl Cancer Inst 2003;95(8):625–7.
17. Fukushima T, Suzuki S, Mashiko M, et al. BRAF mutations in papillary carcinomas of the thyroid. Oncogene 2003;22(41):6455–7.
18. Kimura ET, Nikiforova MN, Zhu Z, et al. High prevalence of BRAF mutations in thyroid cancer: genetic evidence for constitutive activation of the RET/PTC-RAS-BRAF signaling pathway in papillary thyroid carcinoma. Cancer Res 2003;63(7):1454–7.
19. Namba H, Nakashima M, Hayashi T, et al. Clinical implication of hot spot BRAF mutation, V599E, in papillary thyroid cancers. J Clin Endocrinol Metab 2003;88(9):4393–7.
20. Soares P, Trovisco V, Rocha AS, et al. BRAF mutations and RET/PTC rearrangements are alternative events in the etiopathogenesis of PTC. Oncogene 2003;22(29):4578–80.
21. Xu X, Quiros RM, Gattuso P, et al. High prevalence of BRAF gene mutation in papillary thyroid carcinomas and thyroid tumor cell lines. Cancer Res 2003;63(15):4561–7.
22. Davies H, Bignell GR, Cox C, et al. Mutations of the BRAF gene in human cancer. Nature 2002;417(6892):949–54.
23. de la Chapelle A, Jazdzewski K. MicroRNAs in thyroid cancer. J Clin Endocrinol Metab 2011;96(11):3326–36.
24. Xing M, Westra WH, Tufano RP, et al. BRAF mutation predicts a poorer clinical prognosis for papillary thyroid cancer. J Clin Endocrinol Metab 2005;90(12):6373–9.
25. Kim TY, Kim WB, Rhee YS, et al. The BRAF mutation is useful for prediction of clinical recurrence in low-risk patients with conventional papillary thyroid carcinoma. Clin Endocrinol (Oxf) 2006;65(3):364–8.
26. Xing M, Alzahrani AS, Carson KA, et al. Association between BRAF V600E mutation and recurrence of papillary thyroid cancer. J Clin Oncol 2015;33(1):42–50.
27. Xing M, Alzahrani AS, Carson KA, et al. Association between BRAF V600E mutation and mortality in patients with papillary thyroid cancer. JAMA 2013;309(14):1493–501.

28. Greider CW, Blackburn EH. Identification of a specific telomere terminal transferase activity in Tetrahymena extracts. Cell 1985;43(2 Pt 1):405-13.
29. Szostak JW, Blackburn EH. Cloning yeast telomeres on linear plasmid vectors. Cell 1982;29(1):245-55.
30. Low KC, Tergaonkar V. Telomerase: central regulator of all of the hallmarks of cancer. Trends Biochem Sci 2013;38(9):426-34.
31. Horn S, Figl A, Rachakonda PS, et al. TERT promoter mutations in familial and sporadic melanoma. Science 2013;339(6122):959-61.
32. Huang FW, Hodis E, Xu MJ, et al. Highly recurrent TERT promoter mutations in human melanoma. Science 2013;339(6122):957-9.
33. Liu X, Bishop J, Shan Y, et al. Highly prevalent TERT promoter mutations in aggressive thyroid cancers. Endocr Relat Cancer 2013;20(4):603-10.
34. Bell RJ, Rube HT, Kreig A, et al. The transcription factor GABP selectively binds and activates the mutant TERT promoter in cancer. Science 2015;348(6238):1036-9.
35. Borah S, Xi L, Zaug AJ, et al. TERT promoter mutations and telomerase reactivation in urothelial cancer. Science 2015;347(6225):1006-10.
36. Bu R, Siraj AK, Divya SP, et al. Telomerase reverse transcriptase mutations are independent predictor of disease-free survival in Middle Eastern papillary thyroid cancer. Int J Cancer 2018;142(10):2028-39.
37. Jin L, Chen E, Dong S, et al. BRAF and TERT promoter mutations in the aggressiveness of papillary thyroid carcinoma: a study of 653 patients. Oncotarget 2016;7(14):18346-55.
38. Landa I, Ganly I, Chan TA, et al. Frequent somatic TERT promoter mutations in thyroid cancer: higher prevalence in advanced forms of the disease. J Clin Endocrinol Metab 2013;98(9):E1562-6.
39. Liu R, Bishop J, Zhu G, et al. Mortality risk stratification by combining BRAF V600E and TERT promoter mutations in papillary thyroid cancer: genetic duet of BRAF and TERT promoter mutations in thyroid cancer mortality. JAMA Oncol 2017;3(2):202-8.
40. Liu X, Qu S, Liu R, et al. TERT promoter mutations and their association with BRAF V600E mutation and aggressive clinicopathological characteristics of thyroid cancer. J Clin Endocrinol Metab 2014;99(6):E1130-6.
41. Melo M, da Rocha AG, Vinagre J, et al. TERT promoter mutations are a major indicator of poor outcome in differentiated thyroid carcinomas. J Clin Endocrinol Metab 2014;99(5):E754-65.
42. Shen X, Liu R, Xing M. A six-genotype genetic prognostic model for papillary thyroid cancer. Endocr Relat Cancer 2017;24(1):41-52.
43. Shi X, Liu R, Qu S, et al. Association of TERT promoter mutation 1,295,228 C>T with BRAF V600E mutation, older patient age, and distant metastasis in anaplastic thyroid cancer. J Clin Endocrinol Metab 2015;100(4):E632-7.
44. Xing M, Liu R, Bishop J. TERT promoter and BRAF mutations cooperatively promote papillary thyroid cancer-related mortality. Thyroid 2014;24(S1):A-131.
45. Xing M, Liu R, Liu X, et al. BRAF V600E and TERT promoter mutations cooperatively identify the most aggressive papillary thyroid cancer with highest recurrence. J Clin Oncol 2014;32(25):2718-26.
46. Griewank KG, Murali R, Puig-Butille JA, et al. TERT promoter mutation status as an independent prognostic factor in cutaneous melanoma. J Natl Cancer Inst 2014;106(9) [pii:dju246].

47. Rusinek D, Pfeifer A, Krajewska J, et al. Coexistence of TERT promoter mutations and the BRAF V600E alteration and its impact on histopathological features of papillary thyroid carcinoma in a selected series of Polish patients. Int J Mol Sci 2018;19(9):2647.
48. Song YS, Lim JA, Choi H, et al. Prognostic effects of TERT promoter mutations are enhanced by coexistence with BRAF or RAS mutations and strengthen the risk prediction by the ATA or TNM staging system in differentiated thyroid cancer patients. Cancer 2016;122(9):1370–9.
49. Liu R, Zhang T, Zhu G, et al. Regulation of mutant TERT by BRAF V600E/MAP kinase pathway through FOS/GABP in human cancer. Nat Commun 2018;9(1):579.
50. Fukahori M, Yoshida A, Hayashi H, et al. The associations between RAS mutations and clinical characteristics in follicular thyroid tumors: new insights from a single center and a large patient cohort. Thyroid 2012;22(7):683–9.
51. Garcia-Rostan G, Zhao H, Camp RL, et al. ras mutations are associated with aggressive tumor phenotypes and poor prognosis in thyroid cancer. J Clin Oncol 2003;21(17):3226–35.
52. Volante M, Rapa I, Gandhi M, et al. RAS mutations are the predominant molecular alteration in poorly differentiated thyroid carcinomas and bear prognostic impact. J Clin Endocrinol Metab 2009;94(12):4735–41.
53. Alzahrani AS, Murugan AK, Qasem E, et al. Absence of EIF1AX, PPM1D, and CHEK2 mutations reported in Thyroid Cancer Genome Atlas (TCGA) in a large series of thyroid cancer. Endocrine 2019;63(1):94–100.
54. Cancer Genome Atlas Research Network. Integrated genomic characterization of papillary thyroid carcinoma. Cell 2014;159(3):676–90.
55. Donghi R, Longoni A, Pilotti S, et al. Gene p53 mutations are restricted to poorly differentiated and undifferentiated carcinomas of the thyroid gland. J Clin Invest 1993;91(4):1753–60.
56. Fagin JA, Matsuo K, Karmakar A, et al. High prevalence of mutations of the p53 gene in poorly differentiated human thyroid carcinomas. J Clin Invest 1993;91(1):179–84.
57. Garcia-Rostan G, Camp RL, Herrero A, et al. Beta-catenin dysregulation in thyroid neoplasms: down-regulation, aberrant nuclear expression, and CTNNB1 exon 3 mutations are markers for aggressive tumor phenotypes and poor prognosis. Am J Pathol 2001;158(3):987–96.
58. Garcia-Rostan G, Tallini G, Herrero A, et al. Frequent mutation and nuclear localization of beta-catenin in anaplastic thyroid carcinoma. Cancer Res 1999;59(8):1811–5.
59. Landa I, Ibrahimpasic T, Boucai L, et al. Genomic and transcriptomic hallmarks of poorly differentiated and anaplastic thyroid cancers. J Clin Invest 2016;126(3):1052–66.
60. Pozdeyev N, Gay LM, Sokol ES, et al. Genetic analysis of 779 advanced differentiated and anaplastic thyroid cancers. Clin Cancer Res 2018;24(13):3059–68.
61. Faam B, Ghaffari MA, Ghadiri A, et al. Epigenetic modifications in human thyroid cancer. Biomed Rep 2015;3(1):3–8.
62. Huang Y, Qu S, Zhu G, et al. BRAF V600E mutation-assisted risk stratification of solitary intrathyroidal papillary thyroid cancer for precision treatment. J Natl Cancer Inst 2018;110(4):362–70.
63. Yang X, Li J, Li X, et al. TERT promoter mutation predicts radioiodine-refractory character in distant metastatic differentiated thyroid cancer. J Nucl Med 2017;58(2):258–65.

64. Ito Y, Miyauchi A, Inoue H, et al. An observational trial for papillary thyroid microcarcinoma in Japanese patients. World J Surg 2010;34(1):28–35.
65. Ito Y, Miyauchi A, Kihara M, et al. Patient age is significantly related to the progression of papillary microcarcinoma of the thyroid under observation. Thyroid 2014;24(1):27–34.
66. Sugitani I, Toda K, Yamada K, et al. Three distinctly different kinds of papillary thyroid microcarcinoma should be recognized: our treatment strategies and outcomes. World J Surg 2010;34(6):1222–31.
67. Liu D, Hu S, Hou P, et al. Suppression of BRAF/MEK/MAP kinase pathway restores expression of iodide-metabolizing genes in thyroid cells expressing the V600E BRAF mutant. Clin Cancer Res 2007;13(4):1341–9.
68. Chakravarty D, Santos E, Ryder M, et al. Small-molecule MAPK inhibitors restore radioiodine incorporation in mouse thyroid cancers with conditional BRAF activation. J Clin Invest 2011;121(12):4700–11.
69. Ho AL, Grewal RK, Leboeuf R, et al. Selumetinib-enhanced radioiodine uptake in advanced thyroid cancer. N Engl J Med 2013;368(7):623–32.
70. Alzahrani AS, Qasem E, Murugan AK, et al. Uncommon TERT promoter mutations in pediatric thyroid cancer. Thyroid 2016;26(2):235–41.
71. Subbiah V, Kreitman RJ, Wainberg ZA, et al. Dabrafenib and trametinib treatment in patients with locally advanced or metastatic BRAF V600-mutant anaplastic thyroid cancer. J Clin Oncol 2018;36(1):7–13.
72. Xing M. Clinical utility of RAS mutations in thyroid cancer: a blurred picture now emerging clearer. BMC Med 2016;14:12.
73. Medici M, Kwong N, Angell TE, et al. The variable phenotype and low-risk nature of RAS-positive thyroid nodules. BMC Med 2015;13:184.

第8章
常规甲状腺切除术治疗原发性甲状腺癌

Benjamin R. Roman, Gregory W. Randolph, Dipti Kamani

关键词

- 甲状腺切除术 ● 甲状腺手术 ● 甲状腺解剖 ● 喉返神经
- 甲状腺癌 ● 术中神经监测

要点

- 常规甲状腺切除术是甲状腺癌最常见、最经得起时间考验和首选的治疗方法。
- 最近的三项进展——美国甲状腺协会2015年新指南、2017年Bethesda分类和NIFTP的引入——进一步完善了甲状腺癌和结节相关手术的适应证。
- 为了判断手术的适应证和范围,并为了与患者共享手术决策和术前咨询,详细的术前评估显得极为重要。
- 尽管外科医生可能有自己的偏好,但常规甲状腺切除术的基本步骤仍然相同。
- 对头颈部解剖学的掌握、一丝不苟的手术以及根据术前确定的疾病范围决策手术,对于取得良好的结果很重要。

引言

2018年,美国预计诊断出53 990例甲状腺癌新病例[1],使其成为女性第5大常见癌症,总人群中排名第12。近几十年来,甲状腺癌的发病率不断上升，据人口水平估计，2016 年新增病例达到 64 300 例[2]。最近的证据表明，甲状腺癌的发病率处于平稳状态[3,4]，而美国癌症协会（American Cancer Society）自 2016 年以来提供的估计报告也进一步证实了这一点。美国新发甲状腺癌中，绝大多数是甲状腺乳头状癌（papillary thyroid cancer，PTC）。今天新发现的甲状腺癌病例中，一半以上是不超过 1.5cm 的 PTC[5]。甲状腺滤泡状癌、甲状腺髓样癌、甲状腺低分化癌和甲状腺未分化癌也属于原发性甲状腺癌，但似乎与甲状腺癌发病率的增加关系不大（甲状腺癌发病率的增加似乎主要归因于乳头状癌发病率的增加）。

手术切除一直是治疗甲状腺癌的传统方法。19 世纪和 20 世纪，手术切除甲状腺的安全性和可靠性由 William Kocher 改进和标准化，并由 William S. Halsted 在美国普及。虽然积极监测是部分 PTC 病例的一种新的合理选择[6,7]，但手术作为主要的治疗手段已经经受住了时间的考验。传统的甲状腺切除术仍然是目前甲状腺癌最常见和首选的治疗策略，具有较少的并发症和可接受的颈部瘢痕，且术后生存率较高，复发率也较低。

本章着重介绍甲状腺癌的常规外科治疗，回顾了长期以来的原则和实践。还将介绍新的争议和技术，包括甲状腺手术适应证的改变，术中喉返神经和喉上神经（superior laryngeal nerve，SLN）和甲状旁腺的处理，甲状腺手术的范围，以及术后随访评估和生活质量改进的重要性。其他章节特别讨论了甲状腺癌的淋巴结和颈部清扫的管理，以及甲状腺切除术的非常规入路方法，包括机器人和其他内镜方法。

适应证

与癌症相关的常规甲状腺切除术通常是出于以下几种原因之一进行的。这些原因包括：①诊断性切除可疑癌结节的甲状腺叶；②经活检证实的甲状腺癌的治疗；③甲状腺腺叶切除术后的"补充甲状腺全切除术"，以方便放射性碘的给药以及简化癌症的随访；④复发性甲状腺癌的治疗；⑤已知致癌基因突变的患者预防性甲状腺切除术。

最近的三项进展进一步完善了与甲状腺癌和结节相关的手术指征。这些措施包括更新的美国甲状腺协会 2015 年甲状腺结节和癌症管理指南，更新的 Bethesda 甲状腺细针穿刺（fine needle aspiration，FNA）活检分类标准，以及将某些先前称为癌症的病变重命名为具有乳头状核特征的非侵袭性滤泡性甲状腺肿瘤（noninvasive follicular thyroid with papillary-like nuclear feature，NIFTP）。

新的美国甲状腺协会 2015 年指南对甲状腺结节的管理建议和指南进行了两项明显更改[7](表 8.1)。首先,高度可疑结节建议仅在直径>1cm 时进行 FNA 活检;换言之,任何直径<1cm 的甲状腺结节即使在影像学上可疑,也不需要进行活检,只要它位于甲状腺腺体内而不贴近被膜即可。其次,首次对部分患者采用了积极监测的管理方法。

表 8.1
ATA 2015 指南中有关甲状腺结节和癌症治疗的重大变化

新 ATA2015 推荐	推荐内容
结节<1cm 无须活检	甲状腺结节诊断 FNA 建议用于: A. 结节最大直径> 1cm,超声高度疑似 B. 结节最大直径> 1cm,超声中度疑似 C. 结节最大直径> 1.5cm,超声低度疑似 甲状腺结节诊断性 FNA 可考虑用于: D. 结节最大直径> 2cm,超声提示恶性可能性低(例如海绵状) 不行 FNA,进行观察也是一种合理的选择,对于以下情况,不需要甲状腺结节诊断 FNA: E. 不符合上述条件的甲状腺结节 F. 结节是纯囊性的
可考虑积极监测	细胞学诊断甲状腺原发性恶性肿瘤几乎总是会导致甲状腺手术但是,在以下情况下,可以将积极监测的管理方法视为立即手术的替代方法: A. 风险极低的患者(例如微小乳头状癌) B. 因并发症导致处于手术风险很高的患者 C. 预期剩余寿命相对较短的患者 D. 患有其他内科或外科问题的患者、必须在甲状腺手术之前解决的患者

ATA,美国甲状腺协会;FNA,细针穿刺

2017 年,Bethesda 甲状腺结节 FNA 活检分类系统从 2009 年的初始版本更新,反映了肿瘤风险的新数据(表 8.2)[8,9]。此外,2017 年版对各类别的常规管理建议进行了基于循证的修改。具体来说,2009 年对 Bethesda Ⅲ结节(不确定意义的异型性或不确定意义的滤泡性病变)的推荐是重复 FNA,而 2017 年是重复 FNA、分子检测或腺叶切除。2009 年对 Bethesda Ⅳ结节(滤泡性肿瘤或可疑滤泡性肿瘤)的建议是手术切除腺叶,而 2017 年则是分子检测或腺叶切除。对于 Bethesda Ⅴ(怀疑恶性)和 Bethesda Ⅵ结节(恶性)的建议一直是手术治疗。2017 年,甲状腺腺叶切除术和甲状腺全切除术被列为两种

手术方式的选择。

2016 年，一个由国际甲状腺病理学家、内分泌学家和外科医生组成的团队为一种传统的临床甲状腺病变创造了一个新的名称 NIFTP[10]。在此之前，该病变曾以"包裹性滤泡型甲状腺乳头状癌"命名。这一团队回顾了该病变的病例，发现与肿瘤未被包裹的病例相比，没有死亡、复发或转移，因此修改了命名。值得注意的是，如果不进行诊断性甲状腺腺叶切除术，NIFTP 的诊断就无法确定，因此病变的更名不会显著改变手术适应证。尽管如此，如表 8.2 所示，它确实会根据 NIFTP 是否被视为癌症而改变术前癌症风险，因此这可能会改变关于手术指征的决策。由于 NIFTP 被指定为非肿瘤病变，NIFTP 的存在将主要影响临床管理，减少诸如补充性甲状腺全切除术、T_4 抑制和放射性碘（radioactive iodine，RAI）治疗等术后治疗的使用[11]。

表 8.2
Bethesda 甲状腺细胞病理组织学报告系统（2009 年和 2017 年版本对比）

诊断类别	(2009)恶性肿瘤风险/%	(2017)恶性肿瘤风险 NIFTP ≠ CA/%	(2017)恶性肿瘤风险 NIFTP=CA/%	(2009)常规管理	(2017)常规管理
Ⅰ 无法诊断或不令人满意	1~4	5~10	5~10	在超声引导下重复 FNA	在超声引导下重复 FNA
Ⅱ 良性	0~3	0~3	0~3	临床随访	临床和超声检查
Ⅲ 意义不明的非典型性或意义不明的滤泡性病变	约 5~15	6~8	约 10~30	重复 FNA	重复 FNA，分子检测或甲状腺腺叶切除术
Ⅳ 滤泡性肿瘤或可疑滤泡性肿瘤	15~30	10~40	25~40	外科甲状腺腺叶切除术	分子检测，甲状腺腺叶切除
Ⅴ 可疑恶性肿瘤	60~75	45~60	50~75	近全甲状腺切除术或甲状腺腺叶切除术	近全甲状腺切除术或甲状腺腺叶切除术
Ⅵ 恶性	97~99	94~96	97~99	近全甲状腺切除术	近全甲状腺切除术或甲状腺腺叶切除术

FNA，细针穿刺

术前评估

在进行甲状腺手术之前，核实手术适应证并评估所需的手术范围是非常重要的。术前仔细评估患者的病史和症状、体格检查结果、超声检查或其他影像学的结果以及细胞学检查（包括分子诊断结果）对于决策至关重要。这些因素有助于决定手术的范围。此外，完善适当的喉部检查以确定声带的术前功能，这可能会影响手术的范围、术前谈话和术中的决策。

手术范围：病史、体格检查、影像学和细胞学

手术范围决策基于对所有有助于诊断/怀疑癌症和疾病范围的信息的总和。病史应包括患者的年龄和性别（20岁以下或60岁以上患恶性肿瘤的风险较高，男性风险较高），甲状腺癌家族史或易患癌症的家族综合征（家族性乳头状癌、考登综合征、2A或2B型多发性内分泌肿瘤）和电离辐射史暴露（特别是童年时期）。对症状的回顾应包括甲状腺肿块迅速增大的病史、新发呼吸性嘶哑和是否存在颈部肿块。

体格检查时，必须注意扪查甲状腺结节，包括结节的大小、硬度和有无与喉部或表面皮肤的固定。侧颈淋巴结转移的检查应集中在胸锁乳突肌内侧2~4区。尤其重要的是喉镜检查声带麻痹（vocal cord paralysis，VCP），本章也会进行讨论。

应关注实验室结果。尽管通常会检测促甲状腺激素水平，但甲状腺球蛋白和甲状腺球蛋白抗体、降钙素和癌胚抗原通常不用于常规甲状腺结节检查。促甲状腺激素升高与恶性肿瘤风险增加有关。

影像学检查通常包括超声检查。超声检查中的实性结节、不规则边缘、微钙化、中心血流和大小异常提示了恶性肿瘤的风险增加。应注意肿瘤甲状腺外侵犯的超声特征，以及可疑的淋巴结转移灶，包括中央区、气管-食管沟和侧颈。建议术前完善计算机断层扫描（CT）检查，可与超声检查互补，尤其是在有淋巴结转移的情况下[12]。PTC的大部分病灶在颈中央区，超声检查看不太清楚，特别是在甲状腺仍在原位的情况下[12]。

FNA细胞学结果和分子诊断也影响结节的恶性风险和计划的手术范围。任何<Bethesda Ⅵ的甲状腺癌诊断，只要没有其他高危发现（VCP、淋巴结转移），通常会选择按照计划的手术范围进行甲状腺叶切除。当甲状腺癌的术前

诊断已确定，或者有其他高危发现提示未来可能需要放射性碘治疗，手术范围就可能包括甲状腺全部切除和适当的淋巴结清扫。细胞病理学和分子诊断方面的考虑将在本书其他章节进行更详细的综述。

术前喉部检查

甲状腺手术前应特别注意检查喉部功能[13]。这很重要，原因如下：① VCP的存在可能不引起声音改变，可能是恶性肿瘤的一个迹象[14]；② VCP的存在影响手术风险和术前谈话；③术前声带功能可能会影响术中的神经监测和手术范围；④术后检查喉功能，无论是为了质量评估还是记录手术并发症，都需要术前基线；⑤另外，从法医学的角度来看，术前声带功能记录有助于避免在纠纷中被误判为医源性 VCP。

一些大型医学和外科学会最近已发布了术前和术后喉检查的相关指南和共识。美国头颈学会共识建议，应对所有神经损伤高风险（术前声音异常、颈部或上胸外科手术史、已知癌灶位于甲状腺背侧）的甲状腺手术患者进行术前喉科检查[15]。耳鼻咽喉科-头颈外科学会建议在声音异常、术前怀疑有肿瘤腺外侵犯或有再次手术时，进行术前喉镜检查，因为这些情况都会使迷走神经和/或喉返神经(recurrent laryngeal nerve，RLN)术中处于损伤的高风险状态[16]。

甲状腺癌手术

成功完成甲状腺手术需要根据手术原则仔细注意手术细节并制订手术计划。外科医生应考虑术中如何管理和监测 RLN，并应特别注意甲状旁腺的保存，喉上神经(superior laryngeal nerve，SLN)的保存，以及癌切除的完整性。术中的其他考虑因素包括适当使用冰冻切片来指导计划中手术的决策。在手术结束时，应仔细记录术中所见。颈部清扫对甲状腺癌的彻底治疗很重要，其他章节对此进行了详细介绍。

步骤与手术原则

患者取仰卧位，颈部伸直，双臂收拢，并垫在患者体侧。头高足低位可以降低静脉压力（图 8.1）。使用术中神经监测(intraoperative nerve monitoring，

IONM)时,在诱导前与麻醉师就气管导管的类型和避免长效麻醉药进行仔细沟通是很重要的[17]。颈部舒展完全,包括颏部、侧颈、肩部和上胸部。即使在一个小的微创甲状腺手术中,这种大面积舒展有利于将切口选在平行于正常皮肤皱褶和对称定位的最佳位置,最佳高度约在环状软骨1指宽度以下。

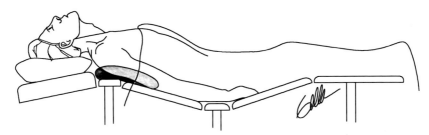

图 8.1 颈部延长的逆向 Trendelenburg 甲状腺切除术
From Randolph GW, editor.Surgery of the thyroid and parathyroid glands.Philadelphia:Saunders;2013;with permission.

甲状腺切除术的切口最好位于或平行于水平皮肤皱褶,以获得最佳的美容效果,理想情况下,位于甲状腺峡部的环状软骨下 1cm 处(图 8.2)。但是,为了将切口置于最深的皮肤皱褶处,也可适当修改切口的高度。无论切除哪个甲状腺叶,切口都要放在中线。外科医生可能在切口长度上有所不同,通常最短的切口为 4cm。由于肿瘤较大、侧区清扫或患者的解剖结构,或根据外科医生对暴露的偏好,也可考虑较长的切口。

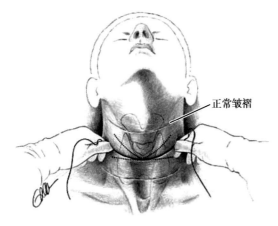

正常皱褶

图 8.2 甲状腺切除术切口在颈部自然皮肤皱褶处有明显的对称性
From Randolph GW, editor.Surgery of the thyroid and parathyroid glands. Philadelphia:Saunders;2013;with permission.

提起颈部上下皮瓣,将颈前静脉前支保留在深面带状肌表面。切开束带肌之间的中线,显示甲状腺峡部、环状软骨和中央区中甲状腺下方的组织。接下来，先手术侧的胸骨舌骨肌被提离甲状腺，露出直接位于甲状腺上方的后外侧胸骨舌骨肌。胸骨甲状腺肌插入甲状腺软骨层，覆盖甲状腺上极。仔细解剖甲状腺上方的肌肉，或肌肉上面的部分，可以暴露甲状腺上极血管和喉上神经的外支。如果胸骨甲状腺肌似乎附着在甲状腺上，则可能有甲状腺癌的腺外侵犯。在这种情况下，肌肉应该留在腺体上，并在其上下两端切开，以使受累的部分肌肉保持与甲状腺的整体粘连。切除带状肌，无论是为了帮助暴露，还是因为可能的恶性浸润，都应该毫不犹豫，因为这一操作对功能或外观没有显著的影响[18]。当解剖进行到侧面时，甲状腺叶可以被拉扯并向内侧旋转，显示甲状腺前外侧表面的甲状腺中静脉，此时可安全结扎(图 8.3)。

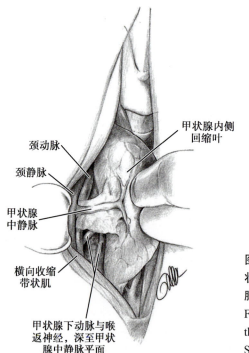

图 8.3 向前内侧牵拉甲状腺，暴露出甲状腺的后表面。这有助于显露甲状腺中静脉，然后将其结扎并分离
From Randolph GW, editor. Surgery of the thyroid and parathyroid glands. Philadelphia: Saunders; 2013; with permission.

下一步根据外科医生的习惯而有所不同。一些医生先处理甲状腺下极和下甲状旁腺，而一些医生先处理甲状腺上极、SLN 和上甲状旁腺。另一些医生则喜欢在将腺体向内侧牵拉以识别 RLN 之前，在下极和上极部分地游离腺体。无论采用何种方法，这些步骤都应识别并保护上、下甲状旁腺，SLN 和 RLN。

熟悉甲状旁腺可能的解剖位置，根据其棕红色斑驳的颜色、特殊的器官形状和与周围脂肪相比的锐利边缘(表 8.3)，识别甲状旁腺。一般来说，甲状旁腺的保存是通过解剖甲状腺包膜来完成的。

表 8.3
甲状旁腺的区别特征

结构	颜色	牢固性	形状	离散滑动	血管门
甲状旁腺	棕褐色、褐色、鲑鱼红	柔软	椭圆形、扁平	是	是
甲状腺	红	是	多变	否	否
脂肪	亮黄	否	非定形的	否	否
淋巴结	白灰到红	是	球形到椭圆形	±	否
胸腺	黄白	否	非定形的	否	否

甲状旁腺的位置与其胚胎迁移途径有关。上甲状旁腺起源于第 4 咽囊，位于甲状腺上极后面，颈部较后/较深。它们位于环状软骨和甲状腺软骨关节的 1cm 范围内，或位于甲状腺下动脉和 RLN 交叉处的 1cm 范围内。下甲状旁腺起源于第 3 咽囊，与上甲状旁腺相比，下甲状旁腺位于颈部较浅/较前的位置（通常与胸腺相连），它们的确切位置更易变化，通常位于甲状腺下极外侧和下方 1cm 范围内。有时，它们保持下降状态，或沿颈动脉分叉与下颈部之间的路径停止下降。Pyrtek 和 Painter[19] 描述了甲状旁腺相对于 RLN 在颈部追踪的平面的特定位置。如果颈部的 RLN 路径显示为冠状面，则下甲状旁腺位于该平面的腹侧或前方，上甲状旁腺位于 RLN 平面的背侧或后方（图 8.4）。SLN 可以通过对上极的细致解剖来保存。在对甲状腺-喉部复合体施加内侧牵引的同时，重要的是将胸骨甲状腺肌的上端侧向牵拉或将该肌的上端分开以获得更大的视觉效果（图 8.5）。SLN 从迷走神经分支，向下延伸到喉部，在喉部分为一个内支和一个外支（SLN 的外支，简称 EBSLN），内支穿过喉部，外支在下缩肌表面，支配环甲肌（图 8.6）。在大约 20% 的病例中，EBSLN 在甲状腺上极（2B 型）的水平或其下方与甲状腺上动脉血管交叉走行，术中极易损伤[20]。EBSLN 经常可以在环甲肌上被找到，或者可以通过电刺激来识别。需要注意的是，20% 的 EBSLN 位于肌肉内走行，因此无法通过视觉识别，神经监测可以通过引起环甲肌抽搐从而 100% 地识别 EBSLN[21]。这样，就可以安全地完成甲状腺上动脉血管的分离、结扎。

熟悉 RLN 的解剖结构、采用精细的解剖技术和术中神经监测技术的应用，都有利于对 RLN 进行显露和保护。IONM 在本章的其他部分中有单独的描述。解剖上，右侧 RLN 自右侧迷走神经发出，勾绕右侧锁骨下动脉后，自胸廓入口进入颈部，其走行比左 RLN 更为倾斜，后者从迷走神经分支，勾绕主动

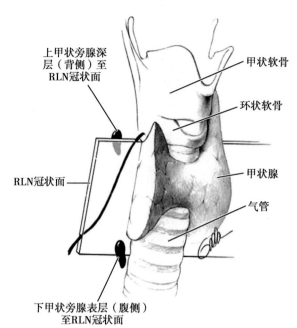

图 8.4 上、下甲状旁腺相对于喉返神经(RLN)所代表的冠状面的各自位置

From Randolph GW, editor.Surgery of the thyroid and parathyroid glands.Philadelphia：Saunders；2013；with permission.

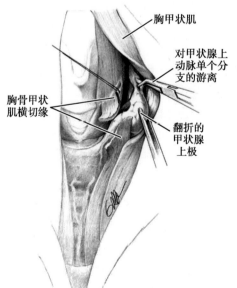

图 8.5 胸骨甲状肌横断提供了更好的暴露上极区,甲状腺上动脉的分支应分别结扎

From Randolph GW, editor.Surgery of the thyroid and parathyroid glands.Philadelphia：Saunders；2013；with permission.

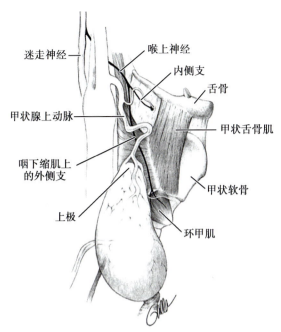

图 8.6 喉上神经从迷走神经分支,然后分为一个进入喉的内侧支和一个外侧支,该外侧支通过咽下缩肌表面以支配环甲肌
From Randolph GW, editor. Surgery of the thyroid and parathyroid glands. Philadelphia: Saunders; 2013; with permission.

脉弓,因此,右侧 RLN 从颈部底部到喉部入口点呈斜向运动,假设其运动过程的最后 1cm 为气管旁位置,左侧 RLN 从颈部底部到喉部入口点的运动更为垂直,在颈部的大部分运动过程中位于气管食管沟的内侧(图 8.7)。RLN 一般在甲状腺的后方,环状软骨的下缘,咽下缩肌的下方与环甲关节后方入喉。大甲状腺肿导致 RLN 移位、喉外 RLN 分支的存在和非返性 RLN 可使 RLN 识别困难[22]。

外科医生有不同的技术来识别和保护该神经(图 8.8)。外侧入路是指在上下极游离后,通过将腺叶向内侧牵引以寻找神经。在这种方法中,神经可以在甲状腺下动脉附近找到,交叉在它的前面或后面。下入路最适合用于再次手术病例或大型甲状腺肿,这涉及"三角"神经,如 Lore 及其同事[23]所述。这种方法的优点是在神经分支之前就找到它,而且在以前的手术中通常是在已解剖过的区域之外。上入路是指先识别入喉处的神经。这种方法的优点是,在靠近甲状软骨下角的位置变化较小,容易触诊。这种方法是鉴别困难病例、再次手术病例或大型甲状腺肿的可靠方法。这种方法的一个缺点是,当被

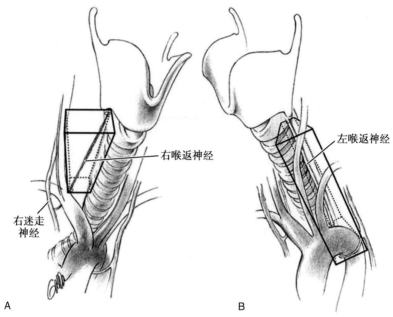

图 8.7 喉返神经在颈部的相对走势:(A)右喉返神经;(B)左喉返神经
From Randolph GW, editor.Surgery of the thyroid and parathyroid glands.Philadelphia:Saunders;2013 ;with permission.

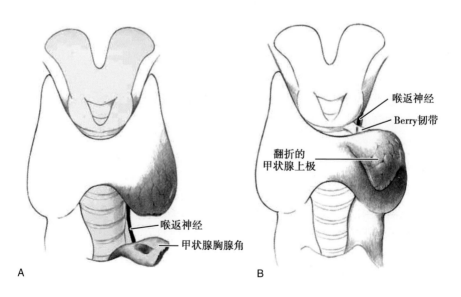

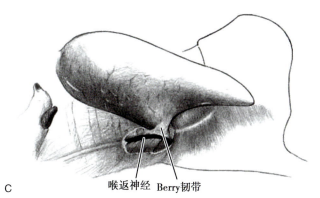

图 8.8　喉返神经的(A)下、(B)上、(C)外侧手术入路
From Randolph GW, editor. Surgery of the thyroid and parathyroid glands. Philadelphia: Saunders; 2013; with permission.

识别时，神经可能已经分支，使未被识别的分支处于危险之中，且这个区域存在 Berry 韧带周围的血管。

切除一侧甲状腺叶后，可进行冰冻切片，并进行对侧叶解剖。这些问题将在本章其他部分单独讨论。手术结束时，应检查甲状腺标本表面是否有甲状旁腺，如经冰冻切片证实为甲状旁腺，应自体移植。将甲状旁腺切碎，放入胸锁乳突肌内，用永久性缝线标记位置，并记录在手术报告中。通过 Valsalva 方法确认有无出血，充分止血，冲洗伤口，然后关闭切口。在关闭切口过程中，注意在中线位置缝合带状肌，以防止气管皮肤粘连。

喉返神经的术中检测

文献中喉返神经损伤和术后声带功能障碍的发生率各不相同，其根本原因包括识别暂时性和永久性麻痹的差异；喉镜检查的方法、时机和完整性；以及高、低手术量外科医生和医院报告的差异。如果由手术量较多的外科医生手术，永久性 RLN 麻痹发生率约 1%~2%[24]。

尽管这些研究报告了使用神经监测仪的患者的 VCP 总体发生率较低，但在这些研究中，差异并不具有统计学意义[25]。这一发现主要是由于数据不足。Dralle 及其同事[26]已经表明，一项充分有力的研究需要 9 000 000 名良性甲状腺肿患者和 40 000 名甲状腺癌患者。值得注意的是，研究表明，在某些高风险手术中，如再次手术、恶性肿瘤手术和大甲状腺肿手术中，神经监测仪可改善术后 VCP 的发生率[27,28]。神经监测仪的潜在优点包括神经识别/神经标测、辅助解剖,术后神经功能预测及损伤部位识别[22]。

IONM 的主要技术是通过气管导管电极进行间歇监测。IONM 的标准化应用是非常重要的,国际神经监测研究小组发表的 IONM 指南对 IONM 的系统应用和解释进行了详细的阐述[29]。IONM 的最新进展包括连续神经迷走神经监测(连续 IONM),在间歇性刺激和 EBSLN 监测之间降低了 RLN 损伤的风险,允许识别所有 EBSLN,包括肉眼无法识别的在肌肉深面走行的 EBSLN[30,31]。

术中冰冻的应用和对侧手术的注意事项

甲状腺手术术中冰冻切片检查可能有一定的益处,但应慎重考虑和决策。冰冻切片对于确认甲状旁腺组织(如,当将缺血的甲状旁腺自体移植到肌肉中时)的有效性已得到公认。同样,冰冻切片对于确认淋巴结转移毫无疑问是有用的,特别是在术中遇到可疑淋巴结时。该技术有助于就所需的淋巴结清扫范围作出决策。

根据冰冻切片结果在术中决定是否切除对侧叶值得商榷。一般来说,在切除甲状腺结节或肿瘤后,可以考虑切除对侧叶,适用情况有几个:①当术后需要放射性碘治疗时;②便于用甲状腺球蛋白水平监测肿瘤复发;③当患者和外科医生决定切除对侧结节时。

使用放射性碘的指征目前已经有所缩窄,导致对侧甲状腺切除术的适应证减少。此外,低风险的甲状腺癌接受半腺叶切除术现在已被广泛接受。由于这种变化,对侧叶切除术中冰冻切片分析和术中决策常被认为是不必要的。即使在术中发现需要术后放射性碘治疗时,通常要决定进行对侧腺叶切除术,而不需要将先切除的腺叶冰冻切片检查。

冰冻切片对于甲状腺良性结节手术意义不大,通常这种情况下,仅计划进行诊断性甲状腺腺叶切除术。如果术中发现甲状腺腺外侵犯,可能需要放射性碘,在进行对侧叶切除术前,术中确认恶性肿瘤是很重要的。一个重要的注意事项是,FNA 上诊断为滤泡和 Hürthle 细胞肿瘤的结节在冰冻切片上不易诊断为恶性,因为通常需要仔细分析包膜和血管的浸润,这需要详尽的病理分析。这种情况与 PTC 相反,PTC 在冰冻切片上更容易诊断。

在进行手术之前,还必须考虑安全性和对侧腺叶切除术的必要性。具体而言,重要的是确认对侧腺叶切除术是适应证,参见本章其他部分。关于安全性,重要的是要在解剖侧确认 RLN 的完整状态,因为双侧 RLN 损伤虽然很少见，但可能需要气管切开术。单侧弱 RLN 信号或可能需要推迟对侧腺叶切除术直至神经恢复。另外，确认同侧的甲状旁腺完整性也很重要。如果两个甲状旁腺都被切除或损坏，而对侧腺叶切除对促进放射性碘的作用并不重要，则应推迟对侧甲状腺切除术。

手术结果记录

在手术报告中仔细记录手术结果是必要的。原因有很多，包括与内分泌科医生沟通与复发风险相关的因素，以帮助作出关于放射性碘治疗的决策。手术记录还可以为未来的手术计划提供相关资料。该记录应包括结节/肿瘤大小、位置、结构浸润和甲状腺外侵犯、切除完整性和淋巴结病变的位置/范围。此外，应记录 RLN、EBSLN 和甲状旁腺的状态。

术后治疗

钙管理

如果仅行腺叶切除术，对侧甲状旁腺不会受到干扰，也不会有低钙血症的风险。然而，甲状腺全切术可导致暂时或永久性低钙血症。外科医生和医疗机构对这种潜在的并发症有不同的处理方法。一种做法是术前评估维生素 D 和钙水平，术后依此预防性口服补钙校正至该水平。另一做法是，检查术后血清钙水平，只有在钙水平较低或有低钙血症症状时才治疗性补充钙和骨化三醇。对于严重的术后低钙血症，除口服补钙外，还可以静脉注射葡萄糖酸钙。只需要常规口服补钙的患者一般可以在 4 周内断服。永久性低钙血症的定义是术后 1 年仍需要药物治疗补钙，是一种罕见并发症。

术后喉部检查

甲状腺手术后嗓音改变并不少见，可能与气管内插管、束带肌或包括环甲肌在内的喉肌损伤或瘢痕有关，也可能与 RLN 或 EBSLN 损伤有关。重要的是要通过喉镜检查来区分这些原因，因为它们的治疗方法各不相同。具体来说，如果存在 RLN 损伤，可以使用一些额外的诊疗手段，但这不在本章的讨论范围内。对所有甲状腺术后患者常规进行喉镜检查的另一个重要原因是这与手术效果评估和质量改善密切相关。许多患者术后不会有任何声音变化，但仔细检查可能会发现声带活动性的功能障碍。外科医生有责任学习这些信息，以便在未来的病例中考虑调整手术技术。

结果衡量和改进

随着外科医生在其职业生涯中的进步，他们要不断学习和改进技术，为患者带来更好的结果。如果无法客观和持续地对其观察手术效果，则不可能获得进步。现在，许多机构都在监管要求以及不断发展的质量衡量和改进环境的指导下进行围手术期质量评估。除收集特定机构或个体的数据外，我们还在不断努力建立国家或地区质量数据注册表，以建立比较基准。如今，欧洲的一些注册机构已被广泛认可，包括由英国内分泌和甲状腺外科医生协会以及北欧甲状腺和甲状旁腺手术质量注册机构维护的注册机构。在美国，专门解决甲状腺手术质量问题的质量注册机构并未得到广泛使用，但将来可能会愈发普及。

（黄 韬）

参考文献

1. American Cancer Society. Cancer facts & figures 2018. Atlanta (GA): American Cancer Society; 2018.
2. American Cancer Society. Cancer facts & figures 2016. Atlanta (GA): American Cancer Society; 2016.
3. Shi LL, DeSantis C, Jemal A, et al. Changes in thyroid cancer incidence, post-2009 American Thyroid Association guidelines. Laryngoscope 2017;127(10):2437–41.
4. Roman BR, Morris LG, Davies L. The thyroid cancer epidemic, 2017 perspective. Curr Opin Endocrinol Diabetes Obes 2017;24(5):332–6.
5. Davies L, Welch HG. Current thyroid cancer trends in the United States. JAMA Otolaryngol Head Neck Surg 2014;140(4):317–22.
6. Tuttle RM, Fagin JA, Minkowitz G, et al. Natural history and tumor volume kinetics of papillary thyroid cancers during active surveillance. JAMA Otolaryngol Head Neck Surg 2017;143(10):1015–20.
7. Haugen BR, Alexander EK, Bible KC, et al. 2015 American Thyroid Association management guidelines for adult patients with thyroid nodules and differentiated thyroid cancer: the American Thyroid Association guidelines task force on thyroid nodules and differentiated thyroid cancer. Thyroid 2016;26(1):1–133.
8. Cibas ES, Ali SZ. The Bethesda system for reporting thyroid cytopathology. Thyroid 2009;19(11):1159–65.
9. Cibas ES, Ali SZ. The 2017 Bethesda system for reporting thyroid cytopathology. Thyroid 2017;27(11):1341–6.

10. Nikiforov YE, Seethala RR, Tallini G, et al. Nomenclature revision for encapsulated follicular variant of papillary thyroid carcinoma: a paradigm shift to reduce overtreatment of indolent tumors. JAMA Oncol 2016;2(8):1023–9.
11. Ferris RL, Nikiforov Y. AHNS series: do you know your guidelines? AHNS endocrine section consensus statement: state-of-the-art thyroid surgical recommendations in the era of noninvasive follicular thyroid neoplasm with papillary-like nuclear features. Head Neck 2018;40(9):1881–8.
12. Lesnik D, Cunnane ME, Zurakowski D, et al. Papillary thyroid carcinoma nodal surgery directed by a preoperative radiographic map utilizing CT scan and ultrasound in all primary and reoperative patients. Head Neck 2014;36(2):191–202.
13. Randolph GW. The importance of pre- and postoperative laryngeal examination for thyroid surgery. Thyroid 2010;20(5):453–8.
14. Randolph GW, Kamani D. The importance of preoperative laryngoscopy in patients undergoing thyroidectomy: voice, vocal cord function, and the preoperative detection of invasive thyroid malignancy. Surgery 2006;139(3):357–62.
15. Sinclair CF, Bumpous JM, Haugen BR, et al. Laryngeal examination in thyroid and parathyroid surgery: an American Head and Neck Society consensus statement: AHNS consensus statement. Head Neck 2016;38(6):811–9.
16. Chandrasekhar SS, Randolph GW, Seidman MD, et al. Clinical practice guideline: improving voice outcomes after thyroid surgery. Otolaryngol Head Neck Surg 2013;148(6 Suppl):S1–37.
17. Macias AA, Eappen S, Malikin I, et al. Successful intraoperative electrophysiologic monitoring of the recurrent laryngeal nerve, a multidisciplinary approach: the Massachusetts Eye and Ear Infirmary monitoring collaborative protocol with experience in over 3000 cases. Head Neck 2016;38(10):1487–94.
18. Phillips DE, Charters P. Strap muscles in thyroid surgery: to cut or not to cut? Ann R Coll Surg Engl 1993;75(5):378.
19. Pyrtek L, Painter RL. An anatomic study of the relationship of the parathyroid glands to the recurrent laryngeal nerve. Surg Gynecol Obstet 1964;119:509–12.
20. Cernea CR, Ferraz AR, Nishio S, et al. Surgical anatomy of the external branch of the superior laryngeal nerve. Head Neck 1992;14(5):380–3.
21. Darr EA, Tufano RP, Ozdemir S, et al. Superior laryngeal nerve quantitative intraoperative monitoring is possible in all thyroid surgeries. Laryngoscope 2014;124(4):1035–41.
22. Randolph GW, editor. Surgery of the thyroid and parathyroid glands. 1st edition. Philadelphia: Saunders-Elsevier Science; 2003.
23. Loré JM Jr, Kim DJ, Elias S. Preservation of the laryngeal nerves during total thyroid lobectomy. Ann Otol Rhinol Laryngol 1977;86(6 Pt 1):777–88.
24. Eisele D. Complication of thyroid surgery. In: Eisele D, editor. Complications in head and neck surgery. St Louis (MO): Mosby; 1993. p. 493–516.
25. Higgins TS, Gupta R, Ketcham AS, et al. Recurrent laryngeal nerve monitoring versus identification alone on post-thyroidectomy true vocal fold palsy: a meta-analysis. Laryngoscope 2011;121(5):1009–17.
26. Dralle H, Sekulla C, Haerting J, et al. Risk factors of paralysis and functional outcome after recurrent laryngeal nerve monitoring in thyroid surgery. Surgery 2004;136(6):1310–22.
27. Randolph GW, Shin JJ, Grillo HC, et al. The surgical management of goiter: part II. Surgical treatment and results. Laryngoscope 2011;121(1):68–76.
28. Chan WF, Lang BH, Lo CY. The role of intraoperative neuromonitoring of recurrent laryngeal nerve during thyroidectomy: a comparative study on 1000 nerves at

risk. Surgery 2006;140(6):866–72 [discussion: 872–3].
29. Randolph GW, Dralle H, Abdullah H, et al. Electrophysiologic recurrent laryngeal nerve monitoring during thyroid and parathyroid surgery: international standards guideline statement. Laryngoscope 2011;121(Suppl 1):S1–16.
30. Phelan E, Schneider R, Lorenz K, et al. Continuous vagal IONM prevents recurrent laryngeal nerve paralysis by revealing initial EMG changes of impending neuropraxic injury: a prospective, multicenter study. Laryngoscope 2014;124(6):1498–505.
31. Barczynski M, Randolph GW, Cernea CR, et al. External branch of the superior laryngeal nerve monitoring during thyroid and parathyroid surgery: International Neural Monitoring Study Group standards guideline statement. Laryngoscope 2013;123(Suppl 4):S1–14.

第9章
颈部淋巴结清扫在甲状腺癌手术治疗中的应用

Ahmad M. Eltelety, David J. Terris

关键词

- 甲状腺切除术 • 颈部淋巴结清扫 • 淋巴结 • 转移 • 甲状腺癌

要点

- 由于影像学的普及,尤其是颈部高分辨率超声检查的应用,甲状腺癌的发病率正逐渐增加。
- 甲状腺乳头状癌是最常见的甲状腺恶性肿瘤。
- 甲状腺癌通常伴发颈部淋巴结转移。
- 长期以来,颈部淋巴结的处理范围在甲状腺癌手术治疗中一直是一个颇有争议的话题。
- 遵循最新循证医学证据进行临床实践可改善患者预后。

引言

随着影像学诊断方法的不断发展,甲状腺结节的患者数量急剧增加[1]。其中大多数甲状腺结节<1cm,且通常无症状。过度检查以及超声引导下细针穿刺活检术的广泛应用导致诊断甲状腺微小乳头状癌患者数量激增。2016年,美国甲状腺癌患者大约为64 300名[2]。甲状腺乳头状癌(papillary thyroid cancer,PTC)是迄今为止最常见的甲状腺恶性肿瘤,在甲状腺恶性肿瘤人群中的占比超过75%[3],容易出现区域颈淋巴结转移。目前文献报道的PTC区域

性颈部淋巴结转移率存在很大差异,在 30%~80%。尽管如此,分化良好的甲状腺癌的预后通常很好,长期生存率超过 90%[4]。

决策制订

颈部中央区淋巴结清扫术

预防性

预防性中央区淋巴结清扫(central neck dissection,CND)是指在没有术前临床、影像学证据或术中病理证明存在颈部淋巴结转移的情况下,切除颈部中央区淋巴结[5]。尽管先前的观点推荐这种方法,但美国甲状腺协会最新指南(2015 年)不主张在肿瘤较小的(T_1 和 T_2)PTC 患者中常规行预防性 CND。尽管对于肿瘤较大的(T_3 和 T_4)PTC 患者,预防性 CND 是可接受的,但事实是,隐匿性的颈部淋巴结转移不太可能成为甲状腺癌患者疾病进展的驱动因素[6]。更重要的是,这些建议都不是基于循证医学 A 级证据的。

值得注意的是,即使是<1cm 的甲状腺微小癌也存在很高的区域淋巴结转移发生率,但这几乎不会影响患者的远期结局和预后[7-9]。此外,尚无来自美国的数据证据表明预防性 CND 会对患者的生存产生影响。从历史上看,日本人曾更积极地处理颈部中央区淋巴结,其改善预后的有限证据支持预防性 CND[10-14]。但是,即使在日本,最近的趋势也是减少积极的手术,甚至不做手术(密切随访)[15]。

15 年前,为了最大限度地减少甲状腺癌复发,初次治疗时对于原发灶和淋巴结多数选择积极的手术方式,而目前的趋势则是复发后由有经验的医师进行中央区淋巴结的再次手术[16-18]。因此,我们无须对绝大多数患者进行颈部中央区淋巴结预防性清扫手术,避免增加喉返神经损伤,尤其是甲状旁腺(parathyroid,PTH)损伤的风险[19-26]。而对于这部分患者,如果不进行中央区的淋巴结清扫,可能永远也不会发现淋巴结转移病灶。

甲状腺髓样癌(medullary thyroid carcinoma,MTC)一般在诊断时临床分期较晚,因此临床上很少发现没有颈部淋巴结转移(cN_0)的情况。外科手术的治疗方法应更为积极,包括常规行颈部中央区淋巴结清扫,即使术前并没有证据证明这些淋巴结发生了转移(cN_0)[27,28]。

治疗性

治疗性 CND 是指在通过术前临床体检、影像学评估、术中扪查或病理活检确认存在淋巴结转移的情况下行颈部中央区淋巴结清扫[5]。有专家共识认为,一旦病理证实中央区淋巴结存在转移,应常规行规范的中央区淋巴结清扫术。仅切除明显肉眼可见的淋巴结(所谓的摘草莓法)已不再被认可。治疗性 CND 可提高患者的生存率并降低患者的复发率[5,29,30]。治疗性 CND 的主要考虑因素是进行单侧还是双侧清扫。Carty 及其同事采用 CND 范围分类系统[5],对中央区淋巴结清扫范围进行了明确的界定,并允许单侧或双侧气管旁淋巴结清扫术。外科医生应详细描述颈部淋巴结清扫的类型,单侧还是双侧,以及详细的清扫范围。

治疗性 CND 通常与全甲状腺切除术(total thyroidectomy,TT)同步进行。如果病变仅限于一侧气管旁淋巴结,则单侧 CND 优于双侧 CND,这有助于降低术后低钙血症(暂时性或永久性)的发生率,并减少双侧喉返神经(recurrent laryngeal nerve,RLN)损伤导致呼吸困难的风险。当两侧气管旁区域都受侵及时,双侧 CND 在肿瘤学上是合适的,因为在这种情况下双侧手术的获益大于手术并发症所致的风险。治疗性 CND 的好处主要是降低疾病复发率,同时避免再次手术可能带来的并发症,也有证据表明治疗性 CND 可延长患者生存[30-32]。

颈侧方淋巴结清扫术

预防性

通常认为,在 PTC 的治疗中,无须进行预防性颈侧方淋巴结清扫术(lateral neck dissection,LND)。尽管临床上颈淋巴结阴性(cN_0)的患者中,有 25% 可能发生颈侧淋巴结微转移,这些微转移极少进展到临床可见的转移。对于这部分患者来说,没有任何证据表明选择性颈侧方淋巴结清扫可以改善患者预后和结局,且即使由经验丰富的手术者进行手术,预防性 LND 的并发症率也超过其获益。

但在处理 MTC 时存在一定程度的争议。目前针对临床无侧方淋巴结转移的 MTC 患者,主要有三种处理策略。对于没有颈侧方淋巴结转移的患者,有一项研究发现颈侧方淋巴结不处理的患者和进行预防性 LND 患者的预后没有统计学差异[33]。其他学者在处理同类患者时采取了更积极的态度。例如 de Groot 及其同事[34]提倡通过行 CND、双侧 LND 和上纵隔淋巴结清扫术来减少局部复发风险。但美国甲状腺协会建议采取谨慎的方法:MTC 患者,若无区域淋巴结转移或全身转移迹象,应行 TT 和 CND,而无须行 LND;若临床有中央区淋巴结转移,但无侧方淋巴结转移征象,也无须行预防性 LND。针对第二种情况,有一部分专家支持进行预防性 LND,为解决这一争议,美国甲状腺协会专家组一致认为：若为家族性 MTC，且降钙素水平高或甲状腺包块可触及，应接受 TT、CND 和双侧预防性 LND 治疗。若为散发性 MTC，且肿瘤>2cm 伴中央区颈淋巴结转移，可以接受 TT、CND 和同侧预防性 LND 治疗。

治疗性

对于已患有 PTC 且存在明显的颈侧区淋巴结转移的患者，推荐使用治疗性 LND。基于 PTC 的常见淋巴转移路径，LND 手术区域通常应包括Ⅱa、Ⅲ、Ⅳ和Ⅴb 区。甲状腺上极的病变倾向于转移至Ⅱ区淋巴结，而其余腺体中的癌细胞则倾向于转移至Ⅲ区和Ⅳ区。Ⅱb 区和Ⅴa 区的淋巴结转移率分别低至 6% 和 11%。癌肿较大或局部晚期（T4 和肿瘤>4cm），以及Ⅳ区存在明确淋巴结转移的患者，发生Ⅴb 区淋巴结转移的风险较高，因此，需要同时进行Ⅴb 区选择性清扫[35,36]。

值得注意的是，淋巴结转移是 45 岁以上患者的独立预后影响因子。在未满 45 岁的患者中，发生淋巴结转移也意味着较高的死亡风险，这些患者被认为是中高危人群[6,13,31,37]。由于患有颈侧淋巴结转移的患者死亡风险较高，大多数患者术后都会接受放射性碘（radioactive iodine，RAI）治疗，并应同时进行 TT[38]。

针对合适的患者合理实施 LND 是安全可行的，并发症较低[39]。侧方淋巴结很少侵犯胸锁乳突肌（sternocleidomastoid，SCM）或神经血管。"摘草莓"等更保守的手术可能导致较高的复发率[40]。尽管 PTC 的淋巴转移方式是从内侧到外侧，但是在相当一部分患者中确实发生了跳跃转移，出现颈部侧区淋巴结转移。因此，对于这部分患者，在没有临床或影像学证据的情况下，预防性 CND 并不是必需的[41]。如果在 TT 和 RAI 后出现肿瘤局部复发，有必要进行全面的颈淋巴结清扫术，以最大限度地减少残留或复发的风险[42]。

可扪及颈侧方转移淋巴结的 MTC 患者有 47% 会出现对侧淋巴结转移。因此，这些患者可以进行双侧 LND，以降低局部复发的风险[27]。

关键的操作技巧

对于颈部淋巴结清扫术全面细致的描述，已超出了本书的范围，为此，读者可以参考其他优秀文献资料[43-45]。笔者仅依据循证数据和个人经验在此分享相关的注意事项和关键步骤。

中央区手术

中央区淋巴结清扫（CND）通常在甲状腺全切（TT）之后进行。清扫始于喉前淋巴结，并向下延伸至气管前淋巴结至无名动脉平面。气管旁淋巴结清扫通常从环状软骨平面开始，向下一直延伸到无名动脉（右侧）和无名动脉与气管的交界处（左侧）。重要的是，右侧气管旁淋巴结可位于 RLN 的后方，这与右侧 RLN 在颈中部的斜行有关，且双侧气管旁淋巴结均可能位于颈动脉的后方。清扫中央区淋巴结，特别是右侧，应充分游离 RLN，从而尽可能减少对 RLN 的牵拉。尽管要求尽可能原位保留甲状旁腺，但现实中很难实现在彻底进行 CND 的同时完美保留下甲状旁腺的血供。上甲状旁腺（特别是位于健侧）通常可以原位保留[22,46]。甲状旁腺功能减退和随之而来的低钙血症是公认的 TT 并发症（在初次手术中发生率在 6.4%~21.6%，再次手术中发生率更高，这是因为瘢痕和纤维化使得甲状旁腺更加难以被识别和保留）；而 CND 与 TT 同时进行会导致甲状旁腺功能减退的发生率增加。所以，从无菌区取走标本之前，应该对标本进行彻底检查，寻找是否存在任何适合自体移植的甲状旁腺组织。术后管理的重点是在无须行实验室评估的前提下，预防性处理低钙血症 3 周[47]。

颈侧区手术

颈侧区清扫（LND）开始于颈阔肌肌皮瓣的游离提吊，这一步骤在单纯的甲状腺切除术中是不需要的。在胸锁乳突肌（SCM）表面切开颈深筋膜，显露清扫范围的侧壁，上界是颌下腺和二腹肌肌腱，下界是锁骨。在胸骨舌骨肌外侧和 SCM 深面内侧区域清扫脂肪淋巴组织，尤其要注意骨骼化颈内静脉。同时应识别和保护副神经。清扫应包含后方 Ⅴb 区水平到前方 SCM 深面的颈前三角区，标本可整块取出或分两次取出[40]。

应在切除的标本上用皮钉标记相应的颈部分区，以便于病理学评估。

再次手术

如果患者甲状腺球蛋白水平升高（在甲状腺球蛋白抗体未升高的情况下），加之形态上有可识别的病灶（通常在超声检查中可见），就需要进行细针穿刺活检。如果证实为恶性，则应考虑再次手术。穿刺洗脱液甲状腺球蛋白测定有助于鉴别转移性甲状腺癌，特别是颈侧区淋巴结转移癌的诊断[17]。回顾先前的手术记录和病理报告可能对计划再次手术有所帮助。特别的关注点应包括 RLN 的功能状态、甲状旁腺的完整性、病变切除的程度,以及发生任何并发症的可能性[16]。

对于中央区再手术,侧后方入路可能有助于避开先前手术形成的瘢痕。可在 SCM 内侧和带状肌外侧,或胸骨舌骨肌和胸骨甲状肌之间的潜在腔隙中分离。应尽量在气管食管沟或在其入喉之前识别 RLN。为了显露需要,或者如果有肿瘤附着,可以切除带状肌。

再次手术时,建议使用喉返神经监测仪,但它不能代替喉返神经的解剖学识别。再次手术中通常可在两个位置识别 RLN。在下咽缩肌下缘的上方可看到喉返神经的远端,如果下方手术区域或纵隔上段广泛肿瘤复发或纤维化,则最好在此区域进行喉返神经定位。与之相反,如果出于同样的原因难以在上缘识别神经,则可以位于手术区域下方的胸廓入口处,在先前手术区域的下方识别神经。重要的是,瘢痕组织可能导致神经在气管前壁处出现位置异常。在这种情况下,神经很容易在该位置被损伤,因此,再次手术分离气管前壁时,应保持高度警惕[48]。

如果是颈侧区复发,通常会进行选择性清扫。高分化甲状腺癌很少转移到Ⅰ区淋巴结,大多数情况下,无须清扫该区域。因此,初次手术应尽可能清扫Ⅱa、Ⅲ、Ⅳ和Ⅴb区淋巴结。在以减少再次复发率为治疗目的时,推荐区域性淋巴结清扫[29]。在极少的情况下,如果发现上纵隔有肿瘤侵犯,可能需要与胸外科医生协同实施(部分或完全)胸骨劈开手术。

并发症:预防和治疗

乳糜瘘

乳糜瘘(也称为乳糜漏)是颈淋巴结清扫术的一种手术并发症,在处理左侧 PTC Ⅳ区转移淋巴结时尤为常见(此处为胸导管汇入颈内静脉的区域)。初始保守治疗包括低脂饮食、全胃肠外营养和绷带加压包扎等。在大多数乳糜液引流量较少的情况下,保守治疗有效。如果保守治疗失败(尤其是当每日乳糜液引流量超过 500ml 时,会有电解质紊乱的风险),则应该采取更积极的干预措施,包括再次手术行胸导管结扎、切口负压治疗,以及使用生长抑素类药物的治疗等。上述治疗方法疗效各有差异[49-51]。

脊髓副神经综合征

肩关节功能障碍是 LND 后的常见并发症,即使在副神经得以保留的情况下。

据报道,行 LND 并保留副神经的患者,肩关节功能障碍发生率在 30%~40%,并有多种临床表现:常见的有肩下垂、持续性隐痛、外展活动范围减少,以及关节僵硬等。尽管神经结构得到保留,但仍可能发生上述综合征,表明存在其他因素导致这种情况的发生。可能的因素包括颈丛神经损伤和暂时性肩胛带肌功能障碍。制动最终会导致关节僵硬和粘连性滑膜炎,而术后早期康复和肩关节被动运动物理治疗可以减轻术后肩关节症状。颈丛神经小剂量肉毒毒素注射已被证明可有效控制某些患者的病情,且不良反应极小[52,53]。

重要血管损伤

尽管不常见,但严重的血管损伤是每位接受颈淋巴结清扫的患者都可能出现的致命并发症之一。优先处理顺序依次是气道,呼吸,循环。液体复苏最好给予大量输血,有时可能需要 O 型阴性血液。一旦血管受损,需要立即采取的步骤包括:断端近端和远端控制,尽早恢复血流,必要时考虑暂时性血管分流。明确的治疗方案包括血管结扎、血管修复和血管旁路手术。根据情况,可能需要血管外科医师处理。介入手术越来越普及,对部分损伤或可能受累的血管进行支架植入术可能是合适的,多学科的努力协作也为患者获得最佳结局提供了可能[54]。

总结

在甲状腺癌的手术治疗中,适应证下进行颈部淋巴结清扫术是必要的。现在很少进行预防性 CND,但是如果患者有中央区淋巴结转移的临床或影像学证据,则必须进行 CND。这可能会增加甲状旁腺功能低下以及因而导致的低钙血症的发生率。LND 应由经验丰富的外科医生进行,并提倡行区域淋巴结清扫以取得最佳的肿瘤学结局。

(徐 琰　齐晓伟　张 毅)

参考文献

1. Jemal A, Siegel R, Ward E, et al. Cancer statistics, 2010. CA Cancer J Clin 2010; 60(5):277–300.
2. Siegel RL, Miller KD, Jemal A. Cancer statistics. CA Cancer J Clin 2016;66(1): 7–30.
3. Sherman SI. Thyroid carcinoma. Lancet 2003;361(9356):501–11.

4. Ort S, Goldenberg D. Management of regional metastases in well-differentiated thyroid cancer. Otolaryngol Clin North Am 2008;41(6):1207–18.
5. Carty SE, Cooper DS, Doherty GM, et al. Consensus statement on the terminology and classification of central neck dissection for thyroid cancer. Thyroid 2009;19(11):1153–9.
6. Haugen BR, Alexander EK, Bible KC, et al. 2015 American Thyroid Association management guidelines for adult patients with thyroid nodules and differentiated thyroid cancer: the American Thyroid Association guidelines task force on thyroid nodules and differentiated thyroid cancer. Thyroid 2016;26(1):1–133.
7. Trivizki O, Amit M, Fliss DM, et al. Elective central compartment neck dissection in patients with papillary thyroid carcinoma recurrence. Laryngoscope 2013;123(6):1564–8.
8. De Carvalho AY, Chulam TC, Kowalski LP. Long-term results of observation vs prophylactic selective level VI neck dissection for papillary thyroid carcinoma at a cancer center. JAMA Otolaryngol Head Neck Surg 2015;141(7):599–606.
9. Shah MD, Hall FT, Eski SJ, et al. Clinical course of thyroid carcinoma after neck dissection. Laryngoscope 2003;113(12):2102–7.
10. Dubernard X, Dabakuyo S, Ouedraogo S, et al. Prophylactic neck dissection for low-risk differentiated thyroid cancers: risk-benefit analysis. Head Neck 2016;38(7):1091–6.
11. Pitoia F, Ward L, Wohllk N, et al. Recommendations of the Latin American Thyroid Society on diagnosis and management of differentiated thyroid cancer. Arq Bras Endocrinol Metabol 2009;53(7):884–7.
12. Perros P, Colley S, Boelaert K, et al. Guidelines for the management of thyroid cancer. Clin Endocrinol (Oxf) 2014;81(s1):1–122.
13. Pacini F, Schlumberger M, Dralle H, et al. European consensus for the management of patients with differentiated thyroid carcinoma of the follicular epithelium. Eur J Endocrinol 2006;154(6):787–803.
14. Takami H, Ito Y, Okamoto T, et al. Therapeutic strategy for differentiated thyroid carcinoma in japan based on a newly established guideline managed by Japanese society of thyroid surgeons and Japanese association of endocrine surgeons. World J Surg 2011;35(1):111–21.
15. Oda H, Miyauchi A, Ito Y, et al. Incidences of unfavorable events in the management of low-risk papillary microcarcinoma of the thyroid by active surveillance versus immediate surgery. Thyroid 2016;26(1):150–5.
16. Pai SI, Tufano RP. Reoperation for recurrent/persistent well-differentiated thyroid cancer. Otolaryngol Clin North Am 2010;43(2):353–63.
17. Scharpf J, Tuttle M, Wong R, et al. Comprehensive management of recurrent thyroid cancer: an American Head and Neck Society Consensus Statement. Head Neck 2016;38(12):1862–9.
18. Clayman GL, Agarwal G, Edeiken BS, et al. Long-term outcome of comprehensive central compartment dissection in patients with recurrent/persistent papillary thyroid carcinoma. Thyroid 2011;21(12):1309–16.
19. Grant CS, Stulak JM, Thompson GB, et al. Risks and adequacy of an optimized surgical approach to the primary surgical management of papillary thyroid carcinoma treated during 1999-2006. World J Surg 2010;34(6):1239–46.
20. Kutler DI, Crummey AD, Kuhel WI. Routine central compartment lymph node dissection for patients with papillary thyroid carcinoma. Head Neck 2012;34(2):260–3.

21. Roh JL, Park JY, Park C II. Total thyroidectomy plus neck dissection in differentiated papillary thyroid carcinoma patients: pattern of nodal metastasis, morbidity, recurrence, and postoperative levels of serum parathyroid hormone. Ann Surg 2007;245(4):604–10.
22. Cavicchi O, Piccin O, Caliceti U, et al. Transient hypoparathyroidism following thyroidectomy: a prospective study and multivariate analysis of 604 consecutive patients. Otolaryngol Head Neck Surg 2007;137(4):654–8.
23. Lee YS, Kim SW, Kim SW, et al. Extent of routine central lymph node dissection with small papillary thyroid carcinoma. World J Surg 2007;31(10):1954–9.
24. Torlontano M, Crocetti U, Augello G, et al. Comparative evaluation of recombinant human thyrotropin-stimulated thyroglobulin levels, 131I whole-body scintigraphy, and neck ultrasonography in the follow-up of patients with papillary thyroid microcarcinoma who have not undergone radioiodine therapy. J Clin Endocrinol Metab 2006;91(1):60–3.
25. Pacini F, Molinaro E, Castagna MG, et al. Recombinant human thyrotropin-stimulated serum thyroglobulin combined with neck ultrasonography has the highest sensitivity in monitoring differentiated thyroid carcinoma. J Clin Endocrinol Metab 2003;88(8):3668–73.
26. Bonnet S, Hartl D, Leboulleux S, et al. Prophylactic lymph node dissection for papillary thyroid cancer less than 2 cm: implications for radioiodine treatment. J Clin Endocrinol Metab 2009;94(4):1162–7.
27. Dackiw APB. The surgical management of medullary thyroid cancer. Otolaryngol Clin North Am 2010;43(2):365–74.
28. Liao S, Shindo M. Management of well-differentiated thyroid cancer. Otolaryngol Clin North Am 2012;45(5):1163–79.
29. Shaha AR. Revision thyroid surgery - technical considerations. Otolaryngol Clin North Am 2008;41(6):1169–83.
30. Agrawal N, Evasovich MR, Kandil E, et al. Indications and extent of central neck dissection for papillary thyroid cancer: an American Head and Neck Society Consensus Statement. Head Neck 2017;39(7):1269–79.
31. Zaydfudim V, Feurer ID, Griffin MR, et al. The impact of lymph node involvement on survival in patients with papillary and follicular thyroid carcinoma. Surgery 2008;144(6):1070–8.
32. Yd P, Smith D, Ld W, et al. The implication of lymph node metastasis on survival in patients with well-differentiated thyroid cancer. Am Surg 2005;71(9):731–5.
33. Pena I, Clayman GL, Grubbs EG, et al. Management of the lateral neck compartment in patients with sporadic medullary thyroid cancer. Head Neck 2018;40(1):79–85.
34. de Groot JWB, Links TP, Sluiter WJ, et al. Locoregional control in patients with palpable medullary thyroid cancer: results of standardized compartment-oriented surgery. Head Neck 2007;29(9):857–63.
35. Lombardi D, Paderno A, Giordano D, et al. Therapeutic lateral neck dissection in well-differentiated thyroid cancer: analysis on factors predicting distribution of positive nodes and prognosis. Head Neck 2018;40(2):242–50.
36. Khafif A, Medina JE, Robbins KT, et al. Level V in therapeutic neck dissections for papillary thyroid carcinoma. Head Neck 2013;35(4):605–7.
37. Adam MA, Pura J, Goffredo P, et al. Presence and number of lymph node metastases are associated with compromised survival for patients younger than age 45 years with papillary thyroid cancer. J Clin Oncol 2015;33(21):2370–5.
38. Nixon IJ, Shaha AR, Patel SG. Surgical diagnosis. Frozen section and the extent

of surgery. Otolaryngol Clin North Am 2014;47(4):519–28.
39. Kupferman ME, Patterson DM, Mandel SJ, et al. Safety of modified radical neck dissection for differentiated thyroid carcinoma. Laryngoscope 2004;114(3): 403–6.
40. Schoppy DW, Holsinger FC. Management of the neck in thyroid cancer. Otolaryngol Clin North Am 2014;47(4):545–56.
41. Fritze D, Doherty GM. Surgical management of cervical lymph nodes in differentiated thyroid cancer. Otolaryngol Clin North Am 2010;43(2):285–300.
42. Wu G, Fraser S, Pai S, et al. Determining the extent of lateral neck dissection necessary to establish regional disease control and avoid reoperation after previous total thyroidectomy and radioactive iodine for papillary thyroid cancer. Head Neck 2012;34(10):1418–21.
43. Walsh NJ, Talukder AM, Terris DJ. Central neck dissection: the five key steps. VideoEndocrinology 2018;5(3).
44. Hughes DT, Doherty GM. Central neck dissection for papillary thyroid cancer. Cancer Control 2011;18(2):83–8.
45. Uchino S, Noguchi S, Yamashita H, et al. Modified radical neck dissection for differentiated thyroid cancer: operative technique. World J Surg 2004;28(12): 1199–203.
46. Ondik MP, McGinn J, Ruggiero F, et al. Unintentional parathyroidectomy and hypoparathyroidism in secondary central compartment surgery for thyroid cancer. Head Neck 2010;32(4):462–6.
47. Singer MC, Bhakta D, Seybt MW, et al. Calcium management after thyroidectomy: a simple and cost-effective method. Otolaryngol Head Neck Surg 2012;146(3): 362–5.
48. Richer SL, Wenig BL. Changes in surgical anatomy following thyroidectomy. Otolaryngol Clin North Am 2008;41(6):1069–78.
49. Kadota H, Kakiuchi Y, Yoshida T. Management of chylous fistula after neck dissection using negative-pressure wound therapy: a preliminary report. Laryngoscope 2012;122(5):997–9.
50. Valentine CN, Barresi R, Prinz RA. Somatostatin analog treatment of a cervical thoracic duct fistula. Head Neck 2002;24(8):810–3.
51. Swanson MS, Hudson RL, Bhandari N, et al. Use of octreotide for the management of chyle fistula following neck dissection. JAMA Otolaryngol Head Neck Surg 2015;141(8):723–7.
52. Salerno G, Cavaliere M, Foglia A, et al. The 11th nerve syndrome in functional neck dissection. Laryngoscope 2002;112(7):1299–307.
53. Wittekindt C, Liu W-C, Preuss SF, et al. Botulinum Toxin A for neuropathic pain after neck dissection: a dose-finding study. Laryngoscope 2006;116(7):1168–71.
54. Tisherman SA. Management of major vascular injury: open. Otolaryngol Clin North Am 2016;49(3):809–17.

第10章
传统机器人内镜甲状腺切除术在甲状腺癌治疗中的应用

Meghan E. Garstka, Ehab S. Alameer, Saad Al Awwad, Emad Kandil

关键词

- 机器人内镜甲状腺切除术 • 甲状腺癌 • 传统的

要点

- 本章详细介绍了用于甲状腺癌治疗的传统机器人内镜下颈外入路的操作技术,这一技术在近年来的文献报道中越来越受到关注。
- 在美国,目前开展的大量机器人甲状腺手术主要集中在少数医学中心,尽管该术式并发症发生率较高,该手术量近期仍有所增加。
- 这些趋势凸显了外科医生为提高手术安全性而了解和学习这一技术的重要性。
- 未来需要大样本多中心研究去探究能从传统机器人内镜甲状腺切除术中获益的甲状腺癌患者。

引言

外科技术在传统甲状腺切除术中的应用,使甲状腺手术朝着微创多元化方向不断发展。21世纪初期,Miccoli及其同事[1]报道了关于微创内镜下甲状腺切除术的研究结果,在美国引起广泛关注[2-4]。外科医师还尝试了采用内镜技术经前胸、乳房或腋窝等颈外入路进行甲状腺手术[5]。这种颈外的"颈部无瘢痕"术式对于许多有美容需求、不想有颈前切口的患者而言无疑是更理想的选择，包括年轻患者和有瘢痕体质或增生性瘢痕病史的患者。然而，关于内镜甲状腺切除术的最初研究表明，这些方法受到了二维视角和非调节的手术器械的限制[5]。而将机器人技术引入甲状腺切除手术，为其提供三维视野和多关节灵活的内镜臂，是有限颈部操作空间的理想选择。Chung 及其同事[6,7]倡导经腋窝入路，Terris 团队[8]提出用于面部提拉术的耳后发际入路，均做了大量早期开拓性工作。

多种机器人辅助手术方式的快速涌现，促使美国甲状腺协会（American Thyroid Association, ATA）在 2016 年发表了关于该术式的共识声明[9]。声明指出，在合适病例中，由经验丰富的甲状腺外科医师进行颈外入路甲状腺手术具有一定的临床价值。声明还建议密切关注相关质控研究结果，严格把握患者的入选标准。在 ATA 发布声明时，美国机器人辅助甲状腺切除术最常用的四种入路是内镜下乳房入路、内镜机器人双侧腋窝-乳房入路、内镜机器人经腋窝入路，以及内镜机器人耳后发际入路。随着经口内镜甲状腺切除术的出现，这些机器人辅助术式入路将被归为传统方法。本章我们将讨论传统机器人内镜甲状腺切除术在甲状腺癌治疗中的应用。

患者选择

通常，在美国最常见的两种传统机器人内镜甲状腺切除术是机器人辅助无充气经腋窝和经耳后发际区的术式，理想患者为体重较轻的体重指数（body mass index，BMI）<30kg/m^2 的病例，然而也有结果显示这些术式仍可用于 BMI>40kg/m^2 的北美患者[10]。这些术式可能更适用于有瘢痕疙瘩或肥厚性瘢痕形成既往史的患者。对于经腋窝入路，患者不能有手术体位相关的解剖或病理上的禁忌证，比如肩袖病或颈椎管狭窄症。对于老年或肥胖患者，应由有经验的外科医生开展这些术式；考虑到学习曲线，对于初学者，推荐使用更严格的患者选择标准。

同样地，综合考虑患者选择和甲状腺病理改变，推荐刚刚开展传统机器人内镜技术的外科医生先尝试甲状腺部分切除术。然而研究报道，熟练的外科医生可以利用这些术式成功施行甲状腺全切术和颈淋巴结清除术[11,12]。因此，随着手术操作复杂性的不断提高，其手术适应证也不断扩大。机器人辅助甲状腺切除术仍有绝对手术禁忌证，包括胸骨后或咽后巨大甲状腺肿、T$_3$ 期甲状腺癌或任何可疑肉眼的肿瘤外侵,以及甲状腺髓样癌[13]。既往报道的相对禁忌证包括:>5cm的肿块、体积>40ml的甲状腺肿、T_2期分化型甲状腺癌、桥本甲状腺炎、Grave病,以及肥胖、有颈部手术史或放射史。尽管如此,许多研究显示这些传统的机器人辅助术式对于桥本甲状腺炎、Graves病,以及进展期甲状腺癌患者是安全可行的[11,12,14-17]。

甲状腺癌和传统机器人内镜手术

来自亚洲的多个中心首先对传统机器人内镜甲状腺切除术进行了报道。2013年,Lee及其同事们[11]指出,接受机器人甲状腺切除术(包括改良根治性颈清扫术)具有与传统开放术式相似的肿瘤学预后和安全性,在颈部不适和肩部残障率发生方面,两者也类似。传统机器人内镜甲状腺切除术具有更好的术后生活质量,包括切口更加美观、颈部感觉异常更少、吞咽不适感发生率更低。2016年,Lee的团队还报道了一项对比机器人辅助下手术及传统开放手术实施甲状腺切除加中央区淋巴结清扫的5年期研究结果,发现两者的长期肿瘤学预后是相似的[12]。2017年,Kim及其同事们[18]对机器人辅助手术和传统开放甲状腺切除在改良根治性颈清术方面进行了比较,结果显示两者具有相似的围手术期和5年期的肿瘤学结局。最近,韩国的Chung教授团队发表了5000例无充气经腋窝甲状腺切除术的数据,其中4767例患者为恶性肿瘤[19]。这项研究显示,通过免充气经腋窝入路的技术可改进颈外入路甲状腺切除术的操作,并已取得满意的手术结果。尽管这项技术的大规模回顾性数据已经发表,但其可重复性仍然受到质疑,合理的学习曲线与经验的积累会使这项技术得到合理的应用。

在近期一项研究中,研究者们针对2015—2017年北美医疗机构中分化型甲状腺癌的西方人群患者,分析了开展机器人辅助甲状腺手术的安全性和可行性[20]。该研究显示作者所在机构进行了144例甲状腺癌手术,其中包括35例(24.3%)机器人辅助的无充气经腋窝入路的手术,两组在失血量、手术时间、并发症发生率、切除标本大小、显微镜下切缘阳性率、清扫的淋巴结数量、患者随访持续时间、临床复发率上的比较均无显著差异。然而,机器人辅助手术的总住院时间更短。研究者认为,在北美人群中,对于分化型甲状腺癌的患者,无充气腋窝入路传统机器人内镜甲状腺切除术是可行的,并且能根治肿瘤,这一结果与亚洲经验类似。然而,在西方人群中,未来需要更大规模的多中心研究来证实这一结论。

经耳后发际线入路（适用于面部提拉术）技术的概述

经耳后发际线入路传统机器人内镜甲状腺切除术的标准步骤如下：

- 患者接受全麻，通过插入带肌电信号的气管导管实现术中喉返神经的监测。
- 手术体位采用仰卧位，双臂固定于手术台两侧。头向健侧旋转20°~30°。枕部发际线需备皮至距切口 1cm 以上。
- 切口的下端平耳后褶皱耳垂的下界，向后上方自然地延伸至枕后发际线的备皮区(图 10.1)。切口行局部浸润麻醉，颈部术区行无菌消毒及铺巾。
- 使用手术刀切开皮肤，电刀分离出颈下皮瓣，从而暴露出胸锁乳突肌；解剖分离沿胸锁乳突肌的前下方进行。
- 首先需要辨识出耳大神经，此处以上可显露出颈外静脉及胸锁乳突肌前缘。如果暴露需要，可离断颈外静脉。
- 沿胸锁乳突肌的前内侧缘解剖至锁骨，显露出由胸锁乳突肌、肩胛舌骨肌以及胸骨舌骨肌组成的肌三角。将肩胛舌骨肌、胸骨舌骨肌、胸骨甲状肌向腹侧牵拉，暴露出同侧甲状腺上极，并分离出上甲状腺蒂。
- 自动式改良甲状腺拉钩(Chung 拉钩)固定于手术台对侧，并向腹侧牵拉带状肌。将一个 Singer 拉钩(Medtronic，美国)或者甲状腺拉钩连接于一个 Greenberg 拉钩(Codman & Shurtleff, Inc，美国)上，并固定在手术台的同侧，用于将胸锁乳突肌牵拉至背侧面。也可以选择改良操作步骤，从胸锁乳突肌的两个头之间创建一个平面。
- 达芬奇机器人系统(Intuitive，美国)置于切口对侧的术区。首先将内镜镜头设置为 30° 向下，置入切口，血管闭合器(双极电凝分离钳或超声刀)以及 Maryland 抓钳分别置于机械臂 2 和机械臂 3，在直视下置入术野。血管闭合器(双极电凝分离钳或超声刀)通常由外科医师的优势手控制。
- 将甲状腺上极向腹侧及下侧牵拉，暴露出甲状腺上血管，并贴近甲状腺被膜进行离断。然后将整个腺体向中间牵拉以便识别气管食管沟内的喉返神经。神经监护仪可用来确认神经的完整性，并沿着神经的走行一直显露至环甲肌的入喉点，鉴别并保留上下位甲状旁腺。
- 随后解剖并离断甲状腺下极，将甲状腺从气管上解剖出来。分离峡部，取出甲状腺。确认喉返神经的完整性,术区止血。
- 如果需要引流,将一个引流管放置在耳后切口的后部。切口分两层闭合,使用可吸收线皮下间断缝合,皮肤则使用可吸收线行间断或连续缝合,或是不可吸收线间断缝合(必须拆线)(图10.2)。
- 必要时,可以在闭合切口时切除多余的皮肤,即可同时行面部除皱手术。

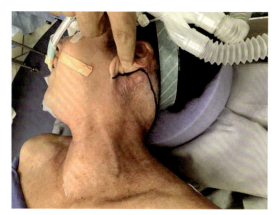

图10.1 经耳后发际入路或面部提拉美容切口的术前外观

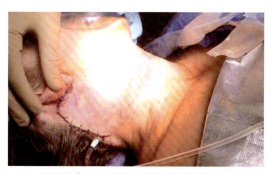

图10.2 经耳后发际入路或面部提拉美容切口的术后外观

经腋窝入路技术的概述

经腋窝入路传统机器人内镜甲状腺切除术的标准步骤如下:
- 患者取仰卧位,进行全身麻醉,用带有肌电信号的气管导管实现术中神经监测。用肩垫使患者颈部略微伸展,将病变侧或甲状腺叶较大侧的手臂放在头侧并在头部上方弯曲后放在改良Ikeda手臂位置(图10.3)。将对侧手臂包裹。研究人员通常使用体感诱发电位(SSEP;

Biotronic,美国)来监测正中神经和尺神经信号(图 10.4)。体位摆好后进行术中超声检查。

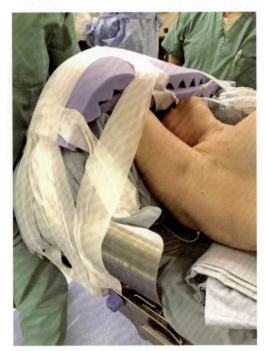

图 10.3　经腋窝甲状腺切除术的改良 Ikeda 手臂体位

- 标记切口的下端位于同侧腋窝的胸骨切迹水平,切口的上端位于同侧腋窝由甲状舌骨膜到腋窝的 60° 角斜线(图 10.5)。
- 连接标记点,沿着胸大肌外侧缘做大约 2 英寸(5.08cm)的纵向标记线。将颈部和前胸消毒铺巾,然后用局部麻醉剂浸润切口部位并切开。
- 利用单极电凝沿着皮下组织进一步解剖,以暴露胸大肌的外侧边界,并向锁骨方向游离以在颈阔肌下平面中形成一个位于胸大肌浅面的皮瓣。这里可能需要用到长头的电刀。
- 带光源的乳房牵开器可方便皮瓣的分离。定位锁骨后进一步向内侧分离胸骨切迹,直至同侧的胸锁乳突肌。识别胸锁乳突肌的胸骨(内侧)头和锁骨(外侧)头。
- 胸锁乳突肌的胸骨头和锁骨头之间的无血管区可用电灼或血管闭合器(vessel sealer)分离建立,并将胸锁乳突肌的胸骨头前拉,暴露肩胛舌骨肌。

第 10 章　传统机器人内镜甲状腺切除术在甲状腺癌治疗中的应用

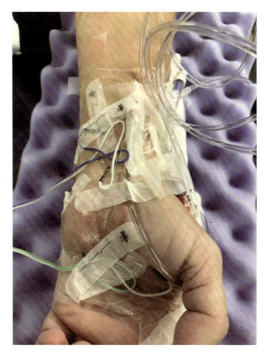

图 10.4　经腋窝入路进行 SSEP 监护的电极

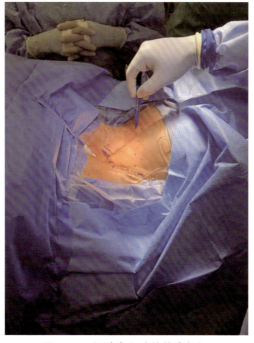

图 10.5　经腋窝入路的体表标识

- 用电灼或血管闭合器分离肩胛舌骨肌最上层结缔组织,暴露甲状腺上极。外科医生在解剖此部位时要小心避免损伤颈内静脉。一旦甲状腺上极暴露后,将 Chung 自动牵开器或改良甲状腺切除牵开器(Marina Medical,美国)安装到手术台的对侧,以向前抬高带状肌(图 10.6)。

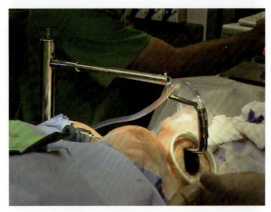

图 10.6　经腋窝入路安装机器人手臂前的皮瓣牵拉

- 达芬奇外科手术机器人从对侧置入手术区域(图 10.7)。将双通道摄像机调至"向下 30°"模式,首先放在切口中间位置。然后,在直视下,将机械臂 2 和机械臂 3 放置在中央摄像头臂的右侧或左侧。接着,在术者的优势侧置入一个血管闭合系统(双极电凝分离钳或超声刀),在对侧臂上放一把 Maryland 分离钳。经机械臂 4 置入抓钳,放在切口的上方,相对于自动牵开器柄位于病变同侧。

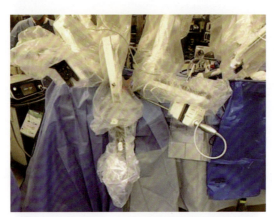

图 10.7　经腋窝入路手术中的机器人手臂安置

- 助手可通过腋下切口放入腔镜吸引或冲洗装置,这也有助于在解剖期间将胸锁乳突肌的锁骨头或气管向下牵拉。助手还负责术中的喉返神经监测操作,以及机械臂的位置的转换和保持。
- 在颈动脉鞘中刺激迷走神经。若考虑到进行双侧解剖或颈部解剖的需要,则可以在迷走神经上放置一个电极以进行连续的神经监测。将甲状腺上极(图 10.8)向内下牵拉,解剖分离甲状腺上血管时紧贴甲状腺,以免损伤喉上神经外支。甲状腺从环甲肌上游离下来,注意识别并保护上位甲状腺旁腺。

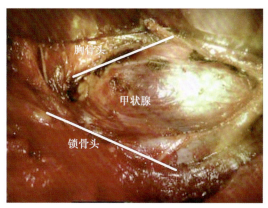

图 10.8　术中甲状腺腺叶局部解剖图

- 将甲状腺向内牵拉,解剖分离甲状腺中静脉。在气管食管沟处寻找识别喉返神经,并仔细分离直至环甲肌。一定要确定喉返神经功能的完整性。
- 解剖分离甲状腺下极。识别并保留下位甲状旁腺。将甲状腺下极从喉返神经内侧解剖切开,并从气管上切除直至到达对侧。将甲状腺叶及峡部分开,将标本取出。
- 如果要进行中央区淋巴结清扫术,沿着喉返神经,将中央区淋巴结完整解剖游离,并和胸腺及甲状腺整块切除。
- 关于全甲状腺切除术,一旦同侧腺叶切除后,就要将对侧腺叶从气管上解剖游离。当到达对侧气管食管沟处时,要刺激并识别喉返神经。解剖并结扎甲状腺上极和下极;监测喉返神经直至环甲膜,将剩下的甲状腺切除并从腋窝切口取出。
- 最后完成喉返神经和迷走神经 R2、V2 信号的测定,确切止血。放置引流管,将腋下切口分为两层缝合,以不连续的皮下缝合和连续的皮内缝合方式闭合切口(图 10.9)。

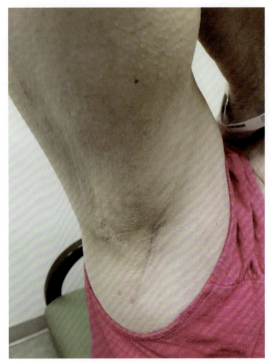

图 10.9　经腋窝入路术式的术后切口愈合后外观

并发症

这里讨论的传统机器人内镜甲状腺手术的并发症不仅包括传统颈部开放手术所观察到的并发症,例如喉返神经损伤、术后疼痛、颈部血肿、伤口感染和低钙血症等,还包括这种远离颈部入路技术所特有的并发症,例如采用经腋窝入路造成的臂丛神经损伤[8]。据报道,暂时性喉返神经麻痹的发生率为1%~3%,永久性损伤发生率约为 0.3%,血肿的发生率约为 1%,而臂丛神经损伤约为 2.2%。臂丛神经损伤的评估可通过使用体感诱发电位(somatosensory evoked potential,SSEP)监测桡神经、尺神经和正中神经的信号。作者所在机构的一项近期研究采用 SSEP 监测技术对 123 位患者进行了 137 例次的经腋窝机器人内镜甲状腺手术的臂丛神经评估,有 7 例患者(5.1%)的信号发生了显著变化,但立即进行手臂复位可将信号完全恢复至基线水平,从而避免发生因术中体位不当导致的臂丛神经损伤[21]。

总结

本章详细介绍的传统机器人内镜甲状腺手术，在近年来不断被越来越多的文献所报道，包括用于甲状腺癌的治疗。自达芬奇手术系统的制造商 Intuitive Surgical Inc 于 2011 年 10 月对该类手术进行技术支持和人员培训以来，美国国内的相关手术量有所增长[22]。目前，美国绝大多数的机器人内镜甲状腺手术都由病例量较少的医学中心完成，这也是该术式的并发症较传统术式有所增加的原因。这些趋势凸显了加强外科医生对这些技术的了解和经验积累的重要性，以最终提高该手术的安全性。未来，需要更多的大样本多中心研究去探索能从机器人内镜甲状腺切除手术中获益的甲状腺癌患者。

（郑传铭　谢　磊）

参考文献

1. Miccoli P, Bellantone R, Mourad M, et al. Minimally invasive video-assisted thyroidectomy: multiinstitutional experience. World J Surg 2002;26(8):972–5.
2. Terris DJ, Gourin CG, Chin E. Minimally invasive thyroidectomy: basic and advanced techniques. Laryngoscope 2006;116(3):350–6.
3. Duke WS, White JR, Waller JL, et al. Endoscopic thyroidectomy is safe in patients with a high body mass index. Thyroid 2014;24(7):1146–50.
4. Duke WS, White JR, Waller JL, et al. Six-year experience with endoscopic thyroidectomy: outcomes and safety profile. Ann Otol Rhinol Laryngol 2015;124(11):915–20.
5. Bomeli SR, Duke WS, Terris DJ. Robotic facelift thyroid surgery. Gland Surg 2015;4(5):403–9.
6. Mohamed HE, Kandil E. Robotic trans-axillary and retro-auricular thyroid surgery. J Surg Oncol 2015;112(3):243–9.
7. Yoon JH, Park CH, Chung WY. Gasless endoscopic thyroidectomy via an axillary approach: experience of 30 cases. Surg Laparosc Endosc Percutan Tech 2006;16(4):226–31.
8. Terris DJ, Singer MC, Seybt MW. Robotic facelift thyroidectomy: patient selection and technical considerations. Surg Laparosc Endosc Percutan Tech 2011;21(4):237–42.
9. Berber E, Bernet V, Fahey TJ 3rd, et al, American Thyroid Association Surgical Affairs Committee. American Thyroid Association Statement on Remote-Access Thyroid Surgery. Thyroid 2016;26(3):331–7.

10. Kandil EH, Noureldine SI, Yao L, et al. Robotic transaxillary thyroidectomy: an examination of the first one hundred cases. J Am Coll Surg 2012;214(4):558–64 [discussion: 564–6].
11. Lee J, Kwon IS, Bae EH, et al. Comparative analysis of oncological outcomes and quality of life after robotic versus conventional open thyroidectomy with modified radical neck dissection in patients with papillary thyroid carcinoma and lateral neck node metastases. J Clin Endocrinol Metab 2013;98(7):2701–8.
12. Lee SG, Lee J, Kim MJ, et al. Long-term oncologic outcome of robotic versus open total thyroidectomy in PTC: a case-matched retrospective study. Surg Endosc 2016;30(8):3474–9.
13. Bhatia P, Mohamed HE, Kadi A, et al. Remote access thyroid surgery. Gland Surg 2015;4(5):376–87.
14. Kandil E, Noureldine S, Abdel Khalek M, et al. Initial experience using robot-assisted transaxillary thyroidectomy for Graves' disease. J Visc Surg 2011;148(6): e447–51.
15. Noureldine SI, Yao L, Wavekar RR, et al. Thyroidectomy for Graves' disease: a feasibility study of the robotic transaxillary approach. ORL J Otorhinolaryngol Relat Spec 2013;75(6):350–6.
16. Kang SW, Chung WY. Transaxillary single-incision robotic neck dissection for metastatic thyroid cancer. Gland Surg 2015;4(5):388–96.
17. Noureldine SI, Jackson NR, Tufano RP, et al. A comparative North American experience of robotic thyroidectomy in a thyroid cancer population. Langenbecks Arch Surg 2013;398(8):1069–74.
18. Kim MJ, Lee J, Lee SG, et al. Transaxillary robotic modified radical neck dissection: a 5-year assessment of operative and oncologic outcomes. Surg Endosc 2017;31(4):1599–606.
19. Kim MJ, Nam KH, Lee SG, et al. Yonsei experience of 5000 gasless transaxillary robotic thyroidectomies. World J Surg 2018;42(2):393–401.
20. Garstka M, Mohsin K, Ali DB, et al. Well-differentiated thyroid cancer and robotic transaxillary surgery at a North American institution. J Surg Res 2018;228:170–8.
21. Huang S, Garstka M, Murcy M, et al. Somatosensory evoked potential: preventing brachial plexus injury in transaxillary robotic surgery. Laryngoscope, in press.
22. Hinson AM, Kandil E, O'Brien S, et al. Trends in robotic thyroid surgery in the United States from 2009 through 2013. Thyroid 2015;25(8):919–26.

第 11 章
经口内镜甲状腺癌手术

Isariya Jongekkasit, Pornpeera Jitpratoom, Thanyawat Sasanakierkul, Angkoon Anuwong

关键词

- 经口内镜甲状腺手术 • 前庭入路 • TOETVA • 甲状腺癌 • 安全性
- 可行性 • 中央区清扫 • 疗效 • 外科技术

要点

- 前庭入路经口内镜甲状腺切除术（transoral endoscopic thyroidectomy, vestibular approach, TOETVA）与开放手术在疗效和术后并发症上无显著差别，前者美容效果明显。
- TOETVA 可应用于大小不超过 2cm 的低危型分化型甲状腺癌。
- TOETVA 在中央区淋巴结清扫无局限性。
- TOETVA 应用于低危分化型甲状腺癌的长期安全性和可行性结果有待进一步研究。

引言

分化型甲状腺癌（differentiated thyroid cancer, DTC）是最常见的甲状腺癌类型。自 1906 年 Emil Theodor Kocher 开始实施甲状腺手术以来，传统开放甲状腺切除术一直是标准的手术方式[1]。然而，对于罹患群体女性为主的甲状腺癌，开放手术在颈前造成明显瘢痕，给女性患者带来困扰。得益于内镜手术的发展,外科医生可以通过远处入路实施甲状腺手术,从而在颈部不留有瘢痕。过去20年出现了各种各样的远处入路手术方式,然而这些手段依然在非颈部区域造成明显的瘢痕。只有经口内镜甲状腺切除术(transoral endoscopic thyroidectomy,TOET)才能真正称为无瘢痕手术。TOET有各种不同的技术方法,但因为并发症发生率低及手术效果好,TOETVA成为最常用的手术方式[2-7]。

TOETVA 的发展

经自然腔道内镜甲状腺手术概念首先由Witzel及其同事提出[8]。他们在2例尸体和10只活猪上完成了经舌下入路TOET。德国和中国学者尝试了很多不同的经舌下入路TOET手术方式[9],但由于并发症发生率很高,不再被应用于临床。

Richmon及其同事首先报道了口腔前庭入路的方法[10]。他们起初实施的是舌下入路经口机器人辅助甲状腺切除术,后来发现把照相设备移至前庭是更好的方式。Nakajo及其同事[11]完成了8例无充气经口镜头辅助颈部手术。Wang及其同事[6]报道了在12例患者上完成二氧化碳充气前庭入路手术。Nakajo和Wang[6]均报道该术式有引起颏神经损伤的并发症。

Anuwong发表了第一篇关于TOETVA不会造成颏神经损伤和术后并发症发生率低的文章[12],60例患者中无一出现颏神经损伤,仅有2例发生暂时性喉返神经损伤,且在随访期间完全恢复。到目前为止,泰国Police General Hospital实施了超过800例TOETVA,该术式的描述日益完善。

尽管很多文献报道了TOETVA在甲状腺和甲状旁腺疾病应用的安全性和可行性,但还缺乏长期随访结局的文献。TOETVA是目前可选择的一项治疗良恶性甲状腺疾病和甲状旁腺疾病的治疗手段,具有很好的外科疗效和美观效果(图11.1)。

TOETVA 在分化型甲状腺癌中的应用价值

很多文献描述了TOETVA和其他内镜甲状腺切除术应用于良性甲状腺结节的适应证,并得出结论,TOETVA应用于<8~10cm良性甲状腺病变是安全的。然而,实际上在不引起甲状腺被摸撕裂前提下,如果想从2~2.5cm切口取出,甲状腺大小应不超过4cm[13]。随着先进影像技术的应用增加和早期筛

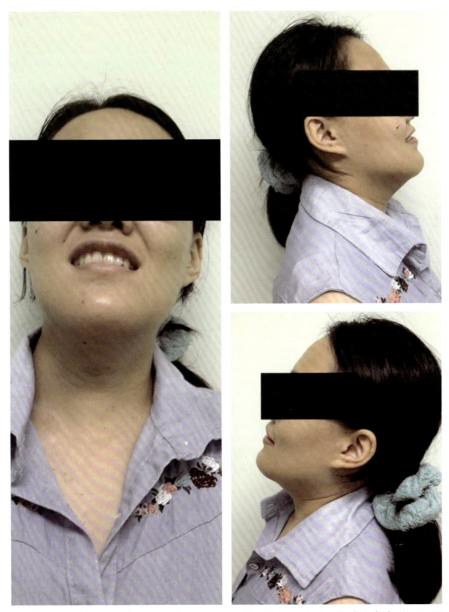

图 11.1　接受 TOETVA 和双颈中央区淋巴结清扫的甲状腺乳头状癌患者术后 7 天颈部外观

术后无并发症,如喉返神经损伤或甲状旁腺功能减低。术后血清 Tg<0.1ng/ml。患者对美容效果满意,颈前区域无瘢痕、无血肿且无擦伤

查,小病灶甲状腺癌的发病率在世界很多地方显著增加,尤其是在亚洲[14-19]。鉴于已知 TOETVA 的局限性和效果及甲状腺疾病自然病史,TOETVA 能够用于治疗小病灶低危 DTC 的治疗。有文献报道表明,TOETVA 可以完成不超过 2cm 的低危型 DTC 的腺叶切除,达到不破坏肿瘤包膜且获取足够病理和肿瘤根治效果的目的[20]。继该文献后,很多文献报道了试图证明 TOETVA 应用于小病灶 DTC 的安全性和可行性,见表 11.1。然而,大部分此类文献是病例系列报道,普遍关注的是术式的新颖性,同时担心肿瘤切除不充分,且缺乏长期随访结果。有几项研究表明,其他经远处入路内镜甲状腺切除术在肿瘤切除的安全性和充分性上与传统开放手术无显著差异。通过比较 TOETVA 系列病例和其他远处入路甲状腺切除病例在术后的血清甲状腺球蛋白水平和术后扫描结果,TOETVA 与其他入路甲状腺切除术在安全性、肿瘤切除充分性上无明显差异[21]。

表 11.1
TOETVA 在甲状腺癌应用的经验

作者,年份	入路	病例数	诊断	手术类型	淋巴结站
Yang 等[38],2015	ETOVA	4	PTC	全甲状腺	中央区清扫
Wang 等[6],2016	TOETVA	10	PTC	腺叶切除	中央区清扫
Anuwong 等[12],2016	TOETVA	2	微小 PTC	腺叶切除	中央区清扫
Dionigi 等[3],2017	TOETVA	2	微小 PTC	腺叶切除	中央区清扫
Wu 等[39],2017	乳腺联合口腔	6	PTC	全甲状腺	中央区清扫
Chai 等[28],2017	TOETVA	10	微小 PTC	腺叶切除	中央区清扫
Anuwong 等[13],2018	TOETVA	26	微小 PTC	腺叶切除	中央区清扫

ETOVA,endoscopic thyroidectomy via oral vestibular approach,口腔前庭入路内镜甲状腺切除术;PTC,pappillary thyroid cancer,甲状腺乳头状癌;TOETVA,transoral endoscopic thyroidectomy,vestibular approach,前庭入路经口内镜甲状腺切除术

较早的研究指出,常规中央区淋巴结清扫(routine central lymph node dissection,RCLD)在 DTC 治疗中很常见,并且对于患者的长期生存率并无益处,但不可否认的是,即使包括<2cm、临床淋巴结阴性的低危甲状腺乳头状癌(papillary thyroid cancer,PTC)的患者在内,也有 80% 至少存在中央区淋巴结的微转移。由于大多数 PTC 生物学行为较为温和、局部复发率低、需要长期的随访(超过 20 年),而且 TOETVA 技术兴起不到 10 年,为了 PTC 患者能够长期获益,笔者推荐对每一位患者均进行 RCLD。喉返神经损伤是不推荐行

RCLD 的主要原因，目前尚无报道说明单侧 TOETVA 会造成永久性喉返神经损伤，因此，我们推荐，应当确保每一位术者行 RCLD[22-27]。在技术方面，开放性甲状腺切除术和 TOETVA 在中央颈淋巴结清扫方面没有显著的差别。最近，Chai 及其同事[28]报道称，在甲状腺乳头状微癌中，进行 TOETVA 中央颈淋巴结清扫出的淋巴结平均数为 2.7±1.7，RLN 均无永久性损伤，7 例患者中仅有 2 例发生了暂时性声带麻痹，并且在 3 个月内全部恢复。

目前，TOETVA 仅在<2cm 的低危 DTC 患者中进行。我们推荐患者通过 TOETVA 行患侧腺叶及峡部的切除术，以减少术后并发症。当患者另一侧腺叶有其他病灶或者患者倾向性选择 TOETVA 的时候，也可以同期通过 TOETVA 行全甲切除以及 RCLD。

TOETVA 的手术方法

适用于 TOETVA 的 DTC 患者选择

TOETVA 适应证：

- 患者是病灶<2cm 的低危 DTC 患者，且影像学上没有包膜外侵犯的证据
- 无颈部手术或放疗史（2 周内或 2 个月以上通过 TOETVA 行补充甲状腺全切术是可行的）

TOETVA 禁忌证：

- 有严重合并症，无法耐受全身麻醉
- 甲状腺髓样癌或未分化癌
- 有侧颈淋巴结受侵证据
- 口腔感染，如脓肿
- 活动性口周和唇部感染，如单纯疱疹病毒感染
- 术前有喉返神经麻痹的证据
- 有颏部硅胶填充物植入史（相对禁忌证）

术前准备

应常规进行术前 B 超定位颈部淋巴结。每位患者均应进行 CT 扫描以明确包膜外侵犯、邻近器官侵犯以及远处转移。术前均应进行纤维喉镜或直接喉镜检查以评估声带功能。数月内如果没有进行口腔检查，则应至口腔诊所进行术前咨询。术前 1 日收治入院。术前给予预防性围手术期抗生素应用

(阿莫西林/克拉维酸1.2g)。

外科技术

患者取仰卧,颈部轻度过伸位。神经检测气管导管经口或经鼻插管。因为大多数外科医生都是右手操作,我们更倾向从左侧进行气管插管,这可以防止器械移动受到限制。无菌巾覆盖上面部。乳头至前额周围的区域用氯己定水溶液消毒。下唇外翻,暴露下前庭。第一个切口在下唇系带与下唇边缘之间距离的2/3处横向、居中切开。第一个切口的长度在1.5~2.5cm,取决于患者甲状腺的大小(图11.2)。使用能量器械切开颏肌至下颌角下缘,以制造颏瓣。将18号Veress气腹针针头穿过第一个切口,将1ml 0.1%肾上腺素溶液和500ml生理盐水注入颈阔肌下平面,称为水性分离。为了完成水性分离,我们通常对每位患者使用约30~50ml的溶液,沿胸锁乳突肌前缘从一侧

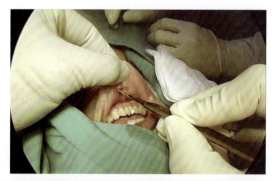

图11.2 摄像头的切口位于下唇内侧到系带距离的2/3

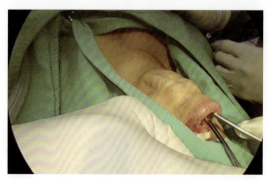

图11.3 使用弯头钳在摄像机端口处扩展隧道。弯头钳的支点应在下巴的尖端,并在颈阔肌下平面扩张隧道

到另一侧再向下到胸骨切迹呈扇形浸润。插入弯血管钳以扩大中心切口。弯钳的支点应放置在下巴的尖端,以达到最佳扩张效果(图 11.3)。钝头剥离棒(Angkoon 剥离棒)插入颈阔肌下平面,沿着浸润区域建腔(图 11.4)。将一根 10mm 的戳卡(Trocar)插入第一个切口,作为摄像头端口。悬挂缝线缝于戳卡头下方 1cm 处,以防止端口前面的皮瓣锐角成角。在口腔前庭的两侧插入两个 5mm 工作戳卡,插入位置位于与切牙假想线成直角的下唇内侧正下方区

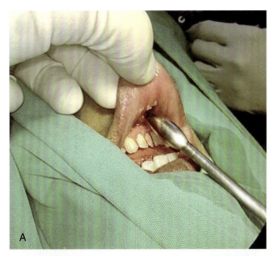

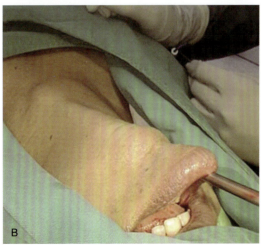

图 11.4　如何应用剥离棒来创建颈阔肌下平面。(A)好的剥离棒的形状头部应接近一个点,但不锋利。(B)如何在两个胸锁乳突肌边界之间以扇形的三个方向使用剥离棒

域内(图 11.5)。再次以与中线切口相同的方式进行水性剥离,但仅向下至下颌骨角水平。两个 5mm 戳卡和摄像头戳卡彼此平行,中间偏差角度很小。我们使用 10mm、30° 的摄像系统。Maryland 分离钳插入两个戳卡中,并在主要术野穿刺纤维组织进入视野。纤维组织也可以通过电灼设备或任何其他类型的血管封闭器械来清除。颈阔肌下间隙延伸到胸锁乳突肌两侧前缘和胸骨切迹。带状肌分离从胸骨切迹至环状软骨水平进行(图 11.6)。从带状肌向甲状腺患侧的侧向分离,至颈动脉鞘为止(图 11.7)。迷走神经通过位于颈动脉鞘外侧的神经监测探针进行监测。即使行全甲切除术,也应使用血管封闭器械来进行峡部切除,以此作为腺体切除的第一步(图 11.8)。我们建议在行峡部切除和 Berry 韧带前半部分切断时,不要超过气管的前 1/3,这样在下一步操作时既保证了腺叶的活动性,又不会引起腺体包膜的意外破裂。可用一额外的横向悬针从外面置入拉开带状肌以获得更好的上极暴露(图 11.9)。当上极暴露完成后,轻柔地分离出甲状腺上动脉、上静脉,把上极的甲状旁腺剥离下

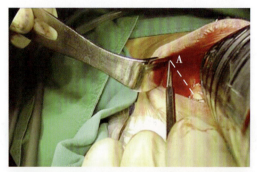

图 11.5　与内唇成直角的切牙假想线,我们在两侧线 A 的末端都放置了 5mm 的戳卡,以防止颏神经受损

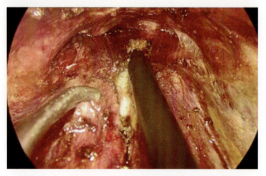

图 11.6　使用 Bovie 电刀于中线分离带状肌

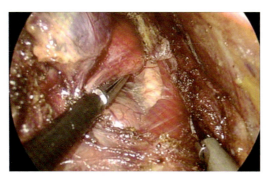

图 11.7　颈动脉是甲状腺的侧向分离的边界。我们在颈动脉的外侧缘测试了迷走神经

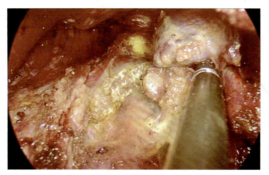

图 11.8　如何完成峡部切除术。我们提起甲状腺，并使用血管封闭器械切开了甲状腺。正确的平面应显示气管前筋膜的白色平面

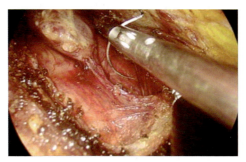

图 11.9　在环状软骨或者上极的水平完成横向悬针

并保留。有时我们能够在这一步看到喉上神经喉外分支(图 11.10),或者也可以通过刺激环甲肌来探查。在保留好上甲状旁腺后,甲状腺上动、静脉分别用血管封切系统或止血夹结扎、横断。夹住甲状腺上极并向上提起有助于显露 Joll space 层面(图 11.11)。

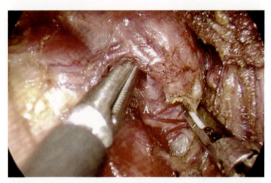

图 11.10　甲状腺上血管与喉上神经(A)外侧分支的关系

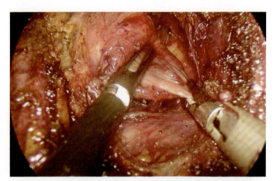

图 11.11　术者左手通过 Joll 空间抓取甲状腺上极,右手通过血管封切系统来控制并分离甲状腺上血管

在横断甲状腺上血管后,下一步是找到喉返神经和下甲状旁腺。找到喉返神经的关键是将正在处理的甲状腺叶拉至另一侧。术中务必在喉返神经入喉处找到喉返神经,并沿其走行向下追踪至甲状腺下极以下(图 11.12)。根据我们的经验,TOETVA 中出现喉不返的概率与传统的开放式甲状腺切除术的发生率相当,为 0~4.76%。术中应当在入喉处的近端和解剖平面的更远端刺激喉返神经,并记录神经信号强度。下甲状旁腺通常位于喉返神经腹侧,在确定并保留喉返神经和下甲状旁腺后,通过血管封切系统从 Berry 韧带上切下患侧甲状腺叶。在此步骤中,我们建议非常小心地将神经和甲状旁腺推离患

侧腺叶,因为与正常的甲状腺相比,这两个结构可能附着更为紧密或具有解剖畸变,因此,我们必须在把患侧甲状腺叶切除干净的同时保证喉返神经与甲状旁腺这两个组织的功能完好。注意不要损伤下方的气管以及神经。为防止横向热量扩散,我们推荐血管密封系统到需保留组织的安全距离为至少 4mm。在完全剥离患侧甲状腺后,将 EndoCatch 袋(标本袋)通过镜头端的戳卡插入,将标本装入袋后与标本袋一起取出,以防止取出时甲状腺包膜破裂。

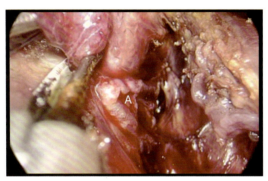

图 11.12 喉返神经(A)从其入喉处沿着甲状腺叶走向胸部

除分离皮瓣的步骤以外,上述的大多数步骤与开放手术无异。中央淋巴结清扫术(central lymph node dissection,CND)的原则也与开放手术相同。在 TOETVA 中,同时进行预防性中央颈清扫术也无任何限制。颈动脉鞘和食道之间的所有脂肪组织和淋巴结都可以顺着喉返神经沿气管和气管食管沟去除。在暴露喉返神经的同时,可沿其走行清扫中央区淋巴结至上纵隔。在判断出甲状旁腺的位置后,上纵隔淋巴结可在切除上胸腺及其周围脂肪组织时一同切除。有时,保留甲状旁腺可能非常困难,因为其与周围脂肪组织或者淋巴结难以区分。因为只处理患侧的甲状腺叶,即使同时损伤了患侧两个甲状旁腺,术后也不一定会导致严重的甲状旁腺功能减退,但仍应重视甲状旁腺的术中保护。我们也可以把怀疑是甲状旁腺的组织送术中快速冰冻,并且在有必要时自体移植回去。中央区淋巴结用一个单独的标本袋取出。

确保在手术结束时止血充分。尽管可以通过在锁骨上方放置另一个 5mm 的戳卡来放置来防出血的情况,但在此手术中几乎不需要引流管。将一 10 号的 Redivac 引流管放入套管针中并且放置在手术床上。于术前与术后分别探测喉返神经与迷走神经的刺激信号强度来确保神经功能的完好。使用 3-0 的鱼骨线连续缝合或者可吸收丝线间断缝合带状肌使其重新靠拢

(图11.13)。使用4-0的可吸收多丝缝合线在颏肌层面缝合中央切口。其他切口在黏膜层及黏膜下层用4-0的可吸收线连续缝合关闭(图11.14)。口腔前庭可用环丁烷溶液冲洗。术后24小时内用几块4cm×4cm的纱布压住颏部(非前颈部)。

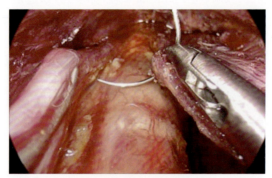

图11.13 在所有标本均已切下并且止血完成后,用4-0的鱼骨线连续缝合带状肌

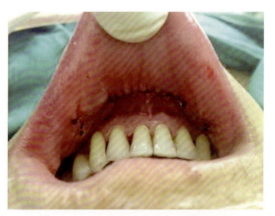

图11.14 术后口腔内的切口缝合关闭

术后护理

通常来说,术后第1周我们建议患者在每天早上、每次进食后,以及每晚睡前用漱口水清洗口腔。可以轻柔地刷牙或者换用较小的儿童牙刷。另外,患者还应当避免过冷或过热的饮品、咳嗽和前颈部按摩。

允许患者在术后立即使用吸管进水(术后第0天)。术后镇痛通常可使用对乙酰氨基酚。在术后第 1 天,患者可在清晨进流食,在晚上进质软食物。在使用口腔镇痛药物充分镇痛并且无发热的情况下,可允许患者出院[29]。

术后并发症以及术后生活质量

术后最重要的并发症是感染,因为手术可能会把口腔中的污染物带进颈部的洁净区。在相关文献回顾中,尚无经口前庭疗法感染的报告。

TOETVA 与开放手术相比,其他术后并发症,比如喉返神经损伤、甲状旁腺功能减退和出血,发生的概率并没有显著差异。同时,腔镜没有限制术中喉返神经监测器械的使用以及用于识别甲状旁腺的吲哚菁绿注射[6,30-33]。Chai 及其同事[28]报道了一系列采用 TOETVA 的 DTC 病例结果。其中 0 例发生术后出血、颏神经损伤、和永久性声带麻痹。10 例中仅有 2 例出现由喉镜证实的一过性声带麻痹,并且在 3 个月中缓解。

据一些研究报道,其他入路的内镜甲状腺手术术后疼痛比开放手术要严重,鉴于皮瓣分离范围要更长、更广。Ha 及其同事[34]对开放甲状腺切除术、无充气内镜下甲状腺切除术,以及机器人腋窝入路的术后颈部疼痛进行了队列研究。按照有无颈部疼痛分类,研究者发现内镜和机器人手术的术后颈部疼痛要比开放手术严重($P=0.026$)。然而三组间的疼痛评分没有显著差异($P=0.2$)。TOETVA 和其他内镜入路相比,其路径最短,皮瓣分离面积最小;与开放手术相比,仅多出了颈部的皮瓣分离。Anuwong 及其同事[4]报道,术后第 1、2、3 天平均疼痛评分分别为 $2.41 \pm 2.04^{[2-7]}$,1.17 ± 1.4,0.47 ± 0.83。

毫无疑问,内镜下甲状腺切除术和开放手术的手术疗效是一致的。正因如此,一切内镜手术的目的应该集中在患者术后的满意程度上。术后生活质量是一个不得不提的方面。和开放手术相比,内镜手术的甲状腺乳头状癌患者在术后 1 个月的情绪功能恢复($P=0.039$)和术后 3 个月的生理功能恢复($P=0.042$)上都有明显提高[35,36]。

随访和监测

根据 2015 年版美国甲状腺协会指南,随访和监测取决于患者进行的是 TOETVA 全切除还是 TOETVA 部分切除,以及患者最初所属的复发风险分层(图 11.15)。

所有患者必须每 6~12 个月做 1 次颈部超声,具体间隔时间取决于复发风险和甲状腺球蛋白水平(表 11.2)。对没有进行 TOETVA 的低危组患者而言,促甲状腺激素必须维持在较低水平(0.5~2mU/L)。如果患者能够维持血清促甲状腺激素在这个目标范围内,那就不一定需要甲状腺激素治疗。

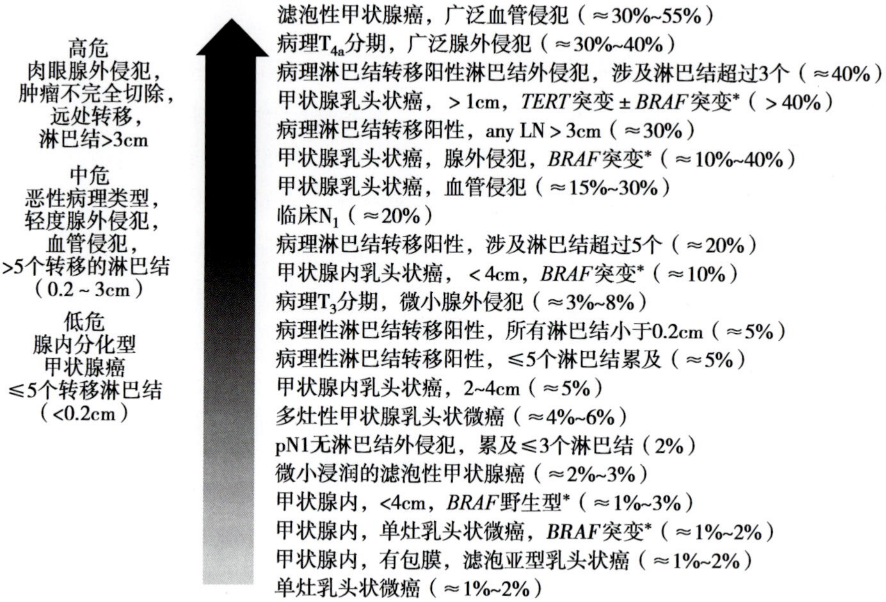

高危
肉眼腺外侵犯,
肿瘤不完全切除,
远处转移,
淋巴结>3cm

中危
恶性病理类型,
轻度腺外侵犯,
血管侵犯,
>5个转移的淋巴结
(0.2~3cm)

低危
腺内分化型
甲状腺癌
≤5个转移淋巴结
(<0.2cm)

滤泡性甲状腺癌,广泛血管侵犯(≈30%~55%)
病理T_{4a}分期,广泛腺外侵犯(≈30%~40%)
病理淋巴结转移阳性淋巴结外侵犯,涉及淋巴结超过3个(≈40%)
甲状腺乳头状癌,>1cm,*TERT*突变 ± *BRAF*突变*(>40%)
病理淋巴结转移阳性,any LN >3cm(≈30%)
甲状腺乳头状癌,腺外侵犯,*BRAF*突变*(≈10%~40%)
甲状腺乳头状癌,血管侵犯(≈15%~30%)
临床N_1(≈20%)
病理淋巴结转移阳性,涉及淋巴结超过5个(≈20%)
甲状腺乳头状癌,<4cm,*BRAF*突变*(≈10%)
病理T_3分期,微小腺外侵犯(≈3%~8%)
病理性淋巴结转移阳性,所有淋巴结小于0.2cm(≈5%)
病理性淋巴结转移阳性,≤5个淋巴结累及(≈5%)
甲状腺乳头状癌,2~4cm(≈5%)
多灶性甲状腺乳头状微癌(≈4%~6%)
pN1无淋巴结外侵犯,累及≤3个淋巴结(2%)
微小浸润的滤泡性甲状腺癌(≈2%~3%)
甲状腺内,<4cm,*BRAF*野生型*(≈1%~3%)
甲状腺内,单灶乳头状微癌,*BRAF*突变*(≈1%~2%)
甲状腺内,有包膜,滤泡亚型乳头状癌(≈1%~2%)
单灶乳头状微癌(≈1%~2%)

图 11.15 疾病复发风险分层

*尽管不建议在最初分层时常规检测 *BRAF* 和/或 *TERT* 突变情况,但 2015 年版美国甲状腺协会指南仍然归纳了以上要点来帮助临床医生在手中有相关资料的情况下完成复发风险分层
Data from Haugen BR, Alexander EK, Bible KC, et al. 2015 American Thyroid Association management guidelines for adult patients with thyroid nodules and differentiated thyroid cancer. Thyroid 2016;26(1):1-133.

表 11.2
按美国甲状腺协会复发危险分层进行不同的术后随访项目

检查项目	6 个月	12 个月	18 个月	24 个月
甲状腺球蛋白	全部*	全部*	全部*	全部*
颈部超声	-	全部*	-	全部*
诊断性放射性碘扫描	-	-	中危	-
CT/MRI	-	高危	-	高危
PET 扫描	-	高危	-	高危

*全部:低危、中危和高危患者

Data from Momesso DP, Tuttle RM. Update on differentiated thyroid cancer staging. Endocrinol Metab Clin North Am 2014;43(2):401-21.

对进行了 TOETVA 全切除的患者，要随访血清甲状腺球蛋白水平，并且在术后进行诊断性的放射性碘全身扫描。如果摄取活性较高，但是没有大量疑似残留甲状腺，建议使用低剂量（30mCi，1Ci=3.7×10^{10}Bq）的放射性碘。不推荐低危组 DTC 患者常规进行清甲。血清甲状腺球蛋白和促甲状腺激素可用作随访的标志物。甲状腺球蛋白不可测的（＜0.2ng/ml）低危组患者，促甲状腺激素应该维持在参考范围的低值（0.5~2mU/L）。但是血清甲状腺球蛋白可测得但处于较低水平的低危患者，促甲状腺激素应该维持在下限或以下（0.1~0.5mU/L）[37]。具体的疗效评估细节将在后文中展开。

TOETVA 补充甲状腺全切除手术

再次手术有时候比较困难，而且由于组织修复的原因，术后并发症的发生概率更高。对所有器官而言（也包括甲状腺），最佳的再次手术时间段为术后 6 周之后或 2 周之内。在最初的 2 周内，手术难度没有增加，分离时粘连不明显，能得到较好的手术结果，没有其他并发症，比如喉返神经损伤、甲状旁腺功能减退[2]。因为 DTC 的发展缓慢，腺叶切除后若有必要进行全甲切除，则全甲切除手术可以推迟 6 周，而疾病的自然进程不会有改变。

讨论

TOETVA 是一种全新的手术方式，能够提供最佳的美容效果。许多研究都证实了这个术式用于良性和恶性肿瘤的安全性和可行性。鉴于这个手术方式近期才出现，仍缺乏长期的随访结果，这种术式用于肿瘤治疗的可靠性仍然需要更多的病例和长期随访来明确，而本章从肿瘤学上展示了其充满安全性和可行性的未来。

（王 宇　嵇庆海）

参考文献

1. Hannan SA. The magnificent seven. Int J Surg 2006;4:187–91.
2. Jitpratoom P, Ketwong K, Sasanakietkul T, et al. Transoral endoscopic thyroidec-

tomy vestibular approach (TOETVA) for Graves' disease: a comparison of surgical results with open thyroidectomy. Gland Surg 2016;5(6):546–52.
3. Dionigi G, Lavazza M, Bacuzzi A, et al. Transoral endoscopic thyroidectomy vestibular approach (TOETVA): from A to Z. Surg Technol Int 2017;30:103–12.
4. Anuwong A, Sasanakietkul T, Jitpratoom P, et al. Transoral endoscopic thyroidectomy vestibular approach (TOETVA): indications, techniques and results. Surg Endosc 2018;32(1):456–65.
5. Le QV, Ngo DQ, Ngo QX. Transoral endoscopic thyroidectomy vestibular approach (TOETVA): a case report as new technique in thyroid surgery in Vietnam. Int J Surg Case Rep 2018;50:60–3.
6. Wang Y, Yu X, Wang P, et al. Implementation of intraoperative neuromonitoring for transoral endoscopic thyroid surgery: a preliminary report. J Laparoendosc Adv Surg Tech A 2016;26(12):965–71.
7. Yi JW, Yoon SG, Kim HS, et al. Transoral endoscopic surgery for papillary thyroid carcinoma: initial experiences of a single surgeon in South Korea. Ann Surg Treat Res 2018;95(2):73–9.
8. Witzel K, von Rahden BH, Kaminski C, et al. Transoral access for endoscopic thyroid resection. Surg Endosc 2008;22:1871–5.
9. Karakas E, Steinfeldt T, Gockel A, et al. Transoralparathyroid sugery, a new alternative or non sense? Langenbecks Arch Surg 2014;399:7415.
10. Richmon JD, Pattani KM, Benhidjeb T, et al. Transoral robotic assisted thyroidectomy a preclinical feasibility study in 2 cadavers. Head Neck 2011;33:330–3.
11. Nakajo A, Arima H, Hirata M, et al. Transoral video-assisted neck surgery (TOVANS). A new transoral technique of endoscopic thyroidectomy with gasless premandible approach. Surg Endosc 2013;27:1105–10.
12. Anuwong A. Transoral endoscopic thyroidectomy vestibular approach: a series of the first 60 human cases. World J Surg 2016;40:491–7.
13. Anuwong A, Ketwong K, Jitpratoom P, et al. Safety and outcomes of the transoral endoscopic thyroidectomy vestibular approach. JAMA Surg 2018;153(1):21–7.
14. Park S, Oh CM, Cho H, et al. Association between screening and the thyroid cancer "epidemic" in South Korea: evidence from a nationwide study. BMJ 2016;355:i5745.
15. Davies L, Welch HG. Increasing incidence of thyroid cancer in the United states, 1973-2002. JAMA 2006;295:2164–7.
16. Kitahara CM, Sosa JA. The changing incidence of thyroid cancer. Nat Rev Endocrinol 2016;12(11):646–53.
17. Lim H, Devesa SS, Sosa JA, et al. Trends in thyroid cancer incidence and mortality in the United States, 1974-2013. JAMA 2017;317(13):1338–48.
18. La Vecchia C, Malvezzi M, Bosetti C, et al. Thyroid cancer mortality and incidence: a global overview. Int J Cancer 2015;136(9):2187–95.
19. Wiltshire JJ, Drake TM, Uttley L, et al. Systematic review of trends in the incidence rates of thyroid cancer. Thyroid 2016;26(11):1541–52.
20. Wu YJ, Chi SY, Elsarawy A, et al. What is the appropriate nodular diameter in thyroid cancer for extraction by transoral endoscopic thyroidectomy vestibular approach without breaking the specimens? A surgicopathologic study. Surg Laparosc Endosc Percutan Tech 2018. https://doi.org/10.1097/SLE.0000000000000563.
21. Razavi CR, Tufano RP, Russell JO. Completion thyroidectomy via the transoral endoscopic vestibular approach. Gland Surg 2018;7(Suppl 1):S77–9.

22. Agrawal N, Evasovich MR, Kandil E, et al. Indications and extent of central neck dissection for papillary thyroid cancer: an American Head and Neck Society Consensus Statement. Head Neck 2017;39(7):1269–79.
23. Gambardella C, Tartaglia E, Nunziata A, et al. Clinical significance of prophylactic central compartment neck dissection in the treatment of clinically node-negative papillary thyroid cancer patients. World J Surg Oncol 2016;14(1):247.
24. Deutschmann MW, Chin-Lenn L, Au J, et al. Extent of central neck dissection among thyroid cancer surgeons: cross-sectional analysis. Head Neck 2016; 38(Suppl 1):E328–32.
25. Chinn SB, Zafereo ME, Waguespack SG, et al. Long-term outcomes of lateral neck dissection in patients with recurrent or persistent well-differentiated thyroid cancer. Thyroid 2017;27(10):1291–9.
26. Lee YC, Na SY, Park GC, et al. Occult lymph node metastasis and risk of regional recurrence in papillary thyroid cancer after bilateral prophylactic central neck dissection: a multi-institutional study. Surgery 2017;161(2):465–71.
27. Zhao W, You L, Hou X, et al. The effect of prophylactic central neck dissection on locoregional recurrence in papillary thyroid cancer after total thyroidectomy: a systematic review and meta-analysis: pCND for the locoregional recurrence of papillary thyroid cancer. Ann Surg Oncol 2017;24(8):2189–98.
28. Chai YJ, Chung JK, Anuwong A, et al. Transoral endoscopic thyroidectomy for papillary thyroid microcarcinoma: initial experience of a single surgeon. Ann Surg Treat Res 2017;93(2):70–5.
29. Anuwong A, Kim HY, Dionigi G. Transoral endoscopic thyroidectomy using vestibular approach: updates and evidence. Gland Surg 2017;6(3):277–84.
30. Vidal Fortuny J, Belfontali V, Sadowski SM, et al. Parathyroid gland angiography with indocyanine green fluorescence to predict parathyroid function after thyroid surgery. Br J Surg 2016;103(5):537–43.
31. Zaidi N, Bucak E, Yazici P, et al. The feasibility of indocyanine green fluorescence imaging for identifying and assessing the perfusion of parathyroid glands during total thyroidectomy. J Surg Oncol 2016;113(7):775–8.
32. Yu HW, Chung JW, Yi JW, et al. Intraoperative localization of the parathyroid glands with indocyanine green and Firefly(R) technology during BABA robotic thyroidectomy. Surg Endosc 2017;31(7):3020–7.
33. Lavazza M, Liu X, Wu C, et al. Indocyanine green-enhanced fluorescence for assessing parathyroid perfusion during thyroidectomy. Gland Surg 2016;5(5): 512–21.
34. Ha TK, Kim DQ, Park HK, et al. Comparison of postoperative neck pain and discomfort, swallowing difficulty, and voice change after conventional open, endoscopic, and robotic thyroidectomy: a single-center cohort study. Front Endocrinol (Lausanne) 2018;9(418):1–6.
35. Lee MC, Park H, Lee BC, et al. Comparison of quality of life between open and endoscopic thyroidectomy for papillary thyroid cancer. Head Neck 2016;3: E827–31.
36. Wang LY, Ganly I. Nodal metastases in thyroid cancer: prognostic implication and management. Future Oncol 2016;12(7):981–94.
37. Haugen BR, Alexander EK, Bible KC, et al. 2015 American Thyroid Association Management guidelines for adult patients with thyroid nodules and differentiated thyroid cancer. Thyroid 2016;26(1):1–133.
38. Yang J, Wang C, Li J, et al. Complete endoscopic thyroidectomy via oral vestib-

ular approach versus areola approach for treatment of thyroid diseases. J Laparoendosc Adv Surg Tech A 2015;25(6):470–6.
39. Wu GY, Fu JB, Lin FS, et al. Endoscopic central lymph node dissection via breast combined with oral approach for papillary thyroid carcinoma: a preliminary study. World J Surg 2017;41(9):2280–2.

第 12 章
分化型甲状腺癌的常规放射性碘治疗

Dorina Ylli, Douglas Van Nostrand, Leonard Wartofsky

关键词

- 放射碘 • 甲状腺癌 • 治疗 • 定义 • 适应证 • 剂量 • 剂量学
- 重组人 TSH

要点

- 放射性碘消融术、放射性碘辅助治疗或碘 -131 治疗是分化良好的甲状腺癌患者疗法中不可或缺的一部分,其治疗剂量可以通过经验剂量法或计算剂量法来决定。
- 重组人促甲状腺激素可用于检测复发 / 残留的甲状腺癌并有助于放射性碘消融,能够替代甲状腺激素撤除,且安全有效。
- 治疗团队应充分了解各种治疗甲状腺癌的方法,并考虑其是否对放射碘剂量有影响,在此基础上再制订最佳的个性化治疗方案。

引言

自 1946 年首次报道甲状腺癌的放射性碘(碘 -131)治疗后[1],放射性碘(radioactive iodine,RAI)就一直被公认为治疗分化良好甲状腺癌(well-differentiated thyroid cancer,WDTC)患者的重要方法。本章的目的是概述放射性碘在 WDTC 治疗中的应用。本章内容如下:①定义;②分期;③选择放射性碘剂量的两种主要方法;④放射性碘消融术、放射性碘辅助治疗或碘 -131

治疗各自的目标;⑤放射性碘消融术、放射性碘辅助治疗或碘-131治疗的适应证;⑥美国甲状腺协会(American Thyroid Association,ATA)和核医学与分子影像学会的指南中所包含的放射性碘治疗的应用建议;⑦重组人促甲状腺激素(recombination human thyroid-stimulation hormone,rhTSH)在放射性碘治疗中的应用;⑧ MedStar 华盛顿医疗中心使用碘-131治疗的方法。

定义

鉴于世界各地的术语差异,以下几个术语的使用定义如下:"放射性碘消融术"是指使用碘-131破坏正常的残留功能性甲状腺组织,其目的是:①有助于解释随后血清甲状腺球蛋白(thyroglobulin,Tg)的水平;②在后续 RAI 全身扫描中提高检测局部区域和/或转移性疾病的敏感性;③使后续碘-131治疗疗效最大化;④有助于消融后扫描发现消融前扫描未发现的其他部位的病灶[2,3]。

"放射性碘辅助治疗"是使用碘-131消灭未知的微小甲状腺癌和/或可疑但未经证实的残留甲状腺癌,从而有可能降低甲状腺癌的复发率和死亡率[2,3]。

"碘-131治疗"是使用碘-131破坏已知的局部和/或远处转移,以达到潜在治愈、降低甲状腺癌的复发率和死亡率和/或疾病缓解的目的[2,3]。

"放射性碘-131治疗"这个术语的使用可能会引起混淆,该术语通常用于泛指残甲消融、辅助治疗或已知的局部或远处转移灶的治疗。尽管许多医生可能认为上述区分是不必要的,但作者认为,术语的区别使用有助于表达时间和治疗的主要目的,并有助于指南的制定和应用。在本文中,剂量(dosage)是指以毫居里(mCi)或贝克勒尔(Bq)为单位的放射性碘的用量,该术语可以与术语"活性"互换使用。术语"剂量"应保留,以表示辐射到器官或肿瘤的吸收剂量,以拉德(rad)或戈瑞(Gy)表示。

分期

当前存在众多分期系统:AMES 系统(年龄、转移灶、肿瘤范围和肿瘤大小),TNM 系统(肿瘤、淋巴结、远处转移),俄亥俄州评分系统,AGES 系统(年龄、组织学等级、肿瘤的范围和大小),MACIS 系统(转移、年龄、切除的完整性、侵袭和肿瘤大小),以及 NTCTCS(美国甲状腺癌治疗合作研究)系统。TNM

系统由美国癌症联合委员会（American Joint Commission on Cancer, AJCC）开发并被纳入 ATA WDTC 管理指南。需要注意的是，在最近的第 8 版 AJCC 癌症分期手册中，TNM 系统有所改变[4,5]。主要变化包括：①将诊断时的年龄界限从 45 岁提高到 55 岁；②从 T_3 的定义中去除局部淋巴结转移和镜下甲状腺外扩散。这些变化预计会下调大量患者的疾病分期，并很可能被纳入下一轮 ATA 指南中[4,5]。

用于放射性碘消融术、放射性碘辅助治疗或碘 -131 治疗的放射性碘剂量（活性）选择

放射性碘的剂量可以通过以下两种方法中的一种来选择：经验剂量法或计算剂量法（图 12.1）。经验剂量法是指根据医生的经验使用固定剂量的放射性碘，这种剂量已经使用了数十年[6-16]，由医生对各种因素的权重进行微调，例如：①使用目的（消融、辅助治疗或碘 -131 治疗）；②肿瘤范围；③组织学分级；④患者年龄；⑤是否存在远处转移；⑥患者是儿童还是成人（框 12.1）。图 12.2 描述了几种用于选择碘 -131 剂量治疗转移性 WDTC[6-12]的经验性方法。

经验剂量法的优点包括：①易于选择剂量；②使用历史悠久；③并发症发生频率和严重程度在可接受范围。因为给药时没有进行治疗前诊断性扫描，另一个潜在的优势是可以避免诊断性使用碘 -131 后继发顿抑的可能性。然而，在给予经验性固定剂量之前改变治疗方法时，关于顿抑的概念以及消融前或治疗前扫描的价值都存在争议。尽管对这些争议的充分讨论不在本章讨论范围之内，但可以说，通过使用碘 -123 或将碘 -131 活性剂量降低至 1~2mCi（0.037~0.074GBq），可以消除或降低顿抑的风险[17]。作者认为，经验性方法的主要缺点是不能确定该剂量是否有治疗作用和 / 或是否会超过关键器官（如骨髓）的辐射剂量阈值。换言之，经验性固定剂量法就其本质而言，并不能确定导致肿瘤死亡的最小有效放射性碘剂量，也无法确定患者可以耐受的最大安全剂量。另一个潜在的局限性是，当经验剂量不够有效且需要一个或更多个后续剂量时，随着时间的推移，这样的多个经验固定剂量总和的疗效可能不及一次性给予总剂量相同的放射性碘，因为分次剂量会降低剂量率（rad/h）。同时，先前的非致死剂量可能会降低后续剂量的有效性。

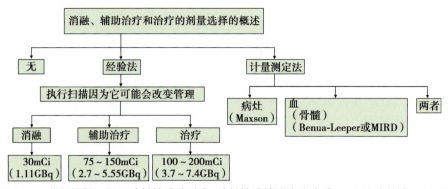

图 12.1 此图概括了用于放射性碘消融术、放射性碘辅助治疗或碘-131 治疗的碘-131 剂量选择的各种方法

框 12.1
影响放射性碘消融术、放射性碘辅助治疗或碘-131 治疗中放射性碘剂量选择的多种因素

- 分期（或者风险）
- 方便性
- 成本
- 设备
- 政府法规
- 年龄
- 组织学
- 手术范围
- 残留甲状腺组织摄碘百分数
- 残留甲状腺组织体积
- 残留甲状腺组织中碘-131 的有效半衰期
- 残留甲状腺组织的几何形状
- 患者对低碘饮食的依从性
- TSH 水平
- 转移的位置（例如，肺部、骨骼、脑部）
- 转移数目
- 转移的大小
- 受累器官数量
- 继发转移的患者体征和症状
- 放射性碘的吸收
- 疾病的放射学证据（例如胸部 X 线片和/或 CT 上的肺内大结节与肺内微小结节）
- 手术切除的可能性
- 转移对先前任何放射性碘治疗的反应（例如体格检查、放射性碘扫描、胸部 X 线片、CT、MRI、超声和/或血清 Tg 水平）

续表

- 放射性碘的总累积剂量
- 基线全血细胞计数和差异预处理，尤其注意粒细胞、淋巴细胞和血小板
- 先前治疗后 3~6 周内绝对中性粒细胞和血小板计数的反应
- 先前治疗后基线绝对中性粒细胞和血小板计数的变化
- 治疗前的肺功能检查结果
- 自上次治疗以来肺功能检查的变化
- 用于评估的骨髓活检（不是转移灶，而是用于评估骨髓中的细胞百分比和脂肪组织百分比）
- 伴随疾病
- 患者的需求

计算剂量学方法可以通过病灶和/或全身剂量学（whole-body dosimetry，WBD）确定。Maxon 等人[18] 及 Thomas 等人[19] 所述的病灶剂量测定法是根据破坏转移病灶所需的辐射吸收剂量所确定的放射碘剂量。基于病灶的计算剂量法的优点是：①选择并给予更高剂量的放射性碘具有更大的杀灭肿瘤作用，可能改善治疗结果；②给予更低、更安全的放射性碘剂量具有一定的肿瘤杀伤作用且减少不良反应；③避免无法获得肿瘤杀伤剂量时的不必要开支和不良反应。缺点包括：①增加了进行剂量测定的成本和不便；②进行剂量测定的设备数量有限。

Benua 和 Leeper[20] 所述的全身剂量学（WBD）试图确定向关键器官传递最大耐受剂量（maximum tolerable dose，MTD）的最大耐受活度（maximum allowable activity，MTA），以防止或减少不可接受的不良事件。最大耐受剂量（MTA）通常是指血液的吸收剂量为 200rad（2Gy），可作为骨髓吸收剂量的替代。医学内照射辐射剂量法已建议将血液吸收剂量 300rad（3Gy）作为最大耐受剂量（MTD）[21]。全身剂量学的优点：①根据最大耐受剂量确定每个患者放射碘的最大耐受活度；②找出高达 20% 的最大耐受活度低于经验固定剂量的患者，否则这些患者可能会被给予超出耐受范围的经验固定剂量[22,23]；③相对于多次小剂量的分次给予，对转移灶给予单次高出 1 倍的放射吸收剂量时具有良好的安全性；④使用历史悠久；⑤与远处转移性部位和严重程度相关的合理的并发症风险。其局限性包括：①增加成本和不便；②因无法准确评估转移灶的吸收剂量而可能在无效的情况下给予最大耐受活度；③诊断剂量碘 -131 可能会引起顿抑；④无法测量除血液以外的器官（例如唾液腺）的最大耐受剂量；⑤进行剂量测定的设施数量有限。为了增加剂量测定的核医学中心的数量，简化的剂量测定方法已经被提出[24-27]。

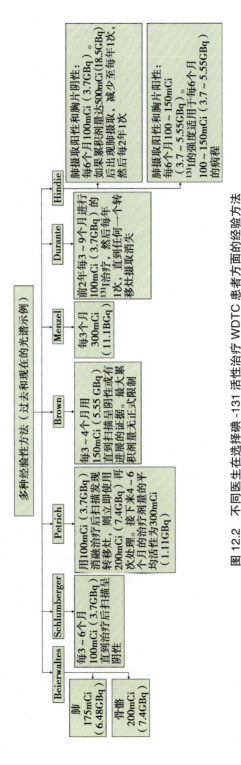

图 12.2 不同医生在选择碘 -131 活性治疗 WDTC 患者方面的经验方法

Adapted from Nostrand D.131-I treatment for distant metastases. In: Wartofsky L, Van Nostrand D, editors. Thyroid cancer: a comprehensive guide to clinical management. 3rd edition. New York: Springer; 2016.p.619; with permission.

与经验疗法相比,尚不清楚计算剂量法是否能提供更好的治疗结局。当仅以消融为目的时,经验剂量破坏残留甲状腺组织的效果应能令人满意。但是,当需要辅助治疗或治疗时,关于经验剂量法和计算剂量法中谁更有效仍存在争议。Klubo-Gwiezdzinska 及其同事[28]已经证明,在局部病灶患者中,接受计算剂量法治疗的患者比接受经验治疗的患者具有更高的完全缓解率。另一方面,Deandreis 及其同事[29]得出结论,经验剂量法和常规使用的全身/血液清除剂量法在总体生存率上没有差异。现有的 ATA 和 SNMMI(Society of Nuclear Medicine and Molecular Imaging,核医学与分子影像学协会)指南尚不支持某种方法优于其他方法[2,30]。但是在骨髓储备降低或肾功能受损等情况下,SNMMI 建议进行剂量测定,以确保达到病灶所需的最高碘-131 剂量的同时,骨髓少于 2Sv(200rem)的照射剂量[30]。SNMMI 推荐在碘-131 用量超过 200mCi 和 55 岁以上患者中进行剂量学测定[30]。

遗憾的是,很难对 WDTC 患者进行经验剂量法和计算剂量法比较的对照良好的前瞻性试验。在获得更多数据之前,医生应了解这两种方法的利弊,并选择一种最适合患者的方法。

放射性碘消融术、放射性碘辅助治疗或碘 -131 治疗的目的

放射性碘消融的多个目标已经被提出,其中包括:①提高后续放射性碘扫描检测转移性疾病的敏感性;②利于后续 Tg 水平的解释;③有可能治疗残余的术后镜下肿瘤;④降低复发率;⑤提高生存率;⑥获得比诊断扫描更敏感的消融后全身扫描结果。ATA 指南指出,消融是"为通过 Tg 和全身放射性碘扫描检测复发性疾病和初步分期提供便利"。辅助治疗的目的是"通过理论上破坏可疑但未经证实的残留疾病来提高无病生存率,特别适用于疾病复发风险较高的患者"[2]。但 SNMMI 指出,其目标是"消除甲状腺切除术后残留的正常组织和假定的残留癌组织"[30]。碘 -131 治疗的目标仍然是"通过治疗高风险患者的持续性疾病来改善疾病特异性生存和无疾病生存"[2]。消融和辅助治疗之间的显著区别已被欧洲核医学协会认可[31]。

放射性碘消融和辅助治疗的适应证

ATA 和 SNMMI 已发布了各自关于消融和辅助治疗指征指南[2,30]。ATA 建议基于 AJCC TNM 分期系统和分层风险,而 SNMMI 则建议基于分期,两个

协会的建议比较见表 12.1。

总之，ATA 指南对消融和辅助治疗进行了明确区分，建议仅在出现不良特征时才对低危患者使用消融，而对中高危患者使用辅助治疗。SNMMI 在消融和辅助治疗之间没有区分，建议对具有高风险特征的 <1cm 的肿瘤和 >1cm 的所有肿瘤中进行消融。

表 12.1
美国甲状腺协会和核医学与分子影像学指南中有关放射性碘消融和辅助治疗的指征

分期/风险分层	建议
ATA 指南	
ATA 低危分化型甲状腺癌患者	甲状腺切除术后不建议行常规 RAI 消融术[a]（推荐率低，证据质量低）
没有其他不良特征的单灶性乳头状微小癌	不建议使用常规 RAI 消融（强烈推荐，证据质量中等）
没有其他不良特征的多灶性乳头状微小癌	不建议行常规 RAI 消融术[a]（推荐率低，证据质量低）
ATA 中危分化型甲状腺癌	应考虑使用 RAI 辅助治疗（推荐率低，证据质量低）
ATA 高危患者	建议进行常规 RAI 辅助治疗（强烈推荐，证据质量中等）
核医学与分子影像学会指南	
最大肿瘤直径 >1cm 的患者	建议进行 RAI 消融
最大肿瘤直径 <1cm 的高危患者[b]	建议进行 RAI 消融
极低危和低危甲状腺癌	RAI 治疗存在争议

[a] 不同的复发风险、疾病随访和患者偏好的特征与 RAI 决策有关；

[b] 侵袭性组织学（丘脑细胞、岛状、弥漫性硬化、高细胞、柱状细胞、小梁、实性和分化差的乳头状癌亚型）、淋巴或血管浸润、淋巴结或远处转移、多灶性疾病、包膜浸润或穿透、甲状腺周围软组织受累，或甲状腺切除术后抗甲状腺球蛋白抗体水平升高（以便可以通过闪烁显像进行监测）

Adapted from Haugen BR, Alexander EK, Bible KC, et al. 2015 American Thyroid Association management guidelines for adult patients with thyroid nodules and differentiated thyroid cancer: the American Thyroid Association guidelines task force on thyroid nodules and differentiated thyroid cancer. Thyroid 2016;26(1):1-133; and Silberstein EB, Alavi A, Balon HR, et al. The SNMMI practice guideline for therapy of thyroid disease with 131I 3.0. J Nucl Med 2012;53(10):1633-51, with permission.

放射性碘治疗的适应证

ATA 和 SNMMI 关于碘 -131 治疗局灶性疾病、肺转移、骨转移、脑转移的指南比较见表 12.2。

表 12.2
ATA、SNMMI 指南中有关放射性碘治疗的适应证

局部疾病		
	ATA	RAI 可用于小病灶的患者,或在大病灶情况下与手术联合使用
	SNMMI	晚期局部病灶或淋巴结转移可以先进行手术治疗,然后再用碘 -131 治疗。一般来说,碘 -131 治疗对于直径>1~2cm 的大块疾病效果较差
远处转移		
	ATA	肺转移 ①肺微小转移:只要病灶继续摄取 RAI 并在临床上有效,建议每 6~12 个月进行 RAI 治疗(强烈推荐,中等质量的证据) ②肺部大结节转移:可以用 RAI 进行治疗,并在证明有客观益处(病变体积减小,Tg 降低)时重复治疗(推荐强度低,证据质量低)
		骨转移 在病灶摄碘的骨转移瘤中,应该使用 RAI 疗法,尽管治愈率很低(强烈推荐,中等质量的证据)
		脑转移 手术切除和 EBRT(外照射放疗)是治疗中枢神经系统转移瘤的主要手段。病灶摄碘的中枢神经系统转移可以考虑 RAI 治疗;在这种情况下,在 RAI 治疗之前推荐立体定向外照射放疗并伴随糖皮质激素治疗(推荐力度较弱,证据质量较低)
	SNMMI	建议使用 RAI 治疗远处转移。骨髓的辐射剂量通常是限制因素。在高活性碘 -131 的情况下,在 50~55 岁以上的患者中,特别是在肾小球滤过率降低且肺转移可能摄取大量碘 -131 的情况下,可以进行剂量测定
无明显的结构性病变		
	ATA	如果没有明显的结构性疾病,甲状腺激素停药后血清 Tg<10g/ml,或使用 rhTSH 时血清 Tg<5ng/ml,则无须进行经验性 RAI 治疗即可随访患者(推荐度低,证据质量低)
		对于影像学检查[解剖学颈部/胸部影像学检查和/或[^{18}F]- 氟代脱氧葡萄糖(^{18}F-FDG)-PET/CT]未能揭示肿瘤来源,但是血清 Tg 水平显著升高,或血清 Tg 水平快速升高,或 TgAb 水平升高的患者,可以考虑采用 RAI 定向治疗

续表

ATA	如果给予经验性 RAI 治疗,且治疗后扫描结果为阴性,则患者应被认为患有 RAI 难治性疾病,不应再接受 RAI 治疗(推荐力度较弱,证据质量较低)
SNMMI	在没有 TgAb 的情况下,升高的血清 Tg 水平或血清 Tg 水平快速升高可能是经验性 RAI 治疗的指征

ATA,美国甲状腺协会;CNS,中枢神经系统;SNMMI,核医学和分子影像学会

Adapted from Haugen BR, Alexander EK, Bible KC, et al.2015 American thyroid association management guidelines for adult patients with thyroid nodules and differentiated thyroid cancer: The American thyroid association guidelines task force on thyroid nodules and differentiated thyroid cancer. Thyroid 2016;26(1):1-133; and Silberstein EB, Alavi A, Balon HR, et al. The SNMMI practice guideline for therapy of thyroid disease with 131I 3.0. J Nucl Med 2012;53(10):1633-51, with permission

消融、辅助治疗和治疗的放射性碘剂量选择

ATA 和 SNMMI 关于消融、辅助治疗和治疗的剂量建议和指南将在后面讨论(表 12.3)。ATA 指南建议术后残甲消融的活度为 30mCi,但对于没有不良特征证据的低风险患者可以免除消融。对于中危或高危患者,根据残留疾病的个体化风险因素,辅助治疗剂量可以为 75~150mCi(2.77~5.55GBq)。对于复发或远处转移,建议碘 -131 经验性治疗剂量为 100~200mCi(3.7~7.4GBq),或通过剂量学计算其活度。SNMMI 指南略有不同,建议术后消融活动为 30~100mCi(1.11~3.7GBq),按经验或剂量法给予碘 -131 治疗的活度不超过 200mCi(7.4GBq)。

表 12.3
ATA 和 SNMMI 关于放射性碘使用的建议比较

消融和辅助治疗

ATA- 消融	①如果进行 RAI 残留消融,则应给予 30mCi(1.11GBq)的低给药活性(强烈推荐,高质量的证据) ②对于怀疑残留量较大的近全甲状腺切除术的患者,可能需要考虑较高的活动(推荐强度低,证据质量低)
ATA- 辅助治疗	通常建议 RAI 剂量最高为 150 mCi(5.55GBq)(弱推荐,低质量证据)
SNMMI	对于术后消融残甲,通常规定其活度范围为 30~100mCi(1.11~3.7GBq),这取决于放射性碘的摄入量和残留的功能性组织的数量

续表

局部病灶	
ATA	①关于一种 RAI 给药方法优于另一种方法（经验剂量法 vs. 全身剂量法 vs. 病灶剂量法）的优势，无法提出任何建议（无建议，证据不足）②经验上，对于 70 岁以上的患者，应避免碘 -131 剂量超过 150mCi（5.55GBq），这些剂量往往可能超过最大可耐受剂量（强烈推荐，中等质量的证据）
SNMMI	对于颈部或纵隔淋巴结甲状腺癌的治疗，RAI 活性范围为 150~200mCi（5.55~7.4GBq）
远处转移	
ATA	肺转移 　微转移 　　- 经验性 RAI 活度为 100~200mCi（3.7~7.4GBq） 　　- 或 70 岁以上患者，100~150mCi（3.7~5.55GBq） 　　- 或由剂量学确定 [a] 　大的转移 　　- 经验量：100~200mCi（3.7~7.4GBq） 　　- 或病灶剂量法 / 全身剂量法 [a] 骨转移 　-RAI 经验量为 100~200mCi（3.7~7.4GBq） 　- 或由剂量测定确定（弱推荐、低质量证据）
SNMMI	对于远处转移的治疗，建议放射性活度为 200mCi（7.4GBq）或更高为了减少严重骨髓抑制的风险，在 48 小时内碘 -131 在体内的滞留量应 <120mCi（4.44GBq），如果存在弥漫性肺转移，则应 <80mCi（2.96GBq），以降低放射性肺炎的风险
没有结构性病变	
ATA	100~200mCi（3.7~7.4GBq）的 RAI 经验活度或剂量学（弱推荐，低质量证据）
SNMMI	150~200mCi（5.55~7.4GBq）的经验性 RAI 活度伴随骨髓剂量测定（如果需要）

[a] 剂量学，应限制全身滞留到 80mci（2.96GBq）在 48 小时和 200cGy 到骨髓

Adapted from Haugen BR, Alexander EK, Bible KC, et al. 2015 American thyroid association management guidelines for adult patients with thyroid nodules and differentiated thyroid cancer: The American thyroid association guidelines task force on thyroid nodules and differentiated thyroid cancer. Thyroid 2016;26(1):1-133;and Silberstein EB, Alavi A, Balon HR, et al. The SNMMI Practice Guideline for Therapy of Thyroid Disease with 131I 3.0. J NuclMed 2012;53(10):1633-51, with permission.

重组人促甲状腺激素(rhTSH)在放射性碘消融、辅助治疗或治疗中的应用

如前所述,几乎所有用于放射性碘消融、辅助治疗的途径都要求患者在甲状腺切除术后或停用 L-T_4 后出现内源性 TSH 水平升高下的甲减。因此,患者须经历 3~6 周的甲减期,并伴有许多不适症状。随着重组人促甲状腺激素 rhTSH(注射用促甲状腺激素 α)的开发,医生可以为患者提供另一种选择,以实现扫描和治疗所必需的血清 TSH 升高[32]。rhTSH 的使用提高了 Tg 的检测和放射性碘扫描的诊断甲状腺癌的敏感性[33]。因此,在检测复发或残留甲状腺癌和保障残甲消融等方面,rhTSH 已成为甲状腺激素撤除的安全和有效的替代方案。

最常见的过程如下:

周一	抽血查 Tg
	rhTSH 注射 0.9mg(肌肉注射)
周二	rhTSH 注射 0.9mg(肌肉注射)
周三	服用 4mCi(0.148GBq)的碘 -131
周四	无处理
周五	抽血查 Tg
	全身碘扫

不可避免的是,将 rhTSH 用途扩展到初始消融或 / 和持续性疾病的后续治疗,都应当检验 rhTSH 作为甲状腺素撤药的替代方法的有效性。

使用重组人促甲状腺激素(rhTSH)准备的消融和辅助治疗

Memorial Sloan Kettering 癌症中心小组率先将 rhTSH 用于消融,并报告说,在使用 rhTSH 消融可见的甲状腺床摄取方面,与停用甲状腺素后的消融效果相当[34]。Bartenstein 及其同事[35]最近的一份报告描述了在 144 名患有 T_4 期原发肿瘤的高危患者中,注射 rhTSH 与停药法的残甲消融率没有差异。一项纳入 1 535 名患者的 meta 分析表明,两种制备方法的消融率相似[36]。虽然缺乏长期随访数据,但最近的回顾性研究表明,在 5~10 年的随访中,使用 rhTSH 患者在消融时获得的最终临床结果非常相似[37]。不过,对使用 rhTSH 治疗转移性疾病的患者尚无长期随访结果。目前,rhTSH 在欧洲被批准用

于转移性疾病患者的碘-131治疗前准备,而美国食品药品管理局(Food and Drug Administration,FDA)尚未批准。

任何一种甲状腺功能残余组织消融方法,通常让患者低碘饮食。但当采用 rhTSH 进行消融前准备时,会刺激患者吸收从甲状腺激素中来源的碘,使血清和尿碘水平会更高。尽管理论上高碘环境可能会降低放射性碘的治疗效果,但前期研究表明 rhTSH 仍可以取得与停用甲状腺素相当的消融效果,这可能会打消我们的顾虑。

ATA 指南对于 rhTSH 应用的建议:①以下情况可以使用:拟行放射性碘残甲消融或辅助治疗的无广泛淋巴结受累的 ATA 低危和中危分化型甲状腺癌(如 T_1~T_3,N_0/N_x/N_{1a},M_0);②以下情况可考虑使用:拟行放射性碘辅助治疗的有广泛淋巴结受累但无远处转移的 ATA 中危分化型甲状腺癌(即 T_1~T_3,N_0/N_x/N_{1a},M_0)。辅助治疗方案与前述相似,连续 2 天肌内注射 rhTSH,每次 0.9mg,第二次注射后 24 小时给予放射性碘。

重组人促甲状腺激素准备后的碘-131 治疗

关于残留或转移性甲状腺癌的后续治疗,使用 rhTSH 制剂代替停用甲状腺素显然是一种美国 FDA 官方批准范围外的使用,很少有研究支持这种使用方法。Klubo-Gwiezdzinska 及其同事[38]回顾性研究了 56 名接受 rhTSH 或撤药准备的远处转移患者,根据生存率、无进展生存率、生化和结构反应以及不良反应,发现两种方法的治疗效果相似。从更专业的角度来看,Plyku 及其同事[39]研究了 4 名同时使用撤药和注射 rhTSH 的患者,观察到停药后单位活度碘-131 的吸收剂量比单纯注射 rhTSH 高,但有限的研究难以得出明确结论。尽管可能在某些合并症(停药和伴随甲状腺功能减退对患者构成重大风险)患者中使用 rhTSH 是出于不得已,但 ATA 指南指出,尚无足够的数据可支持推荐该做法。rhTSH 的另一个适应证是,伴发垂体功能低下的患者停药后无法升高其内源性 TSH 的罕见情况,或患有广泛转移性灶持续分泌甲状腺激素而抑制垂体 TSH 分泌的罕见情况。

MedStar 华盛顿医院中心方法

对于那些要用碘-131 消融的患者,作者通常使用 30mCi(1.11GBq)的经验剂量。但是,对于无不良特征的低危患者,通常可以推迟消融。如果需要辅助治疗,则根据临床情况推荐经验性或剂量学剂量。如果没有碘-123 扫描

(消融前)前的转移证据,且该扫描未显示框 12.2 中的任何发现,则可以为成年患者提供 75~150mCi(2.78~5.55GBq)的经验剂量。对于儿童患者,根据体重和体表面积,遵循表 12.4 中规定的雷诺修饰因子来制订剂量方案[40]。但是,专为儿童或成人设计的经验性剂量,可根据框 12.1 所述的一种或多种因素作进一步调整。对于患有弥漫性肺部摄取、明显远处转移或骨髓储备有限的儿童,使用全身剂量计算最大安全剂量十分重要。确保在不存在摄碘肺弥漫性肺转移瘤时对血液的吸收剂量不超过 200rad(2Gy),在给药后 48 小时的全身滞留量不超过 120mCi(4.44GBq);而存在摄碘肺弥漫性肺转移瘤时,给药后 48 小时的全身滞留量不超过 80mCi(2.96BGq)[41]。还可根据在诊断性扫描中发现的甲状腺床摄取程度以及残留甲状腺组织区域的数量和大小来调整成人剂量(图 12.3)。其他文章已对此进行了更详细的讨论[42]。

当患者的消融前扫描显示框 12.2 中的情况时,建议可以选择以下处理方案:①可以增加经验剂量;②可以采用全身剂量计算法计算所需剂量;③推迟消融或治疗直至进一步的评估或治疗后。进一步的评估通常从颈部超声和 / 或 MRI 成像、胸部 CT、^{18}F-FDG-PET 扫描和细针穿刺细胞学检查可疑病灶开始。对于肿瘤细胞学检查呈阳性的患者,可能建议进行额外的手术治疗。

对于第一次预处理扫描之前有已知转移的患者,或对随访期间 Tg 水平升高,已知或强烈怀疑局部复发或远处转移性疾病的患者,作者采用全身剂量学方法。在有肺转移的患者中,给药剂量在 48 小时内不超过 80mCi(2.96GBq)全身滞留量,所有其他患者中,在 48 小时内不超过 120mCi(4.44GBq)全身滞留。在 1~2mCi(0.037~0.074GBq)范围内使用较低的碘 -131 诊断剂量可避免任何明显的顿抑。选择的最终碘 -131 治疗剂量不超过最大允许活性和全身滞留的阈值。可以根据框 12.1 中所列的一种或多种因素来个性化和减少所选剂量。

框 12.2
消融前扫描的实用程序

甲状腺床或颈部淋巴结的碘摄取模式和百分比可能改变治疗或消融 / 治疗剂量

▲ 单个区域 5%~30% 的摄取,建议考虑额外的手术或修改 RAI 的剂量。
▲ 单个区域的低摄入量低于 1%,建议修改 RAI 的经验剂量。
▲ 与颈部转移一致的 RAI 摄取方式提示:①用 MR 或高分辨率超声进一步评估;②额外细针穿刺,手术或同时进行;和 / 或③使用较大的经验剂量。

续表

可能改变患者在 RAI 治疗前的评估和 / 或处理的远处转移
▲ 肺中的局部或弥散性摄取可能需要使用 CT 平扫进行进一步评估、肺功能测试和剂量测定,以确定最大可耐受的剂量并不会超过可接受的 48 小时体内滞留量。后者可以相对于经验剂量增加或减少剂量,并且尽可能避免急性放射性肺炎和肺纤维化的可能性。
▲ 提示骨转移的区域,可能需要进一步 CT、手术、更大的经验性剂量、剂量学和 / 或其他治疗方式(例如转移瘤切除、随后的外部放射疗法或射频消融)的协调评估。
▲ 头部的局灶性摄取可能需要对大脑进行磁共振成像。如果病灶区域是脑转移,那么可以考虑手术。如果进行体外放射治疗(如,伽玛刀)及 RAI,则应减少经验性剂量,并在碘 -131 治疗之前,先应用类固醇、甘油和 / 或甘露醇治疗。

Adapted from Atkins F, Van Nostrand D. Radioiodine whole body imaging. In: Wartofsky L, Van Nostrand D, editors. Thyroid cancer: a comprehensive guide to clinical management. 3rd edition. New York: Springer; 2016. p.145; with permission.

表 12.4
雷诺修正因子(儿童治疗时的剂量选择)

因子	体重 /kg	人体表面积 /m²
0.2	10	0.4
0.4	25	0.8
0.6	40	1.2
0.8	55	1.4
1	77	1.7

体表面积 $=0.1 \times$ 体重 $(kg)^{0.67}$

Adapted from Van Nostrand D. Radioiodine treatment for distant metastases. In Wartofsky L, Van Nostrand D, editors: Thyroid cancer: a comprehensive guide to clinical management. 3rd edition. New York: Springer; 2016. p.620; with permission.

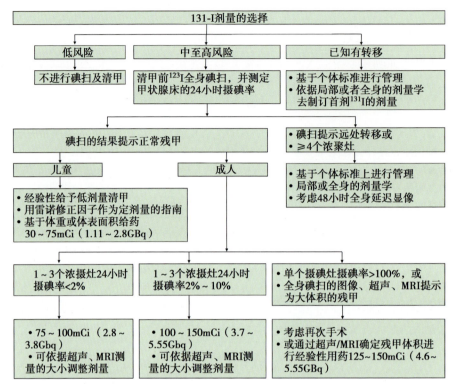

图 12.3 作者在 MedStar 华盛顿医院中心选择 131-I 剂量进行消融、辅助治疗或 WDTC 患者治疗的方法概述

WBS，全身扫描

Adapted from Van Nostrand D. Radioiodine ablation. In: Wartofsky L, Van Nostrand D, editors. Thyroid cancer: a comprehensive guide to clinical management. 2nd edition. Totowa (NJ): Humana Press; 2006.p.611-2; with permission.

总结

无论碘 -131 的剂量是通过经验法还是计算剂量学方法确定的，放射性碘消融术、放射性碘辅助治疗或碘 -131 治疗仍然是 WDTC 患者治疗中不可缺少的组成部分。随着对各种方法的透彻了解以及可能改变放射性碘剂量的许多因素的考虑，治疗团队应该制订最佳、合理的个性化治疗计划。

补充说明

作为对本节内容的补充，应该理解消融前扫描的应用价值，因为其提供了重要的信息,这些信息可能是:①在给予放射性碘消融剂量之前改变患者的治疗方式(框 12.2);②可能会改善结果。尽管消融前扫描不能在所有情况下提供意料之外的重要信息,但是所获得的信息可能改变总体的治疗策略,付出合理的成本及其引起的少许不便是值得的[43]。

(李 丹 吕中伟)

参考文献

1. Seidin SM, Marinelli LD, Oshry E. Radioactive iodine therapy effect on functioning metastases of adenocarcinoma of the thyroid. JAMA 1946;132:838–47.
2. Haugen BR, Alexander EK, Bible KC, et al. 2015 American thyroid association management guidelines for adult patients with thyroid nodules and differentiated thyroid cancer: the American thyroid association guidelines task force on thyroid nodules and differentiated thyroid cancer. Thyroid 2016;26(1):1–133.
3. Van Nostrand D. The benefits and risks of I-131 therapy in patients with well-differentiated thyroid cancer. Thyroid 2009;19(12):1381–91.
4. Tuttle RM, Haugen B, Perrier ND. Updated American Joint Committee on Cancer/tumor-node-metastasis staging system for differentiated and anaplastic thyroid cancer (eighth edition): what changed and why? Thyroid 2017;27(6):751–6.
5. Amin MB, Edge S, Greene F, et al, editors. AJCC cancer staging manual. New York: Springer; 2017.
6. Beierwaltes WH, Rabbani R, Dmuchowski C, et al. An analysis of ablation of thyroid remnants" with I-131 in 511 patients from 1947-1984: experience at University of Michigan. J Nucl Med 1984;25:1287–93.
7. Schlumberger M, Challeton C, De Vathaire F, et al. Radioactive iodine treatment and external radiotherapy for lung and bone metastases from thyroid carcinoma. J Nucl Med 1996;37:598–605.
8. Petrich T, Widjaja A, Musholt TJ, et al. Outcome after radioiodine therapy in 107 patients with differentiated thyroid carcinoma and initial bone metastases: side effects and influence of age. Eur J Nucl Med 2001;28:203–8.
9. Brown AP, Greening WP, McCready VR, et al. Radioiodine treatment of metastatic thyroid carcinoma: The Royal Marsden hospital experience. Br J Radiol 1984;57:323–7.
10. Menzel C, Grunwald F, Schomburg A, et al. "High-Dose" Radioiodine therapy in advanced differentiated thyroid carcinoma. J Nucl Med 1996;37:1496–503.
11. Hindié E, Melliere D, Lange F, et al. Functioning pulmonary metastases of thyroid cancer: does radioiodine influence the prognosis? Eur J Nucl Med Mol Imaging 2003;30:974–81.
12. Durante C, Haddy N, Baudin E, et al. Long-term outcome of 444 patients with distant metastases from papillary and follicular thyroid carcinoma: benefits and limits of radioiodine therapy. J Clin Endocrinol Metab 2006;91(8):2892–9.
13. Castagna MG, Cevenini G, Theodoropoulou A, et al. Post-surgical thyroid ablation with low or high radioiodine activities results in similar outcomes in interme-

diate risk differentiated thyroid cancer patients. Eur J Endocrinol 2013;169(1): 23–9.
14. Mallick U, Harmer C, Yap B, et al. Ablation with low-dose radioiodine and thyrotropin alfa in thyroid cancer. N Engl J Med 2012;366(18):1674–85.
15. Verburg FA, Mäder U, Reiners C, et al. Long-term survival in differentiated thyroid cancer is worse after low-activity initial post-surgical 131I therapy in both high- and low-risk patients. J Clin Endocrinol Metab 2014;99(12):4487–96.
16. Schlumberger M, Leboulleux S, Catargi B, et al. Outcome after ablation in patients with low-risk thyroid cancer (ESTIMABL1): 5-year follow-up results of a randomized, phase 3, equivalence trial. Lancet Diabetes Endocrinol 2018;6(8): 618–26.
17. Van Nostrand D. Stunning: does it exist? a commentary. In: Wartofsky L, Van Nostrand D, editors. Thyroid cancer: a comprehensive guide to clinical management. New York: Springer; 2016. p. 243–5.
18. Maxon HR, Thomas SR, Hertzbert VS, et al. Relation between effective radiation dose and outcome of radioiodine therapy for thyroid cancer. N Engl J Med 1983; 309:937–41.
19. Thomas SR, Maxon HR, Kereiakes JG. In vivo quantitation of lesion radioactivity using external counting methods. Med Phys 1976;3:253–5.
20. Benua RS, Leeper RD. A method and rationale for treating metastatic thyroid carcinoma with the largest safe dose of I-131. In: Medeiros-Neto G, Gaitan E, editors. Frontiers in thyroidology. Vol. 2. New York: Plenum Medical Book Co; 1986. p. 1317–21.
21. Dorn R, Kopp J, Vogt H, et al. Dosimetry-guided radioactive iodine treatment in patients with metastatic differentiated thyroid cancer: largest safe dose using a risk-based approach. J Nucl Med 2003;44:451–6.
22. Kulkarni K, Van Nostrand D, Atkins FB, et al. The frequency with which empiric amounts of radioiodine "over-" or "under-" treat patients with metastatic well-differentiated thyroid cancer. Thyroid 2006;16:1019–23.
23. Tuttle RM, Leboeuf R, Robbins RJ, et al. Empiric radioactive iodine dosing regimens frequently exceed maximum tolerated activity levels in elderly patients with thyroid cancer. J Nucl Med 2006;47:1587–91.
24. Hanscheid H, Lassmann M, Luster M, et al. Blood dosimetry from a single measurement of the whole body radioiodine retention in patients with differentiated thyroid carcinoma. Endocr Relat Cancer 2009;16:1283–9.
25. Van Nostrand D, Atkins F, Moreau S, et al. Utility of the radioiodine whole-body retention at 48 hours for modifying empiric activity of 131-iodine for the treatment of metastatic well-differentiated thyroid carcinoma. Thyroid 2009;19:1093–8.
26. Jentzen W, Bockisch A, Ruhlmann M. Assessment of simplified blood dose protocols for the estimation of the maximum tolerable activity in thyroid cancer patients undergoing radioiodine therapy using 124I. J Nucl Med 2015;56:832–8.
27. Atkins F, Van Nostrand D, Moreau S, et al. Validation of a simple thyroid cancer dosimetry model based on the fractional whole-body retention at 48 hours post-administration of (131)I. Thyroid 2015;25(12):1347–50.
28. Klubo-Gwiezdzinska J, Van Nostrand D, Atkins F, et al. Efficacy of dosimetric versus empiric prescribed activity of 131I for therapy of differentiated thyroid cancer. J Clin Endocrinol Metab 2011;96(10):3217–25.
29. Deandreis D, Rubino C, Tala H, et al. Comparison of empiric versus whole-body/blood clearance dosimetry-based approach to radioactive iodine treatment in patients with metastases from differentiated thyroid cancer. J Nucl Med 2017;58(5):

717–22.
30. Silberstein EB, Alavi A, Balon HR, et al. The SNMMI practice guideline for therapy of thyroid disease with 131I 3.0. J Nucl Med 2012;53(10):1633–51.
31. Verburg FA, Aktolun C, Chiti A, et al, EANM and the EANM Thyroid Committee. Why the European Association of Nuclear Medicine has declined to endorse the 2015 American Thyroid Association management guidelines for adult patients with thyroid nodules and differentiated thyroid cancer. Eur J Nucl Med Mol Imaging 2016 Jun;43(6):1001–5.
32. Ringel MD, Burgun SJ. Recombinant human thyrotropin. In: Wartofsky L, Van Nostrand D, editors. Thyroid cancer: a comprehensive guide to clinical management. New York: Springer; 2016. p. 119–29.
33. Ladenson PW. Recombinant thyrotropin for detection of recurrent thyroid cancer. Trans Am Clin Climatol Assoc 2002;113:21–30.
34. Robbins RJ, Larson SM, Sinha N, et al. A retrospective review of the effectiveness of recombinant human TSH as a preparation for radioiodine thyroid remnant ablation. J Nucl Med 2002;43(11):1482–8.
35. Bartenstein P, Calabuig EC, Maini CL, et al. High-risk patients with differentiated thyroid cancer T4 primary tumors achieve remnant ablation equally well using rhTSH or thyroid hormone withdrawal. Thyroid 2014;24(3):480–7.
36. Tu J, Wang S, Huo Z, et al. Recombinant human thyrotropin-aided versus thyroid hormone withdrawal-aided radioiodine treatment for differentiated thyroid cancer after total thyroidectomy: a meta-analysis. Radiother Oncol 2014;110(1):25–30.
37. Sabra MM, Tuttle RM. Recombinant human thyroid-stimulating hormone to stimulate 131-I uptake for remnant ablation and adjuvant therapy. Endocr Pract 2013;19(1):149–56.
38. Klubo-Gwiezdzinska J, Burman KD, Van Nostrand D, et al. Radioiodine treatment of metastatic thyroid cancer: relative efficacy and side effect profile of preparation by thyroid hormone withdrawal versus recombinant human thyrotropin. Thyroid 2012;22(3):310–7.
39. Plyku D, Hobbs RF, Huang K, et al. Recombinant human thyroid-stimulating hormone versus thyroid hormone withdrawal in 124I PET/CT-based dosimetry for 131I therapy of metastatic differentiated thyroid cancer. J Nucl Med 2017;58(7):1146–54.
40. Reynolds JC. Comparison of I-131absorbed radiation doses in children and adults; a tool for estimating therapeutic I-131 doses in children. In: Robbins J, editor. Treatment of thyroid cancer in children, DOE/EH-0406, US Department of Commerce Technology Administration, National Technical Information Service. Springfield, Virginia; 1994. p. 127–35.
41. Francis G, Waguespsk SG, Bauer AJ, et al. Management Guidelines for the Children with thyroid nodules and differentiated thyroid cancer. Thyroid 2015;25(7):716–59.
42. Van Nostrand D. Remnant ablation, adjuvant and treatment of locoregional metastasis with I^{131}. In: Wartofsky L, Van Nostrand D, editors. Thyroid cancer: a comprehensive guide to clinical management. 3rd edition. New York: Springer; 2016. p. 611–2.
43. Van Nostrand D. To perform or not to perform radioiodine scans prior to 131 Remnant Ablation? PRO. In: Wartofsky L, Van Nostrand D, editors. Thyroid cancer: a comprehensive guide to clinical management. New York: Springer; 2016. p. 245–54.

第13章
甲状腺微小乳头状癌的处理

Juan P. Brito, Ian D. Hay

关键词

- 甲状腺乳头状癌 ● 微小癌 ● 处理 ● 共同临床决策

要点

- 甲状腺的发病率增加主要可能是由于体检发现甲状腺微小癌的增多。
- 甲状腺微小癌患者应该根据肿瘤生物学特性和患者自身情况而个体化治疗。
- 共同临床决策是一种帮助临床医师对甲状腺微小癌患者进行个体化诊治的重要方法。

流行病学

全球甲状腺癌的发病率都在升高。近30年来,美国甲状腺癌的发病率增长了超过3倍,从之前的4.9/10万上升至2011年的14.7/10万[1]。增长主要来源于甲状腺乳头状癌(papillary thyroid cancer,PTC),特别是<1cm的甲状腺微小乳头状癌(papillary thyroid microcarcinoma,PTM)[2]。图13.1展示了梅奥医学中心(Mayo Clinic)1974—2013年甲状腺癌肿瘤大小所占比例的变化[3]。≤1cm甲状腺癌的平均年度增长百分比为9%,1~2cm肿瘤的年增长率为5%,2~4cm肿瘤的年增长率为4.5%,4cm以上肿瘤的年增长率为6%。事实上,估计有39%的甲状腺癌属于PTM[4]。图13.2展示了梅奥医学中心

1936—2015 年所有 PTC 按照大小进行的分类。其中 5%~10% 的 PTM 是在因甲状腺良性疾病行甲状腺切除术或因其他不相关疾病死亡而进行尸检的患者中发现的[5,6]。由于越来越多甲状腺微小癌在年纪较大的患者中被检出,目前,美国 45 岁以上患者最常见的甲状腺癌类型即是 PTM[7]。

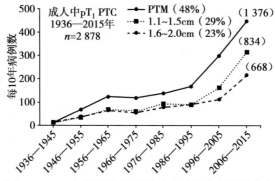

图 13.1　80 年间甲状腺癌肿瘤大小(肿瘤的最大直径)比例的变化。数据来源于 1936—2015 年梅奥医学中心 2 878 名 pT_1 期成年甲状腺癌患者

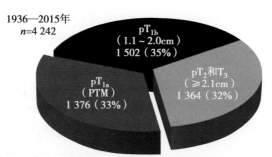

图 13.2　1936—2015 年梅奥医学中心 4 242 例成年甲状腺癌肿瘤大小比例分布。可见这 80 年间 33% 的肿瘤属于微小癌(≤1cm)

最近美国甲状腺学会(American Thyroid Association,ATA)关于甲状腺结节处理指南的修改可能会影响目前甲状腺癌发病率的变化趋势。指南推荐,所有 ≤1cm 的甲状腺结节不应该进行活检,除非超声或临床表明有潜在的侵袭性(如甲状腺外侵犯、声带麻痹),以上特征往往是典型 PTM 所不具备的[8]。因此,很有可能更多实际是 PTM 的甲状腺结节不再进行活检,导致甲状腺癌的发病率降低。虽然关于指南的修订是否影响 PTM 的检出率还没有明确证据,但最近一项分析指出,甲状腺癌发病率的年度百分比变化在过去的几年有所降低[9,10]。

症状和临床表现

鉴于 PTM 的大小，这类肿瘤通常不会导致临床症状，它们通常在患者进行非甲状腺专科检查（如颈部核磁）或因甲状腺良性疾病切除甲状腺时偶然发现。一项最近的研究指出，包括 PTM 在内的甲状腺癌可以在无症状的患者中仅仅通过颈部触诊而发现。实际上，触诊通常不能识别出 PTM，但可以发现其他结节并促使患者进行甲状腺超声。最后，在广泛进行甲状腺癌筛查的国家，发现 PTM 最常用的手段是甲状腺超声筛查[11]。

传统治疗选择

甲状腺手术

手术治疗是 PTM 患者传统治疗的基石。手术干预包括双侧腺叶切除（bilateral lobar resection，BLR），即切除整个甲状腺，另一种方式是仅切除病灶所在的一侧腺叶（图 13.3）。虽然没有临床试验比较不同术式的影响，但是 PTM 非常低的病死率强烈提示了这一比较很可能不会有显著的差异（图 13.4）。事实上，在梅奥医学中心 83 年的随访中，仅有 4 名 PTM 患者因此致死。因此，两种干预的主要区别与其甲状腺癌复发风险、随访监测、手术并发症及甲状腺素替代治疗等有关。全甲状腺切除的支持点包括甲状腺癌的多灶性（约 30%）[12]以及全甲状腺切除术后更好地进行术后随访（包括甲状腺球蛋白肿瘤标记物测量）[13]。另一方面，甲状腺腺叶切除术支持点在于肿瘤的多灶性并不导致额外的临床相关疾病。这一论点的证据在于两种干预手段的复发风险相似，并且都很低（<5%）[14]。腺叶切除还能使余下的 50%~60% 的

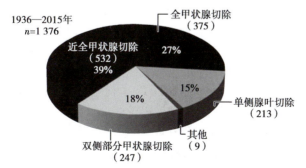

图 13.3 1936—2015 年梅奥医学中心 1 376 名初次行甲状腺癌手术患者的甲状腺切除范围。可见仅 15% 的患者行单侧腺叶切除

患者免去甲状腺素替代治疗,该替代治疗会使患者余生每日都服药并增加长期、频繁监测甲状腺功能的负担。最重要的一个支持腺叶切除术的论据在于患者并不都能得到有经验的甲状腺外科医生的治疗。甲状腺手术最重要的两个并发症(声带麻痹和甲状旁腺功能减低)都直接和手术范围以及手术医生的经验相关。全甲状腺切除术后暂时性或永久性声带损伤以及甲状旁腺功能减低的发生率约为 1% 和 2%,而单侧腺叶切除的并发症风险通常是暂时的,比例在 0~1%[15]。以上数据都是来自第三级医疗中心的数据,都是由经验丰富的外科医生来完成手术。最近,基于人群的研究表明,这一估计实际上显著高估了缺乏手术经验的医疗中心的医疗质量[11]。梅奥医学中心回顾了 1936—2015 年共 1376 名 PTM 患者的研究,发现单侧腺叶切除和双侧腺叶切除、近全或全甲状腺切除患者的 20 年局部复发率并无显著性差异(图 13.5)。

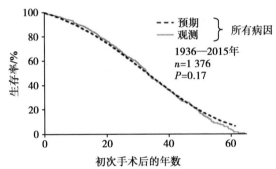

图 13.4 梅奥医学中心 80 年间 1 376 名行根治性手术(图 13.3)的 PTM 患者,预期与观测全因生存曲线。可见两者无显著差异(P=0.17)

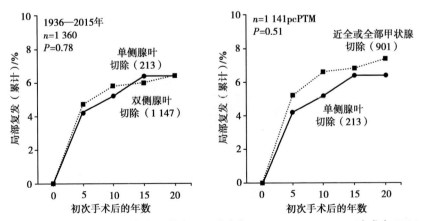

图 13.5 1936—2015 年梅奥医学中心可治愈(potentially curable, PC)成人 PTM 患者,术后 20 年随访局部复发率比较。可见 213 例腺叶切除术的患者与全甲状腺切除(左图)或近全甲状腺切除(右图)患者之间均没有显著性差异

放射性碘同位素消融

对于进行全甲状腺切除的患者,放射性碘治疗(radioactive iodine,RAI)是处理甲状腺残余组织(以帮助监测)和降低甲状腺癌复发风险的一种选择[16]。RAI 通常在复发风险较高的患者身上应用,但鉴于 PTM 的低致死率和致残率,是否进行放射性碘消融(radioiodine remnant ablation,RRA)仍然是有争议的[17]。已经有几项系统综述尝试去评价 RAI 的获益。虽然纳入的研究有显著的异质性,但可注意到甲状腺癌复发的相对风险值(relative risk,RR)因此下降了 5%~20%[18]。因此,对于一个 10 年复发风险为 50% 的高风险甲状腺癌患者而言,使用 RAI 会使这一风险降至 40%。而另一方面,对于一个 10 年复发风险不到 5% 的极低风险甲状腺癌患者而言,绝对风险仅下降 1% 甚至更少。这一微小获益与治疗成本和治疗后负担(例如,治疗所需的影像学检查、治疗前低碘饮食、治疗前停用甲状腺素引起的甲状腺功能低下症状,以及治疗后的隔离等)的比较使得一些指南不建议在 PTM 患者身上应用 RAI[19]。1956—2015 年,1 287 名就诊于梅奥医学中心的 PTM 患者中,仅有 15% 使用了 RRA(图 13.6)。375 例淋巴结阳性的 PTM 患者,手术后(不论甲状腺腺叶切除、近全或全甲状腺切除)使用 RRA 并没有使 20 年局部复发率有所获益(图 13.7)。

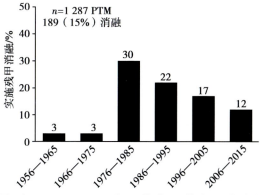

图 13.6 1956—2015 年于梅奥医学中心诊治的 1 287 名成人 PTM 患者进行 RRA 的比例。可见 1976—2015 年 RRA 越来越有选择性地使用

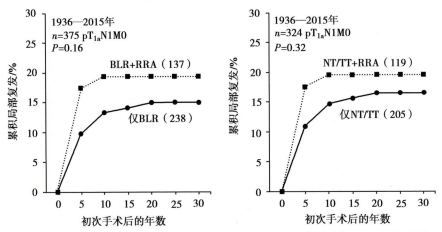

图 13.7　1936—2015 年淋巴结阳性的成年 PTM 患者在术后进行 RRA 不能有效降低局部复发率。左图为甲状腺腺叶切除术后，右图为近全或全甲状腺切除术后（near-total or total thyroidectomy，NT/TT）

促甲状腺素抑制治疗

促甲状腺素抑制治疗（thyrotropin suppression treatment，TST）的主要目的是预防和治疗甲状腺功能减退症状。不过，为了避免肿瘤可能因促甲状腺激素（thyroid-stimulating hormone，TSH）的刺激而继续生长，患者常常会被要求服用超过替代剂量的药物[20]。为了支持这种做法，一项纳入了 4 174 名高分化甲状腺癌患者的 meta 分析显示，TST 可以减少疾病进展、复发和死亡的风险（RR=0.73，CI 0.6~0.88）[21]。不过，这一获益更多见于比 PTM 死亡与复发风险更高的患者[22]。一项纳入了 2 936 名甲状腺癌患者的前瞻性多中心研究数据表明，TST 抑制极低浓度（<0.1mU/L）并不能改善低风险甲状腺癌（包括 PTM）患者的总生存[23]。类似地，一项 RCT 研究比较了 TST 对低风险 PTC 患者预后的影响，结果表明在平均随访了 6.9 年后，复发率和死亡率没有显著性差异[24]。鉴于有限的有效性，TSH 抑制治疗可能的不良反应（医源性甲亢、房颤或骨折[25]）和治疗负担（频繁的监测和调整），ATA 指南不建议对 PTM 患者进行 TSH 抑制治疗[8]。作为取代，建议 PTM 患者在接受 TST 时仅把 TSH 保持在正常低水平即可（TSH 0.5~2.0mU/L）。

更新的管理选择

积极随访监测

在过去的近 10 年,与惰性前列腺癌一样,积极随访监测(密切监测症状和肿瘤超声特征,后期必要时选择性行手术干预)已经在 PTM 患者身上应用[15]。已经有 3 项观察性研究表明积极监测对 PTM 患者是安全且可取的[26-28]。2015 年,ATA 指南将积极随访监测作为 PTM 患者手术干预的一种替代选择。关于积极随访监测背后的证据、实施方法、应用范围的研究,本章将不再讨论。本章仅探讨积极随访监测作为 PTM 患者管理时的决策过程(见后续讨论)。

超声引导下经皮酒精消融

超声引导下经皮酒精消融(ultrasound-guided percutaneous ethanol ablation,UPEA)是在超声引导和局部麻醉下直接将 95% 的酒精注射入肿瘤内[29]。自 1991 年以来,该技术已在梅奥诊所有效地用于处理术后乳头状癌、Hürthle 细胞癌和髓样癌的颈部淋巴结的转移治疗。该技术在 2013 年发表的一项局部晚期乳头状癌(肿瘤最大径>1cm)的长期随访研究中得到了验证,Hay 等[30]报道称这项技术相较于手术管理是安全、有效、经济的。自 2010 年以来,该研究小组使用 UPEA 来控制 PTM($cT_{1a}N_0M_0$)的原发肿瘤,并经常在门诊局部麻醉下使用该方法消除肿瘤。根据最近在 2018 年欧洲甲状腺学会和 ATA 会议上的报告,迄今为止,14 名 PTM 患者中的 16 个经活检证实的肿瘤病灶已得到治疗。颈部有轻微压痛但仅持续数小时,没有因声带麻痹而出现声音嘶哑的受试者。随访时间为 15~95 个月(平均 4.2 年),未发现受试者出现颈部淋巴结转移。所有肿瘤体积均缩小,肿瘤相关的多普勒血流信号均消失,16 个肿瘤病灶中位体积缩小 82%(范围 48%~100%)。在最新的随访后,10 个肿瘤(62%)仍能识别,在这些病例中,中位体积缩小 76%。5 位受试者的 6 个局部病灶(38%)在超声检查中未再报告。UPEA 术后血清甲状腺球蛋白水平无明显变化。作者认为,这项正在进行的队列研究已经证明,对于那些不愿进行手术和积极监测的患者,UPEA 可以成为 PTM 患者的一种廉价、安全和耐受性良好的替代微创治疗[31]。

射频和激光消融

射频和激光消融是一种经皮的图像引导下手术,利用热能量来消除原位肿瘤。这个过程被认为与酒精消融相比,该手术可提供更可预测和更清晰的肿瘤坏死区域,肿瘤坏死面积更好确定[32]。射频消融已被用于治疗甲状腺良性大结节,以及甲状腺切除术后的局部复发灶[33]。鉴于其已被证明在这些甲状腺相关适应证中是安全有效的,这一技术最近被用于治疗部分 PTM 患者。Zhang 及其同事们[34]报道,在 92 例患者的 98 个 PTM 中,经射频消融后,肿瘤体积平均缩小率在 6 个月、12 个月和 18 个月分别为 0.47,0.19,0.08。所有结节中,有 10 个在 6 个月内消退,有 23 个在 12 个月内消退。尽管有 1 例患者有中度疼痛,4 例患者出现暂时性声嘶,但是在后续随访中均未发现可疑的淋巴结转移。

经皮射频消融(percutaneous laser ablation,PLA)已经在 PTM 患者中测试。Zhou 等[35]在 30 例患者中使用了 PLA。其中 1 例消融不完全,进行了二次消融。PLA 在消融后 12 个月有效缩减了肿瘤体积,从 44mm³ 到 9.1mm³。在最新的随访中(平均时长 13.2 个月,范围 12~24 个月),10 例(33.3%)消融区域消失,20 例(66.7%)消融区域残留瘢痕样改变。治疗后的肿瘤未再生长,未出现局部复发或远距离转移。与 UPEA 相似,射频消融可能仅适用于部分选择后的患者,仅应在具备相关技术和专业知识的医疗中心开展。

目前的争议

甲状腺微小乳头状癌过度治疗

在过去的几十年中,随着甲状腺癌的发病率迅速增加,越来越多的人开始意识到,许多接受治疗的 PTM 患者的死亡风险并不高,因为死亡率和复发率都很低。最近的观察研究表明,尽管大多数甲状腺微小乳头状癌的患者也可能受益于腺叶切除术,但全甲状腺切除术的比例在美国有所增加[36]。图 13.8 显示 1936—2015 年梅奥诊所 PTM 手术的变化:在最近 20 年(1996—2015 年),最常见的初始外科手术是全甲状腺切除术,占 1936—2015 年所有 PTM 外科手术的 27%。相比之下,在过去的 30 年里,美国的腺叶切除术比例一直相当稳定(在梅奥诊所过去的 80 年里仅占所有手术的 15%)。

然而,许多甲状腺手术是由缺乏经验的甲状腺外科医生进行的。以人群为基础的研究指出,手术相关并发症发生率与甲状腺术者每年操作手术数量有关,即主刀每年超过 25 例甲状腺手术的医生,比少于 25 例的外科医生给患者带来的预后更佳(手术并发症更少,住院日数更少)。每年主刀 2~5 例的外科医生发生甲状腺并发症的概率为 68%,主刀 6~10 例时,并发症发生率为 42%,11~15 例时为 22%,16~20 例为 10%,21~25 例为 3%。本研究还注意到,

1998—2009 年接受全甲状腺切除术的约 1.7 万名患者中,年手术量中位数为 7 例(51% 的外科医生每年进行 1 例)。结果显示,包括 PTM 患者在内的绝大多数甲状腺癌患者在小手术量的医疗中心承担着更高的不良事件风险[37]。

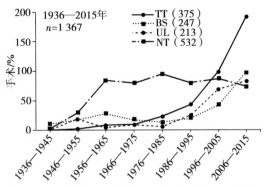

图 13.8 在过去 80 年梅奥诊所治疗的 1 367 名成人 PTM 患者中,不断变化的外科手术比例表明,TT 是 1996—2005 年和 2006—2015 年这 20 年间最常见的成人 PTM 手术方式

BS,双侧甲状腺次全切除术;NT,甲状腺近全切除术;TT,全甲状腺切除术;UL,单侧腺叶切除术

与甲状腺切除术手术量增加类似,在美国,过去 10 年间使用放射性碘治疗低风险甲状腺癌的比例也增加了[38]。1983—2009 年,美国患者接受 RAI 治疗 PTM 的比例从 8% 增至 42%[39],该趋势与梅奥诊所的实践不相符(图 13.6)。PTM 和其他低风险甲状腺癌病变中 RAI 的使用率较高,与更低的社会经济水平(例如无保险、贫困、失业者[38]),主要决策者的专业(核医学医生相较内分泌、外科医生更可能用 RAI[40]),医疗机构(非教学机构比教学机构更多使用 RAI)有关[41]。在 2009 年,ATA 首次明确反对 PTM 术后行 RAI,而这一指南建议略微影响了 RAI 在美国的使用比例[8]。PTM 患者接受 RAI 的比例从 2009 年前的 42% 降至 2009 年后的 32%。10% 的下降比例远大于在肿瘤直径>1.1cm 的患者接受 RAI 的比例的下降,后者从 69% 降至 68%,仅下降了不足 2 个百分点[38]。这些结果提示,PTM 术后行 RAI 仍在美国的临床实践中广泛应用,尽管指南不推荐以上做法。

PTM 患者过度的手术治疗和术后 RAI 治疗可能反映了甲状腺癌一刀切的做法的延续。这种方法不论个体肿瘤的复发率和致死率,均采用相同的治疗方法。关于对甲状腺微小癌复发风险、手术并发症以及发病率的快速增加等研究表明，通用的治疗方法并不存在。相反，应在初始治疗中采用涵盖疾病风险，尊重患者的生物学特征、价值观和背景的个体化治疗方案。

个体化治疗的必要性

临床医生和 PTM 患者有多种治疗选择。目前，还没有比较不同治疗方案疗效的研究，虽然每一种方案都提供了选择该方案的条件和依据。这使得为每个患者选择最佳治疗方案变得相当困难。因此，最好有一个在技术上可行、由患者和临床医生共同评估选择治疗方法的依赖因素，以指导实际临床决策。

什么是技术上可行的？

不是所有的 PTM 病变都是相同的，病变特征将决定哪些治疗适合患者。了解哪些治疗对患者有效的最重要的工具是对患者颈部进行可靠和高质量的超声评估。在评估过程中，临床医生需要注意肿瘤病灶的位置，直径，多中心，与甲状腺被膜、气管和食管的距离。最理想的肿瘤[42]是直径 ≤10mm、无超声证据显示其多中心且距离甲状腺被膜至少 3~5mm，这种情况下，所有的治疗方案均可选择。然而，这种理想的肿瘤并不常见。Griffin 等[15]进行了一项回顾性分析，他们于 2003—2012 年在杜克大学医学中心对 243 名甲状腺癌患者进行了 PTC 手术。这个队列中有 27 名受试者患有 PTM，但无一人为前面提到的"理想"肿瘤。他们注意到，肿瘤通常位于甲状腺周边。类似地，Tuttle 等[28]随访了 291 名直径 ≤1.5cm 的 PTC 患者，中位随访时长为 25 个月，积极随访监测，他们注意到只有 4.5% 的肿瘤符合"理想"肿瘤。这些发现提示 PTM 的表现通常会限制治疗选择。

如何个体化治疗选择

在讨论 PTM 患者可用和可能的治疗选择时，重要的是要了解患者的想法和需求，以及在具体情况下什么是最适合的。年轻的 PTM 患者可能非常重视避免长期密切随访监测，因此，腺叶切除术是最佳选择。一个 76 岁的透析患者可能对摘除甲状腺的重视程度较低，而对保守治疗如 UPEA 或主动监测的重视程度更高。为了进行有意义的对话，患者需要了解每种治疗选择的好处、坏处、成本和对日常生活的影响。临床医生需要传达这些复杂的信息，并在有限的时间内，在临床接触中了解患者的偏好。这对双方来说都是一项艰巨的任务。为了促进这一过程,临床医生应被鼓励采用共享决策(shared decision-making,SDM)的方法。

SDM 是一种临床医生依据现有的循证医学证据和患者讨论不同治疗方案,并找到明智而可行的治疗选择的方法[43]。使用工具和辅助决策可以协助 SDM 进程(图 13.9 和图 13.10)。这些工具可帮助临床医生使用有序图标阵列或象形图来表示全面的信息,以展示治疗方案的风险和性质[43]。Brito 等[44] 开发了一项工具来帮助临床医生和 PTM 患者作出治疗决定。甲状腺癌治疗选择(thyroid cancer choice,TCC)依赖于甲状腺癌专家、患者及临床医生的信息输入,包括:①人群中甲状腺癌发生频率的估计;②治疗选择,包括密切随访监测,甲状腺手术(腺叶切除术 vs. 全甲状腺切除术);③每种治疗选择的死亡、转移、肿瘤生长、不良事件的风险;④计划随访的方式和频率;⑤每种选择的自付费用;⑥各种治疗选择对妊娠的影响。该工具的纸质版已应用于韩国,并已在一项前瞻性观察研究中测试,以评估其对治疗选择的影响。研究人员发现,在 220 名 PTM 患者中,在治疗过程中,较不使用 TCC 的临床医生和患者更愿意选择密切随访监测(RR 1.16,95% CI 1.04~1.09)。虽然这一结果表明该

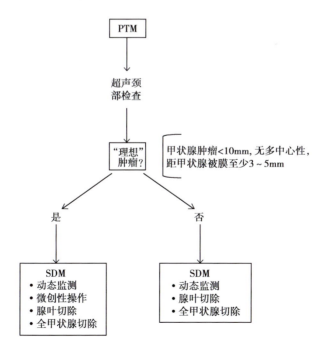

图 13.9 甲状腺微小癌的治疗策略
SDM,共享临床决策

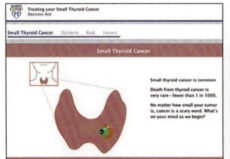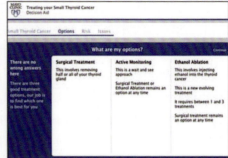
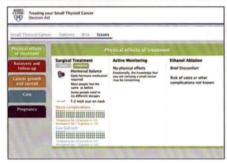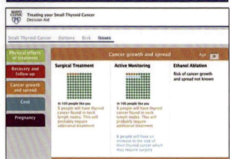

图 13.10 辅助甲状腺癌治疗选择的电子系统的截图

工具可以增加密切随访监测的接受度,但仍需要更多和更严格的研究来证实这一发现。治疗决策的个体化不仅需要基于患者的背景和价值观,还要基于肿瘤的生物学特性。一些遗传学研究已开展或正在开展,以确定具有某些预后价值的特定突变,从而帮助患者和临床医生作出决策。在所有已知的 PTC 患者的遗传突变中,*BRAF V600E* 加上端粒逆转录酶(TERT)突变组合与侵袭性临床病理结果、肿瘤复发和死亡相关[45]。在一个 1 051 名受试者的队列中,有 30 名受试者死亡。在所有 1 051 名受试者中,6%(n=66)有 *BRAF V600E* 和 *TERT* 复合突变,这 66 名受试者中有 25%(n=15)死亡,占本队列中甲状腺癌特异性死亡的一半。在对临床因素进行调整后,这些双重突变患者的死亡风险仍然显著[46]。这些在 PTC 队列中的发现是否可以外推至 PTM 尚不清楚。然而,这些突变存在时不大可能表现为 PTM[47],因而限制了其预后价值。因此,目前的证据并不支持使用这些遗传标记来辅助决策。未来的分子生物学研究可能有助于区分那些更容易生长和转移的 PTM 和在甲状腺内保持生物学沉默的 PTM。

随访监测

甲状腺癌随访监测的目的是发现临床相关的甲状腺癌复发,减少治疗和检测的负担。最常用的两种检测方法是颈部超声和肿瘤标志物血清甲状腺球蛋白。然而,这些检测的频率根据所采用的治疗方法而有所不同。对于接受全甲状腺切除术的患者,术后 6 周~3 个月的初始随访包括甲状腺素、肿瘤标志物甲状腺球蛋白水平的评估。对于接受腺叶切除术的患者,尚未发现监测甲状腺球蛋白有帮助。在最近的一项包含 PTM 的 208 名低风险甲状腺癌患者的研究中,患者接受腺叶切除术并长期随访甲状腺球蛋白水平,研究发现患者甲状腺球蛋白水平在术后逐渐增加,而与是否复发无关,结果并没有显著性差异。术后 6~12 个月应进行颈部超声评估。如果在前 2 年的随访期间临床检查和实验室检测没有获得疾病的证据,甲状腺癌复发的可能性<1%,未来的随访次数可以减少[48]。对于积极随访监测的患者,随访应是长期的,应每 6 个月进行 1 次颈部超声检查。对于接受微创治疗的患者,随访应根据当地医院流程进行,在最初 5 年可能类似于密切随访监测的随访方式。由于 PTM 患者复发风险低,因此,重组 TSH 刺激甲状腺球蛋白检测、全身 RAI 扫描或者 FDG-PET 扫描的临床意义有限或没有必要[8]。

(王朝阳　金立超　刘绍严)

参考文献

1. Davies L, Welch HG. Current thyroid cancer trends in the United States. JAMA Otolaryngol Head Neck Surg 2014;140(4):317.
2. Davies L, Morris LG, Haymart M, et al, on behalf of the AACE Endocrine Surgery Scientific Committee. American Association of Clinical Endocrinologists and American College of Endocrinology disease state clinical review : the increasing incidence of thyroid cancer. Endocr Pract 2016;21(6):686–96.
3. Hay ID, Johnson TR, Kaggal S, et al. Papillary Thyroid Carcinoma (PTC) in children and adults: comparison of initial presentation and long-term postoperative outcome in 4432 patients consecutively treated at the Mayo Clinic during eight decades (1936–2015). World J Surg 2018;42(2):329–42.
4. Lim H, Devesa SS, Sosa JA, et al. Trends in thyroid cancer incidence and mortality in the United States, 1974-2013. JAMA 2017;317(13):1338.
5. Harach HR, Franssila KO, Wasenius VM. Occult papillary carcinoma of the thyroid. A "normal" finding in Finland. A systematic autopsy study. Cancer 1985;56(3):531–8.
6. Martinez-Tello FJ, Martinez-Cabruja R, Fernandez-Martin J, et al. Occult carcinoma of the thyroid. A systematic autopsy study from Spain of two series performed with two different methods. Cancer 1993;71(12):4022–9.
7. Hughes DT, Haymart MR, Miller BS, et al. The most commonly occurring papillary thyroid cancer in the United States is now a microcarcinoma in a patient older than 45 years. Thyroid 2011;21(3):231–6.

8. Haugen BR, Alexander EK, Bible KC, et al. 2015 American Thyroid Association management guidelines for adult patients with thyroid nodules and differentiated thyroid cancer: the American Thyroid Association guidelines task force on thyroid nodules and differentiated thyroid cancer. Thyroid 2016;26(1):1–133.
9. Morris LG, Tuttle RM, Davies L. Changing trends in the incidence of thyroid cancer in the United States. JAMA Otolaryngol Head Neck Surg 2015;91(2):165–71.
10. Haymart MR, Davies L. South Korean thyroid cancer trends: good news and bad. Thyroid 2018;28(9):1081–2.
11. Brito JP, Al Nofal A, Montori VM, et al. The impact of subclinical disease and mechanism of detection on the rise in thyroid cancer incidence: a population-based study in Olmsted County, Minnesota during 1935 through 2012. Thyroid 2015;25(9):999–1007.
12. Wu AW, Nguyen C, Wang MB. What is the best treatment for papillary thyroid microcarcinoma? Laryngoscope 2011;121(9):1828–9.
13. Merdad M, Eskander A, De Almeida J, et al. Current management of papillary thyroid microcarcinoma in Canada. J Otolaryngol Head Neck Surg 2014;43:32.
14. Sung MW, Park B, An SY, et al. Increasing thyroid cancer rate and the extent of thyroid surgery in Korea. PLoS One 2014;9(12):1–10.
15. Griffin A, Brito JP, Bahl M, et al. Applying criteria of active surveillance to low-risk papillary thyroid cancer over a decade: how many surgeries and complications can be avoided? Thyroid 2017;27(4):518–23.
16. R Michael Tuttle M. Controversial issues in thyroid cancer management. J Nucl Med 2017;008748:1–31.
17. Tulchinsky M, Binse I, Campenn A, et al. Radioactive iodine therapy for differentiated thyroid cancer : lessons from confronting controversial literature on risks for secondary malignancy. J Nucl Med 2018;59(5):723–5.
18. Hu G, Zhu W, Yang W, et al. The effectiveness of radioactive iodine remnant ablation for papillary thyroid microcarcinoma: a systematic review and meta-analysis. World J Surg 2016;40(1):100–9.
19. Schvartz C, Bonnetain F, Dabakuyo S, et al. Impact on overall survival of radioactive iodine in low-risk differentiated thyroid cancer patients. J Clin Endocrinol Metab 2012;97(5):1526–35.
20. Brabant G. Thyrotropin suppressive therapy in thyroid carcinoma: what are the targets? J Clin Endocrinol Metab 2008;93(4):1167–9.
21. Brito JP, Hay ID, Morris JC. Low risk papillary thyroid cancer. BMJ 2014;348:g3045.
22. Biondi B, Cooper DS. Benefits of thyrotropin suppression versus the risks of adverse effects in differentiated thyroid cancer. Thyroid 2010;20(2):135–46.
23. Diessl S, Holzberger B, Mäder U, et al. Impact of moderate vs stringent TSH suppression on survival in advanced differentiated thyroid carcinoma. Clin Endocrinol (Oxf) 2012;76(4):586–92.
24. Sugitani I, Fujimoto Y. Does postoperative thyrotropin suppression therapy truly decrease recurrence in papillary thyroid carcinoma? A randomized controlled trial. J Clin Endocrinol Metab 2010;95(10):4576–83.
25. Papaleontiou M, Hawley ST, Haymart MR. Effect of thyrotropin suppression therapy on bone in thyroid cancer patients. Oncologist 2016;21(2):165–71.
26. Ito Y, Miyauchi A, Kihara M, et al. Patient age is significantly related to the progression of papillary microcarcinoma of the thyroid under observation. Thyroid 2014;24(1):27–34.

27. Sugitani I, Toda K, Yamada K, et al. Three distinctly different kinds of papillary thyroid microcarcinoma should be recognized: our treatment strategies and outcomes. World J Surg 2010;34(6):1222–31.
28. Tuttle RM, Fagin JA, Minkowitz G, et al. Natural history and tumor volume kinetics of papillary thyroid cancers during active surveillance. JAMA Otolaryngol Head Neck Surg 2017;10065(10):1015–20.
29. Hay ID, Charboneau JW, Reading CC. Percutaneous ethanol injection for treatment of cervical lymph node papillary thyroid carcinoma. AJR Am J Roentgenol 2002;178(3):699–704.
30. Hay ID, Lee RA, Davidge-Pitts C, et al. Long-term outcome of ultrasound-guided percutaneous ethanol ablation of selected "recurrent" neck nodal metastases in 25 patients with TNM stages III or IVA papillary thyroid carcinoma previously treated by surgery and131I therapy. Surgery 2013;154(6):1448–55.
31. Hay ID, Lee R, Morris J, et al. Ultrasound-guided percutaneous ethanol ablation for selected patients with papillary thyroid microcarcinoma: a novel, effective and well tolerated alternative to neck surgery or observation; 87th Annual Meeting of the American Thyroid Association. Victoria (BC), October 18–22, 2017.
32. Cervelli R, Mazzeo S, De Napoli L, et al. Radiofrequency ablation in the treatment of benign thyroid nodules: an efficient and safe alternative to surgery. J Vasc Interv Radiol 2017;28(10):1400–8.
33. Chung SR, Suh CH, Baek JH, et al. Safety of radiofrequency ablation of benign thyroid nodules and recurrent thyroid cancers: a systematic review and meta-analysis. Int J Hyperthermia 2017;33(8):920–30.
34. Zhang M, Luo Y, Zhang Y, et al. Efficacy and safety of ultrasound-guided radiofrequency ablation for treating low-risk papillary thyroid microcarcinoma: a prospective study. Thyroid 2016;26(11):1581–7.
35. Zhou W, Jiang S, Zhan W, et al. Ultrasound-guided percutaneous laser ablation of unifocal T1N0M0 papillary thyroid microcarcinoma: preliminary results. Eur Radiol 2017;27(7):2934–40.
36. Welch HG, Doherty GM. Saving thyroids — overtreatment of small papillary cancers. N Engl J Med 2018;379(4):308 10.
37. Adam MA, Thomas S, Youngwirth L, et al. Is there a minimum number of thyroidectomies a surgeon should perform to optimize patient outcomes? Ann Surg 2017;265(2):402–7.
38. Marti JL, Davies L, Haymart MR, et al. Inappropriate use of radioactive iodine for low-risk papillary thyroid cancer is most common in regions with poor access to healthcare. Thyroid 2015;25(7):865–6.
39. Roman BR, Feingold JH, Patel SG, et al. The 2009 American Thyroid Association guidelines modestly reduced radioactive iodine use for thyroid cancers less than 1 cm. Thyroid 2014;24(10):1549–50.
40. Haymart MR, Banerjee M, Yang D, et al. The role of clinicians in determining radioactive iodine use for low-risk thyroid cancer. Cancer 2013;119(2):259–65.
41. Haymart MR, Banerjee M, Yang D, et al. Variation in the management of thyroid cancer. J Clin Endocrinol Metab 2013;98(5):2001–8.
42. Brito JP, Ito Y, Miyauchi A, et al. A clinical framework to facilitate risk stratification when considering an active surveillance alternative to immediate biopsy and surgery in papillary microcarcinoma. Thyroid 2016;26(1):144–9.
43. Kunneman M, Montori VM, Castaneda-Guarderas A, et al. What is shared deci-

sion making? (and what it is not). Acad Emerg Med 2016;23(12):1320–4.
44. Brito JP, Moon JH, Zeuren R, et al. Thyroid cancer treatment choice: a pilot study of a tool to facilitate conversations with patients with papillary microcarcinomas considering treatment options. Thyroid 2018;28(10):1325–31.
45. Xing M, Liu R, Liu X, et al. BRAF V600E and TERT promoter mutations cooperatively identify the most aggressive papillary thyroid cancer with highest recurrence. J Clin Oncol 2014;32(25):2718–26.
46. Liu R, Bishop J, Zhu G, et al. Mortality risk stratification by combining *BRAF* V600E and *TERT* promoter mutations in papillary thyroid cancer. JAMA Oncol 2017;3(2):202.
47. Melo M, Da Rocha AG, Vinagre J, et al. TERT promoter mutations are a major indicator of poor outcome in differentiated thyroid carcinomas. J Clin Endocrinol Metab 2014;99(5):754–65.
48. Momesso DP, Vaisman F, Yang SP, et al. Dynamic risk stratification in patients with differentiated thyroid cancer treated without radioactive iodine. J Clin Endocrinol Metab 2016;101(7):2692–700.

第14章
低危甲状腺乳头状微小癌的保守治疗

Akira Miyauchi，Yasuhiro Ito

关键词

- 甲状腺乳头状微小癌 • 密切随访 • 指南 • 不良事件 • 医疗花费
- 疾病进展率

要点

- 大部分低危的甲状腺乳头状微小癌保持稳定。
- 库马医院对患者进行了长达10年的密切随访,结果显示仅8.0%的患者出现肿瘤增大(定义为 ≥3mm),3.8%的患者出现新发淋巴结转移。
- 包括接受手术的患者在内,未发现肿瘤相关的复发或远处转移,也未观察到甲状腺乳头状微小癌的特异性死亡事件。
- 对于甲状腺乳头状微小癌的患者,密切随访应作为首选。

背景

甲状腺乳头状微小癌(papillary thyroid microcarcinoma,PTMC)是指 ≤10mm 的甲状腺乳头状癌(papillary thyroid carcinoma,PTC)。对因其他肿瘤死亡的患者进行尸体解剖,可发现 PTC 的发病率较高。此外,超声检测到3~10mm 的甲状腺癌的比例为 0.5%~5.2%[1]。Takebe[2]教授团队研究发现,日本进行甲状腺超声或超声定位下甲状腺细针穿刺细胞学检查(fine-needle aspiration cytology,

FNAC)的成年女性中,PTMC 检出率高达 3.5%,与既往尸检研究结果一致,且比当时所报道的日本成年女性甲状腺癌的发病率高出 1 000 倍以上(3.1/10 万人);由此拉开了全球甲状腺癌发病率增长的序幕[3-6]。美国在 1973—2009 年期间,甲状腺癌的发病率增长了 2.4~2.9 倍[3,4],其主要原因是医学诊断技术的不断进步和发展,使得原本可能与患者相安无事的无害性 PTMC 被检出。无独有偶,韩国在 1993—2011 年期间启动了甲状腺癌全国筛查项目,所得数据显示甲状腺癌的发病率增长了 15 倍[5]。在这些国家中,尽管甲状腺癌的发病率大幅增加,但肿瘤相关的死亡率却没有相应上升。因此,我们认为,目前对于微小 PTC 存在过度诊断和过度治疗的情况。

对低危甲状腺乳头状微小癌患者进行密切随访最早起源于日本

上文提到许多 PTMC 患者终身无症状而不知其疾患。由于尸检和流行病学筛查发现 PTMC 的发病率显著高于临床诊断,Miyauchi 教授[7]团队认为,大部分的 PTMC 是稳定的,只有少部分患者会出现进展,因此,对于 PTMC 患者,首先采取观察策略,在积极随访的过程中,若患者出现具有临床意义的肿瘤进展再进行手术也不失为治疗进程中的一次积极尝试。确诊 PTMC 后立即手术对于患者来说可能弊大于利。早在 1993 年,就有学者提出并展开临床试验项目,建议用临床密切随访来替代立即手术。此后 2 年,东京癌症研究院附属医院也开展了类似的临床试验[8]。框 14.1 为日本研究者关于低危甲状腺乳头状微小癌密切随访的总结。

框 14.1
日本研究者关于低危甲状腺乳头状微小癌密切随访的总结

1、大部分低危的 PTMC 处于休眠状态或呈惰性生长,小部分日益缩小。

2、迄今为止,在随访期间内,未观察到任何低危 PTMC 患者发生远处转移或甲状腺癌特异性死亡。

3、在密切随访过程中,即使 PTMC 出现进展再接受手术治疗,也无一例患者出现危及生命的复发或甲状腺癌相关性死亡。

4、与 PTC 不同,低危 PTMC 患者即使年龄较大,也较少发生进展。

5、尽管一小部分患者在妊娠过程中 PTMC 有所进展,但在分娩后再进行手术也为时不晚。

续表

6、对于立即手术的患者而言，即使是经验丰富的甲状腺外科医师亲自手术，术后发生喉返神经麻痹和甲状旁腺功能减退症等并发症的概率也远远高于密切随访的患者。

7、10年随访发现，手术患者的总体医疗费用是非手术患者的4.1倍。

8、肿瘤的进展与患病时的年龄成负相关。

密切随访的禁忌证

密切随访虽然具有优越性，但并不适用于所有的PTMC。密切随访的禁忌证主要分为两类(表14.1)。第一类是具有高危因素的PTMC，比如诊断时即发现淋巴结和/或远处转移(较罕见)，肿瘤侵犯喉返神经导致声带麻痹，以及病理提示高危亚型。第二类是肿瘤浸润气管或喉返神经。具有以上两类特点的PTMC未必存在较高的侵袭性，但并不推荐随访。Ito教授[9]团队强调，甲状腺癌和气管表面形成的角度是气管浸润的重要因素(图14.1)。在他们的研究中，24%(12/51)的PTMC直径≥7mm，并和气管表面形成钝角，出现了气管浸润，这样就需要切除气管软骨和黏膜(图14.2A)。而286例直径≥7mm的PTMC，与气管表现形成锐角或近似直角则无明显的气管浸润(图14.2B)。

表 14.1
甲状腺乳头状微小癌密切随访的禁忌证

分类	禁忌证
高危风险	①诊断时即伴有淋巴结和/或远处转移 ②喉返神经或气管的浸犯表现 ③高危病理亚型(比如高细胞亚型PTC或低分化甲状腺癌)
不适合密切随访的肿瘤特征	①肿瘤侵犯气管 ②肿瘤侵犯喉返神经

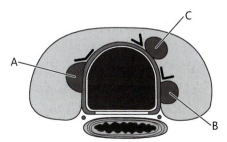

图14.1 肿瘤和气管形成的角度与气管浸润密切相关。(A)钝角；(B)近似直角；(C)锐角

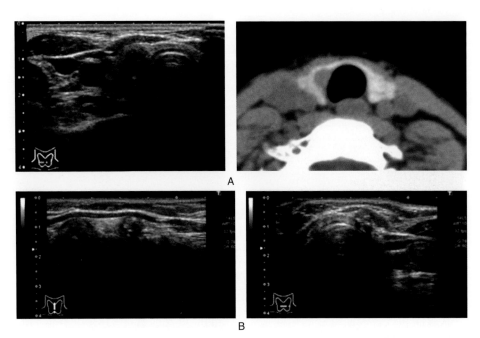

图 14.2 （A）上部两张图：PTMC 与气管所形成的典型钝角（右图：超声检查，左图：CT 平扫）。该患者需要进行气管软骨切除。（B）下部两张图：PTMC 与气管所形成的典型锐角（超声检查；右图：矢状面往左扫描。左图：横断面扫描）。因无气管浸润，故可根据患者意愿决定是否进行手术

喉返神经浸润的可能性与肿瘤和喉返神经之间是否存在正常的甲状腺组织有关（图 14.3）。98 个直径 ≥7mm 的 PTMC 病例中，有 9% 的患者肿瘤与喉返神经中间缺少正常的甲状腺组织（图 14.4），出现了喉返神经的浸润，需要进行局部或部分切除。而在 776 个直径 ≥7mm 的 PTMC 病例中，肿瘤与喉返神经中存在正常的甲状腺组织，则无一例患者出现喉返神经的浸润。<7mm 的 PTMC 没有表现出气管或喉返神经的浸润。局限于甲状腺腺叶内（图 14.5A）的肿瘤患者是密切随访的最佳人选；此外，甲状腺前叶或侧叶存在极微甲状腺外浸润（图 14.5B 和图 14.5C）并非密切随访的禁忌证。肿瘤的多病灶和分化型甲状腺癌家族史也非禁忌证。尽管这些均为低危因素，但对于这些患者而言，行甲状腺全切治疗弊大于利，

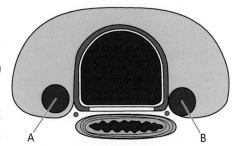

图 14.3 （A）肿瘤和喉返神经中间存在正常的甲状腺组织。（B）肿瘤和喉返神经中间缺少正常的甲状腺组织。是否存在正常的甲状腺组织与喉返神经浸润密切相关

因为可能会发生喉返神经麻痹及甲状旁腺功能减退症等并发症。

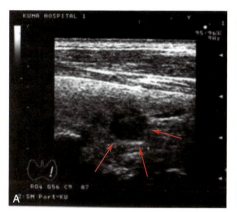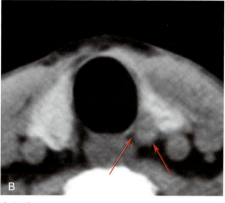

图 14.4 （A）这是一例左侧声带麻痹患者，超声影像显示左侧甲状腺腺叶背部低回声团块影。（B）该患者颈部 CT 显示左侧喉返神经缺少正常的组织边缘，即肿瘤和喉返神经之间无正常的甲状腺组织。箭头所指表示肿瘤从左侧甲状腺叶背部侵犯喉返神经

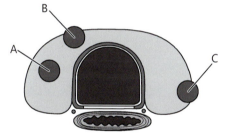

图 14.5 （A）肿瘤局限在甲状腺腺叶内，建议随访。位于甲状腺前叶（B）和侧叶（C）的肿瘤，伴有轻微腺外浸润，可以密切随访，但并非最佳选择

对低危的甲状腺乳头状微小癌进行密切随访

在库马医院，推荐对超声显示直径超过 5mm 伴可疑恶性征象的结节在超声引导下行 FNAC。2016 年，日本乳腺和甲状腺协会出台首个有关甲状腺结节 FNAC 适应证的指南。指南建议，直径超过 5mm 的甲状腺结节，若超声具有明显恶性征象，则应行 FNAC[10]，未行 FNAC 的患者于其他医生处就诊时，医生可能会建议其行非必要的手术治疗。FNAC 已被业界公认为最可靠的"金标准"。美国甲状腺学会（ATA）2015 年版指南参考了来自日本库马医

院[1,7,9]和癌症研究院附属医院[8]有关密切随访带来的友好结局后,更新了关于疑似恶性结节进行 FNAC 的标准,将结节最大径线的最低值由 0.5cm 提高到 1cm,并支持对低风险 PTMC 进行密切随访(除非出现临床显性转移或局部侵袭)[11]。

在库马医院内,临床医生一般会同时提供给低危 PTMC 患者两种治疗选择:密切随访或手术治疗。然而,在观察到低危 PTMC 患者采取密切随访相较立即手术的良好结局后(见后文),密切随访已跃身成为库马医院针对此类患者的一线管理方案。此外,一些医生建议,在随访过程中,通过补充左甲状腺素将患者的促甲状腺激素(thyroid stimulating hormone,TSH)维持在正常低值。

对于选择密切随访的低危 PTMC 患者,建议 6 个月以后复查甲状腺超声,此后每年复查 1 次。如果甲状腺结节最长直径增加 ≥3mm,则认为结节处于增长状态。此时,可建议患者行手术治疗。一般说来,对直径<13mm 的 PTMC 仍然建议随访,但若在此过程中怀疑淋巴结浸润,可以考虑超声定位下 FNAC,以及检测甲状腺球蛋白水平以进一步证实。如有淋巴结浸润,则建议行甲状腺全切除术并清扫淋巴结。

日本研究:PTMC 在密切随访期间发生进展

2003 年,库马医院的学者发表了国际上首篇 PTMC 密切观察结果的论文。文章报道,超过 70% 的患者在观察期间病灶稳定[12]。2010 年,Ito 教授[13]团队的研究显示对 PTMC 患者随访 10 年后,肿瘤增长 ≥3mm 的比例是 15.9%,而出现淋巴结转移的患者比例是 3.4%。若患者一经诊断后首先采取手术治疗,他们可能接受的只是患侧甲状腺切除术,而未做预防性淋巴结清扫。因此,即使迅速启动手术,也无法避免淋巴结转移,很可能还需要二次手术。而据文献报道,接受单次手术和二次手术的患者,其预后相当[14]。2014 年发表于 Thyroid 杂志上的一项纳入 1 235 例患者的研究显示,经过 10 年的随访,发现只有 8% 的患者超声提示肿瘤增大(>3mm),临床确认的淋巴结转移比例仅为 3.8%[15]。此外,该研究还报道肿瘤进展与年龄成负相关。多因素回归分析发现,年龄 ≤40 岁是肿瘤进展的独立危险因素,而家族史和多病灶对于低危 PTMC 的预后并无统计学意义。这一结果与 PTC 形成了鲜明的对比,在 PTC 中,患者年龄偏大是预后不良的重要因素[16]。家族史和多病灶并非 PTMC 进行密切随访的禁忌证,与上述研究所得结果一致。库马医院的研究进一步显示，即使 PTMC 患者在密切随访的过程中出现了轻微进展，再进行手术，也未发现任何患者出现肿瘤复发或特异性死亡。

早在 1995 年，日本癌症研究院医院就开展了对低危 PTMC 患者进行密切随访的研究。在对 230 例患者共计 300 个 PTMC 病灶进行长期随访的过程中，研究者发现只有 7% 出现了肿瘤增大，1% 出现了淋巴结转移[8]。此外，超声结果显示血流丰富和缺少粗大钙化与 PTMC 生长相关[17]。

日本内分泌外科医师协会与日本甲状腺外科学会已将推荐对低危 PTMC 患者进行密切随访写入首版指南中[18]；在 2018 年发表的第 2 版指南也延续了该项建议。

密切随访过程中肿瘤进展率的评估

尽管在是否延误手术时机方面，密切随访也备受争议，但 Ito[15]教授团队的研究结果则给业界吃了一颗定心丸——肿瘤的进展率与年龄成负相关。也就是说，在随访 10 年后，PTMC 患者的肿瘤进展率有所下降。Miyauchi 教授团队进一步将患者按年龄进行阶梯分组（20~70 岁），评估患者在随访期间的肿瘤进展率[19]。以 10 岁为一个阶梯，评估肿瘤进展率（增长 ≥3mm 和/或淋巴结转移）。由此，提出三种假设：假设 A，不同年龄阶段的 PTMC 都可以出现疾病进展；假设 B，最初接受手术治疗的患者出现肿瘤进展，而其他患者肿瘤无进展；假设 C，疾病进展的实际概率介于假设 A 和假设 B 估算的值之间的情况。假设 C 被认为出现的可能性最大。结果显示，20 岁、30 岁、40 岁、50 岁、60 岁和 70 岁的肿瘤进展率分别是 48.6%、25.3%、20.9%、10.3%、8.2% 和 3.5%[19]。也就是说，在 20 多岁的患者中，接近一半的患者会出现肿瘤的进展，继而需要接受手术治疗，其余患者的肿瘤是稳定的。延迟手术的患者无肿瘤复发或特异性死亡。虽然年轻的 PTMC 患者容易出现肿瘤进展，但不危及生命，研究者认为他们仍然可以作为密切随访的对象。而年长的患者则较少出现肿瘤进展，不太需要手术治疗。

密切随访与立即手术的不良事件对比

对患者和医生来说，手术切除 PTMC 似乎要比密切随访来得简单和方便。然而韩国开展的一项全国性流行病学调查研究显示，因甲状腺癌的井喷式增长导致的手术量增加及术后一系列的并发症的出现，相比并未改善的死亡率更引起了业界的广泛关注[5]。Oda 教授团队研究了来自库马医院的 2 153 例低危 PTMC 患者，其中 45% 的患者诊断后立即接受了手术治疗，另有 55% 的患者一开始就选择密切随访[20]。两组患者的预后都比较理想。但即便是由经验丰富的甲状腺外科医生亲自手术，术后不良事件也无法避免（一过性/永久性声带麻痹或甲状旁腺功能减退、术后需服用甲状腺素和遗留手术瘢痕等）[20]。据研究报道，一过性声带麻痹的发生率为 4.1%，永久性声带麻痹的发生率为 0.2%，而一过性和永久性甲状旁腺机能减退症的发生率分别为 16.7% 和 1.6%。如果由年轻医生主刀，不良事件的发生率会更高，且有 66.1% 的患者会被告知术后需服用左甲状腺素替代治疗。以上结果证实，对于低危 PTMC 患者来说，密切随访优于手术治疗。

密切随访期间妊娠患者的管理

妊娠期间女性会分泌大量的人绒毛膜促性腺激素（human chorionic gonadotropin, HCG）。该激素与 TSH 有共同的 α 亚基，可以刺激滤泡细胞增生。因此，妊娠可能促进 PTMC 恶化。既往文献报道，在 9 例妊娠合并 PTMC 的患者中，4 例出现了肿瘤增长[21]。随后 Ito 教授[22]团队研究了 51 例妊娠合并 PTMC 的患者，结果显示只有 4 例（8%）患者出现了肿瘤增长。其中 2 例患者在分娩后接受了手术治疗，术后无复发。剩下 2 例患者产后 PTMC 稳定，故而继续保持密切随访。由此可见，妊娠合并 PTMC 的患者若出现肿瘤增长，可在分娩后再接受手术治疗。年轻的 PTMC 患者可以考虑怀孕，在 PTMC 治疗决策的危险分层中，她们属于适合的观察候选人[23]。

密切随访期间甲状腺素抑制治疗

近期一项研究报道，相比于中年或老年患者，年轻的 PTMC 患者更容易出现肿瘤进展[15]。尽管该研究样本量较小，但在研究中，当患者的 TSH 均控制在正常低值后未发现任何患者出现肿瘤进展[15]。Sugitani 教授[24]团队的研究发现 PTMC 进展与 TSH 水平并不相关，而韩国的研究与之相左，认为肿瘤的进展与 TSH 水平成正相关[25]。目前尚无有关在 PTMC 中进行 TSH 抑制治疗的对照研究，此领域（尤其是在年轻患者中）仍有待深入探索。

密切随访和立即手术的医疗费用对比

医疗费用无论是对患者抑或整个社会来说都是非常重要的问题。在日本，由于医疗体制的不同，几乎所有的临床治疗措施都会在医疗保险系统内进行。Oda 教授[26]团队比较了手术组和密切随访组的患者 10 年内的总体医疗费用（包括诊断、初次手术、二次手术、复发手术、检查和用药），结果显示，手术组总体的医疗费用是随访组的 4.1 倍。来自我国香港的研究结果与之不谋而合[27]。

病理学

Hirokawa 教授[28]团队对因淋巴结浸润（11 例）、肿瘤增大（18 例）和其他与非进展相关的原因（160 例）而切除的 PTMC 手术标本进行了组织病理学研究，发现腺内扩散的比例分别为 36.4%、22.2% 和 2.5%；出现砂粒体的比例分别是 18.2%、5.6% 和 1.3%；Ki-67 表达超过 5% 的比例分别为 9.1%、50.0% 和 5.0%。因此，研究者得到结论，腺内扩散和砂粒体的出现与淋巴结转移有关，而高 Ki-67 表达与肿瘤增大相关。

BRAF 基因突变与 *TERT* 启动子突变

Xing 教授[29]团队研究显示，当 *BRAF* 基因突变和 *TERT* 启动子突变共存时，提示 PTC 预后较差。Yabuta 教授[30]团队对因淋巴结转移（5 例）、肿瘤增大（10 例）和其他与非进展相关的原因（11 例）而切除的 PTMC 手术标本进行了基因突变研究，发现其 *BRAF* 基因突变率分别是 80%、70% 和 64%，但并无患者出现 *TERT* 启动子突变。因此，对于 PTMC 基因突变的检测似乎并不能提示其预后。

其他国家对于低危甲状腺乳头状微小癌的密切随访情况

2012 年，Michael Tuttle 教授参观了日本库马医院，并观摩了 PTMC 的随访流程，随即回到纽约 Memorial Sloan Kettering 癌症中心开展了继日本之后的第二个 PTMC 密切随访项目。Tuttle 教授的同事 Brito 教授[23]团队建议根据患者的肿瘤的危险程度来决定是否进行密切随访。按照肿瘤特征、患者特征和医疗小组特征将患者归为理想、合适和不合适进行随访三个组别。

2017 年,Tuttle 教授团队[31]发表了第一篇美国甲状腺癌密切随访前瞻性研究论文。他们证实了之前日本学者的研究结论,即诊断时的年龄较小是肿瘤生长的独立危险因素。在密切随访的 284 例患者中,有 12.7% 的患者肿瘤体积增大超过 50%,80.2% 的患者无变化,6.7% 的患者肿瘤体积缩小>50%。此外,他们的研究还发现,有 3.8% 的患者在检测到肿瘤直径增加后(≥3mm),肿瘤体积也随之增大。

最近,Memorial Sloan Kettering 癌症中心与韩国研究团队共同开展了一项名为"甲状腺癌治疗选择"的研究,主要针对 PTMC 的两种治疗选择(手术和密切随访),患者被分到寻求医生帮助组和自行选择组中参与调研[32]。结果显示,参与讨论寻求医生帮助的患者选择密切随访的可能性更高。

两项来自澳大利亚的研究就密切随访这一举措对医生进行了调研,发现很多医生更倾向于选择手术[33,34]。但是,此项调研开展于日本学者的研究发表之前,医生们在调研的时候对手术的不良事件以及密切随访的益处并不了解[20]。在库马医院的研究发表后,相比立即手术,医生们则更愿意选择密切随访。

韩国的一项研究对因主观意愿拒绝手术,或者并存其他恶性肿瘤或高危并发症而不能手术的微小 PTC 患者进行了回顾,共纳入了 192 例患者,中位随访 30 个月后,发现 27 例(14%)患者出现了肿瘤体积增长超过 50%,其中 24 例(13%)患者进行了手术治疗[35]。

讨论

早在 1993 年,库马医院即开始了对低风险 PTMC 的密切随访,如今,密切随访已经成为日本和美国指南中推荐的一种治疗方案[11,18]。而在库马医院,密切随访已经成为目前低危 PTMC 首选治疗方式。然而,人们接受这一方案用了将近 20 年的时间,即便是在库马医院内,也并未获得所有医生的认可。1993—1997 年,选择密切随访的患者只有 30%,但是随着时间的推移,选择密切随访的患者比例在不断增加,截至 2014 年已达到 88%[36]。自行选择密切随访的患者比例和接受主治医生建议而选择密切随访的患者比例之间存在显著的差异。由于目前还缺乏具有说服力的证据,这种现象可能在新的比较权威的随访共识制定之后才能得到合理解决。我们希望能有更快的方式获得足够的证据来证明密切随访的安全性及优势。

我们必须重视仍然存在的一些重要的临床问题,首先是增大的 PTMC 肿瘤的测量问题。库马医院采用超声检查来测量每一个 PTMC 的三维直径,但这种方法无法评估结节的深度,因为粗大钙化会造成回声增强影响测量。而在长直径方面,结节的变化是容易测量的,直径增长 ≥3mm 即可认为 PTMC 在增长。对于这部分患者,仍可以密切随访,直到 PTMC 长到 13mm 才考虑推荐进行手术治疗。Tuttle 教授团队[31]提出,超声监测到肿瘤体积增大超过 50% 便可以早期定义肿瘤增长,而非采用最大直径增长 ≥3mm 的标准。他们的研究显示,在随访 2 年和 5 年时,PTMC 的最大直径增长 ≥3mm 的概率分别是 2.5% 和 3.8%,体积增大超过 50% 的概率分别是 11.5% 和 24.8%。如果一个 PTMC 从 6mm×6mm×6mm 增长到了 7mm×7mm×7mm,那么代表它在体积上增大了 59%,但是这种方法过于敏感,也过分关注 PTMC 大小和体积的变化。因此,对于这部分患者来说,最适合手术的时机依然不明确。在日本两家医院的研究中,即使 PTMC 长直径增长 >3mm,也无一例患者出现远处转移和甲状腺癌特异性死亡。

其次,对于 PTMC 患者来说,我们需要减轻患者的心理负担。同时,这也可能是 2015 年版 ATA 指南不推荐对 1cm 以下的无恶性征象的甲状腺结节行 FNAC 的原因[11]。"甲状腺癌治疗选择"这一项目旨在推广 PTMC 患者与其主治医生之间的交流[32],很多接受这个项目的患者倾向于选择密切随访。虽然该项目并未评估 PTMC 患者的心理健康状态,但通过与其主治医生的讨论可以在一定程度上减轻患者的焦虑,这有助于维持肿瘤稳定。当患者在选择治疗方案的时候,医生务必要将所有的重要信息告知患者。医生需要具备专业的临床交流能力并对这类常见的疾病有正确的认识,以确保能给予患者正确的指导。

最后,我们希望给大家带来一个简便易行的治疗策略:在进行 FNAC 之前,编写有关 PTMC 的小册子,向患者提供其含义的简短解读。希望能通过此种方法帮助低危 PTMC 患者合理选择治疗方案。截至目前,低危 PTMC 患者选择密切随访的比例已增至 95%。为减少正在接受密切随访的患者的焦虑情绪,我们准备开展一项健康宣教,通过充分告知患者密切随访相较于手术的安全性和优势,来尽可能地减轻这部分患者的焦虑和担忧。

总结

经过 25 年的数据沉淀,研究者们已经充分证实了在 PTMC 患者中首先进行密切随访较立即手术具有更显著的安全性和优势。由于大部分的 PTMC 比较稳定，即使在密切随访中发现肿瘤增长再接受手术治疗也不失为一个良好选择，故而密切随访应作为低危 PTMC 的首选治疗措施。

（黄玥晔　曲　伸）

参考文献

1. Ito Y, Miyauchi A. A therapeutic strategy for incidentally detected papillary microcarcinoma of the thyroid. Nat Clin Pract Endocrinol Metab 2007;3:240–8.
2. Takebe K, Date M, Yamamoto N, et al. Mass screening for thyroid cancer with ultrasonography. KARKINOS 1994;7:309–17 [in Japanese].
3. Davies L, Welch HG. Increasing incidence of thyroid cancer in the United States, 1973-2002. JAMA 2006;295:2164–7.
4. Davies L, Welch HG. Current thyroid cancer trends in the United States. JAMA Otolaryngol Head Neck Surg 2014;140:217–22.
5. Ahn HS, Kim HJ, Welch HG. Korea's thyroid-cancer "epidemic" – screening and overdiagnosis. N Engl J Med 2014;371:1765–7.
6. Vaccarella S, Franceschi S, Bray F, et al. Worldwide thyroid-cancer epidemic? The increasing impact at overdiagnosis. N Engl J Med 2016;375:614–7.
7. Miyauchi A, Ito Y, Oda H. Insights into the management of papillary microcarcinoma of the thyroid. Thyroid 2018;28:23–31.
8. Sugitani I, Toda K, Yamada K, et al. Three distinctly different kinds of papillary thyroid microcarcinoma should be recognized our treatment strategies and outcomes. World J Surg 2010;34:1222–31.
9. Ito Y, Miyauchi A, Oda H, et al. Revisiting low-risk thyroid papillary microcarcinomas resected without observation: was immediate surgery necessary? World J Surg 2016;40:523–8.
10. Ver 3. In: Japan Association of Breast and Thyroid Sonology, editor. Guidebook on ultrasound diagnosis of the thyroid. Tokyo: Nankodo; 2016. p. 50 [in Japanese].
11. Haugen BR, Alexander EK, Bible KC, et al. 2015 American Thyroid Association management guidelines for adult patients with thyroid nodules and differentiated thyroid cancer: The American Thyroid Association Guidelines Task Force on thyroid nodules and differentiated thyroid cancer. Thyroid 2016;26:1–133.
12. Ito Y, Uruno T, Nakano K, et al. An observation trial without surgical treatment in patients with papillary microcarcinoma of the thyroid. Thyroid 2003;13:381–7.
13. Ito Y, Miyauchi A, Inoue H, et al. An observation trial for papillary thyroid microcarcinoma in Japanese patients. World J Surg 2010;34:28–35.
14. Miyauchi A. Clinical trials of active surveillance of papillary microcarcinoma of the thyroid. World J Surg 2016;40:516–22.
15. Ito Y, Miyauchi A, Kihara M, et al. Patient age is significantly related to the progression of papillary microcarcinoma of the thyroid under observation. Thyroid 2014;24:27–34.

16. Ito Y, Miyauchi A, Kihara M, et al. Overall survival of papillary thyroid carcinoma patients: a single-institution long-term follow-up of 5897 patients. World J Surg 2018;42:615–22.
17. Fukuoka O, Sugitani I, Ebina A, et al. Natural history of asymptomatic papillary thyroid microcarcinoma: time-dependent changes in calcification and vascularity during active surveillance. World J Surg 2016;40:529–37.
18. Takami H, Ito Y, Okamoto T, et al. Therapeutic strategy for differentiated thyroid carcinoma in Japan based on a newly established guideline managed by Japanese Society of Thyroid Surgeons and Japanese Association of Endocrine Surgeons. World J Surg 2011;35:111–21.
19. Miyauchi A, Kudo T, Ito Y, et al. Estimation of the lifetime probability of disease progression of papillary microcarcinoma of the thyroid during active surveillance. Surgery 2018;163:48–52.
20. Oda H, Miyauchi A, Ito Y, et al. Incidences of unfavorable events in the management of low-risk papillary microcarcinoma of the thyroid by active surveillance versus immediate surgery. Thyroid 2016;26:150–8.
21. Shindo H, Amino N, Ito Y, et al. 2014 Papillary thyroid microcarcinoma might progress during pregnancy. Thyroid 2014;24:840–4.
22. Ito Y, Miyauchi A, Kudo T, et al. Effects of pregnancy on papillary microcarcinoma of the thyroid re-evaluated in the entire patients series at Kuma Hospital. Thyroid 2016;26:156–60.
23. Brito JP, Ito Y, Miyauchi A, et al. A clinical framework to facilitate risk stratification when considering an active surveillance alternative to immediate biopsy and surgery in papillary microcarcinoma. Thyroid 2016;26:144–9.
24. Sugitani I, Fujimoto Y, Yamada K. Association between serum thyrotropin concentration and growth of asymptomatic papillary thyroid microcarcinoma. World J Surg 2014;38:673–8.
25. Kim HI, Jang HW, Ahn HS, et al. High serum TSH level is associated with progression of papillary thyroid microcarcinoma during active surveillance. J Clin Endocrinol Metab 2018;103:446–51.
26. Oda H, Miyauchi A, Ito Y, et al. Comparison of the costs of active surveillance and immediate surgery in the management of low-risk papillary microcarcinoma of the thyroid. Endocr J 2017;64:59–64.
27. Lang BH, Wong CK. A cost-effectiveness comparison between early surgery and non-surgical approach for incidental papillary thyroid microcarcinoma. Eur J Endocrinol 2015;173:367–75.
28. Hirokawa M, Kudo T, Ota H, et al. Pathological characteristics of low-risk papillary thyroid microcarcinoma with progression during active surveillance. Endocr J 2016;63:805–10.
29. Xing A, Liu R, Liu X, et al. BRAF V600E and TERT promoter mutations cooperatively identify the most aggressive papillary thyroid cancer with highest recurrence. J Clin Oncol 2014;32:2718–26.
30. Yabuta T, Matsuse M, Hirokawa M, et al. TERT promoter mutations were not found in papillary thyroid microcarcinomas that showed disease progression on active surveillance. Thyroid 2017;27:1206–7.
31. Tuttle RM, Fagin JA, Minkowitz G, et al. Natural history and tumor volume kinetics of papillary thyroid cancers during active surveillance. JAMA Otolaryngol Head Neck Surg 2017;143:1015–20.
32. Brito JP, Moon JH, Zeuren R, et al. Thyroid Cancer Treatment Choice: a pilot study

of a tool to facilitate conversations with patients with papillary microcarcinomas considering treatment choice. Thyroid 2018. https://doi.org/10.1089/thy.2018.0105.
33. Nickel B, Brito JP, Barratt A, et al. Clinicians' view on management and terminology for papillary thyroid microcarcinoma: a qualitative study. Thyroid 2017;27:661–71.
34. Nickel B, Brito JP, Moynihan R, et al. Patients' experiences of diagnosis and management of papillary thyroid microcarcinoma: a qualitative study. BMC Cancer 2018;18:242.
35. Kwon H, Oh HS, Kim M, et al. Active surveillance for patients with papillary thyroid microcarcinoma: a single center's experience in Korea. J Clin Endocrinol Metab 2017;102:1917–25.
36. Ito Y, Miyauchi A, Kudo T, et al. Trends in the implementation of active surveillance for low-risk papillary thyroid microcarcinomas at Kuma Hospital: Gradual increase and heterogeneity in the acceptance of this new management option. Thyroid 2018;28:488–95.

第15章
甲状腺癌的激素抑制治疗

Bernadette Biondi, David S. Cooper

关键词

- 甲状腺癌 • 左旋甲状腺素 • 促甲状腺激素 • 心血管系统 • 骨
- 死亡率

要点

- 甲状腺激素抑制治疗可降低分化型甲状腺癌患者的血清促甲状腺激素水平,该方法有望改善患者的预后。
- 除了进展期的患者,没有充分证据表明TSH抑制能改善预后。
- 甲状腺激素抑制疗法产生的医源性甲状腺功能亢进症可导致包括骨质疏松、骨折和心血管疾病在内的不良结局,包括心房颤动。
- 甲状腺激素抑制治疗的使用应基于疾病的初始风险和对疾病状态的动态评估。尽可能使用最低剂量的甲状腺激素。

引言

甲状腺激素抑制治疗的基本原理是垂体分泌的促甲状腺激素(thyroid-stimulating hormone,TSH)能影响甲状腺癌细胞的生长和发育[1]。多项流行病学研究表明较高的血清TSH水平(即使在正常范围内),可能与甲状腺结节恶变风险增加以及甲状腺癌侵袭性增强有关[2-5]。这一理论在小鼠模型中得到了验证:通过调节甲状腺激素受体信号转导通路,促使血清TSH水平持续升高,最终导致这些小鼠患转移性甲状腺癌的概率增加[6]。在另一个小鼠模型中,通过敲入致癌基因 *BRAF V600E* 突变以诱导甲状腺癌,其基因组中 TSH 受体基因被敲除的小鼠甲状腺癌进展显著变缓[7]。由于缺乏 TSH 受体表达,这些动物也有很高的血清 TSH 水平。虽然这些小鼠仍会发生甲状腺癌,但其疾病侵袭性低于表达野生型 TSH 受体小鼠的甲状腺癌。这表明,尽管 TSH 可能不是甲状腺癌发生的必要条件,但是其与甲状腺癌的持续与发展有关。此外,在具有 *V600E* 突变的动物中,抑制 TSH 水平并不能阻止甲状腺癌的扩散,这可能是由于肿瘤使 TSH 受体的表达出现了继发性改变[8]。该观察结果可能支持以下观点:TSH 抑制治疗在晚期甲状腺癌患者的治疗中可能价值有限(请参阅后文的讨论)。

临床研究

所有接受甲状腺全切除术的患者以及极少数接受腺叶切除术的患者都需要甲状腺激素治疗以维持正常的血清 TSH 水平。相反,至少从理论上讲,TSH 抑制疗法的原理是:低于正常水平的血清 TSH 可能会抑制 DTC 的生长和扩散。为验证这一观点,2002 年,研究者对 10 项 20 世纪 70—90 年代发表的研究结果进行了荟萃分析,结论是,甲状腺激素抑制治疗可有效降低甲状腺癌发病率和死亡率($RR=0.71$,$P<0.05$),减少不良事件(包括疾病进展/复发和死亡)的发生[9]。然而,这些较早的研究未必将 TSH 替代疗法与 TSH 抑制疗法区分开,且缺乏现代技术(例如超声和甲状腺球蛋白测量)来充分检测小范围的复发。但是,最近发表的两篇后续研究[10,11]得出结论:积极的血清 TSH 抑制治疗可使存在远处转移的患者生存获益,尽管其中一项研究的归因生存率并没有统计学差异[10]。重要的是,在另一项研究中[11],与血清 TSH 水平仅被抑制到<0.1mU/L 的患者相比,血清 TSH 水平完全被抑制(<0.03mU/L)并存在转移的患者没有进一步的生存获益。

美国甲状腺癌协会的国家甲状腺癌治疗合作研究组的研究表明,积极的 TSH 抑制疗法对复发风险低的患者无价值,但对高危患者有益[12,13]。最新的一项前瞻性队列研究纳入近 5 000 名受试者,平均中位时间为 6 年,TSH 抑制程度中等。结果表明,与血清 TSH 水平在正常范围至升高范围内相比,血清 TSH 水平始终维持在低于正常(0.1~0.4mU/L)到正常范围内可使处于疾病各个阶段的患者获得更好的结果[14],但随访 5 年后,并未发现抑制 TSH 的其他益处。这与荷兰的一项早期研究一致,后者的研究显示,通过 9 年的随访,血清 TSH 水平抑制在均值<2mU/L 的个体与血清 TSH 水平保持在均值>2mU/L

的个体，在复发率和死亡率上无显著差异[15]。在关于甲状腺癌 TSH 抑制治疗的唯一一项随机前瞻性研究中，400 名日本受试者随机接受左甲状腺素（LT$_4$）治疗，以将血清 TSH 水平维持在参考范围内，或者维持血清 TSH 水平＜0.01mU/L[16]。在平均随访了近 7 年后，即使单独对高复发风险的受试者进行分析，两组之间的无病生存率也没有差异[16]。

最新的美国甲状腺协会（American Thyroid Association, ATA）指南推荐对低风险 DTC 患者应用甲状腺全切除术或腺叶切除术[17]。许多接受腺叶切除术的患者将不再需要用甲状腺激素替代疗法维持血清 TSH 水平。近期，Park 及其同事对 1 818 例接受腺叶切除术的甲状腺癌患者的进行了回顾性分析[18]，发现使用甲状腺激素维持血清 TSH 水平≤2.0mU/L 对无复发生存没有益处。此外，即使在那些未接受 LT$_4$ 治疗的研究对象中，TSH＜2mU/L 和 TSH 水平在 2~4.5mU/L 的两组人群的无复发生存率之间也没有差异。但他们的动态风险分层存在差异，与接受甲状腺激素治疗以将其 TSH 水平维持在 2mU/L 以下的腺叶切除的受试者相比，未接受甲状腺激素的受试者具有生化不确定反应的概率更大（17.2% vs. 9.4%）[18]。但是，应谨慎解读这项研究，因为所有接受了腺叶切除术的受试者也都接受了预防性的同侧中央区淋巴结清扫术，这在美国通常是不进行的。

通常，要达到正常 TSH 水平，每日的 LT$_4$ 剂量需要在 1.6~1.8μg/kg，而抑制血清 TSH 则需要 2.0~2.2μg/kg 的剂量。但是，患者的剂量需求有很大的个体差异性，并且取决于多个因素，包括体重指数、合并药物的使用，以及药物的生物利用度等。

利用左甲状腺素进行促甲状腺激素抑制治疗的不良反应

多年来，所有 DTC 的患者都可能在甲状腺手术和放射性碘（radioactive iodine, RAI）消融后接受过量的 LT$_4$ 剂量，从而有意将血清 TSH 抑制在不可检测的水平（灵敏的第三代测定法可测得 TSH＜0.01mU/L）[19,20]。在这些患者中，血清游离甲状腺素（FT$_4$）浓度通常处于参考范围的上限或明显升高[21-23]。这种被称为外源性（exogenous, Exo）亚临床甲亢（SHyper）的疾病可能与甲亢的症状和体征有关，也可能导致心理、社会和身体生活质量受损[20,24-28]，以及对心脏和骨骼的不良影响，包括增加心血管（cardiovascular, CV）发病率和死亡率，以及增加骨质疏松症和骨折的风险[19]。

心血管疾病的发病率和死亡率

多项回顾性研究报告称,长期 TSH 抑制治疗可增加心率和左心室质量 (left ventricular mass,LVM)[20,29-31],导致心肌劳损[30]和舒张功能受损[32-34],并降低动脉弹性[35]、心脏储备和运动能力[36,37]。尽管这些研究都没有根据 TSH 抑制水平对 CV 形态和功能进行分层评估,但 LVM 的升高与 TSH 抑制持续时间的相关性高于其与循环甲状腺激素水平的相关性。这些结果表明,由轻微甲状腺激素过量引起的长期血液动力学超负荷和持续的运动亢进状态是这种向心性心脏重塑的主要决定因素[19,38]。应用 β 受体拮抗剂[30,39]或恢复甲状腺功能[38]后,可以逆转 CV 形态和功能的不良改变。心房颤动(atrial fibrillation,AF)和血栓前状态是 DTC Exo SHyper 患者最重要的不良事件,是导致心血管疾病(cardiovascular disease,CVD)相关住院风险增加的原因[40]。一项针对长期接受 TSH 抑制疗法的受试者的人群研究表明,CVD 和心律失常的风险随年龄增长而增加[41]。同样,在两项分别对 136 名[42]和 518[43]名受试者进行的回顾性研究中,老年组的房颤患病率更高(18% vs. 8%,60 岁以上 vs. 60 岁以下)[42]。房颤的风险为 17.5%,显著高于按性别和年龄调整的预测风险[42]。

相反,一项前瞻性研究称在 756 名低风险和中度风险受试者中,血清 TSH 水平 ≤ 0.4mU/L 和 > 0.4mU/L 时的 AF 风险相当[44]。同样,在另外两项研究中,TSH 水平与 AF 的发生之间也没有相关性[43,44]。有趣的是,房颤的风险独立于传统的风险因素,却与 RAI 的累积剂量相关[43]。这些数据表明,RAI 对心脏炎症、氧化应激或纤维化具有潜在作用,因为钠 - 碘共转运蛋白基因在心脏组织中表达[45]。所有这些数据表明,高龄、TSH 抑制的持续时间以及合并症的发生,可能是与 Exo SHyper 患者 CV 不良预后相关的主要因素。

DTC 患者的 CV 死亡率和全因死亡率数据不一致[40,46-49]。在一项大型回顾性研究中,与对照组相比,患有 DTC 的受试者的 CV 死亡风险增加了 3.3 倍,全因死亡率增加了 4.4 倍[46]。这些风险与年龄、性别和 CV 事件风险因素无关。TSH 的几何平均值每降低 1 倍,CV 死亡风险增加 3.1 倍,两者独立相关[46]。对于 RAI 治疗,尽管 RAI 治疗组的 CVD 发病率高于对照组和未经治疗组,但在进行 RAI 消融的患者(累积 RAI 剂量为 100mCi)中,全因死亡率的风险与累积 RAI 剂量无相关性[40]。因此,不同程度的 TSH 抑制的潜在作用以及 RAI 治疗对 CV 事件发病率和死亡率的影响仍有待研究。

骨质疏松症的风险

过量的甲状腺激素可通过缩短骨骼重塑周期并加速骨骼更新而对骨骼重塑产生重要影响[50]。另一方面，TSH 是骨转换的负调节剂，对骨吸收具有特定的抑制作用[51,52]。Exo SHyper 对骨转换的影响在横断面和纵向研究中存在矛盾。评估 TSH 抑制疗法对 DTC 患者的骨矿物质密度（bone mineral density，BMD）的两个综述表明，抑制 TSH 并不影响男性或绝经前女性的 BMD，而绝经后女性则有骨质流失的风险[53,54]。

同样，两个 meta 分析[55,56]显示，在 Exo SHyper 的绝经后妇女中，出现 BMD 降低，年骨量减少 0.91%[55]。一些研究报道称，骨小梁评分测量[57]或高分辨率断层 CT 扫描[58,59]显示，TSH 抑制疗法可影响骨小梁的微结构。TSH 抑制治疗也可能与放射性椎体骨折相关，该现象可见于大约 1/3 患 DTC 的妇女，并且与治疗时间、TSH 抑制程度和患者年龄有关[60]。

对低风险或中度风险的 DTC 受试者的一项前瞻性研究表明，与未接受抑制治疗的受试者相比，抑制疗法后 TSH<0.4mU/L 的受试者的骨质疏松症的发生率更高（RR=2.1，P=0.05），且长期用 LT_4 进行 TSH 抑制治疗的 DTC 患者，其术后骨质疏松的发病率较高[44]。TSH 抑制的持续时间被认为是一个重要的因素。在一项随机对照研究中，女性受试者被随机分配接受 TSH 抑制治疗或不接受治疗，其中接受 TSH 抑制治疗的研究对象在术后 1 年开始出现 BMD 明显下降。此外，研究者在年龄较大的受试者（>50 岁）中观察到 BMD 显著降低，而在较年轻的受试者（<50 岁）中未观察到 BMD 的降低。据报道，TSH 抑制治疗持续 5 年后，受试者的 BMD 明显下降，尤其是那些年龄较大且术前 BMD 较低的受试者[61]。一直到术后 5 年，未接受 TSH 抑制的受试者的 T 分数均无显著降低[61]。所有这些结果表明，长期 TSH 抑制疗法与骨质流失有关，在老年患者和绝经后妇女中尤为明显。

骨折风险

与一般人群相比，LT_4 治疗期间血清 TSH 水平<0.1mU/L 的绝经后妇女发生骨质疏松性骨折的风险高 2~4 倍。在 70 岁或以上的老年人中，LT_4 与骨折风险成强烈的剂量反应关系[62]。多项研究和 meta 分析（包括前瞻性研究）已证实亚临床甲状腺激素过量与骨折风险之间的相关性，这些研究主要针对

绝经后妇女[41,62-68]。它们大多证实了 TSH 抑制持续时间与骨折风险增加之间的相关性。SHyper 中轻度的甲状腺激素过量对于肌肉力量、重量和去脂体重有不良影响,可能也与老年患者认知障碍相关,并导致治疗期间患者骨折的风险增加[69]。

游离甲状腺素水平升高与心血管风险的影响

Exo SHyper 患者的总 T_3 或游离 T_3 水平常位于参考范围的中下部分,继而出现 T_4/T_3 比值的增加[13-16]。因此,由于严重程度和循环甲状腺激素水平的差异,内源性和 Exo SHyper(由 Graves 病或毒性结节性甲状腺肿引起)在生化方面不具有可比性[69]。这可能表明,内源性和 Exo SHper 对于心血管系统和骨骼结构的不良影响作用机制不同。一些研究报道表明,就 AF 和 CV 死亡率而言,在参考范围内高血清 FT_4 水平可能与老年患者的不良健康结局相关[70-73]。当血清 FT_4 在参考范围的最高 1/4 时,老年受试者 AF 和 CV 的发病率和死亡率可能会增加[70-73]。此外,在参考范围内的 TSH 低值和 FT_4 高值与正常绝经后妇女髋部骨折风险增加 22%~25% 相关[74]。需要进行前瞻性研究来评估增加的 T_4/T_3 比值对 DTC 患者的 CV 和骨骼风险的作用。

外源性亚临床甲状腺功能亢进症的治疗

需要进行大规模的随机对照研究以证明 TSH 抑制治疗对心脏和骨骼影响的因果关系,并评估 TSH 标准化对 CV 风险和骨折的疗效。没有研究曾经评估过 β 受体拮抗剂对 CV 死亡率的影响,即使这些药物可以改善与普通人群发病率增加相关的 CV 参数。阿仑膦酸盐治疗可以预防接受甲状腺素替代治疗的甲状腺癌患者的骨小梁丢失[75]。但是,应考虑 AF 的潜在风险并进行风险收益评估[76]。

甲状腺激素治疗的建议

鉴于有证据表明积极进行 TSH 抑制对复发和死亡风险较低的低危甲状腺癌患者几乎没有益处,并且考虑到这种疗法的潜在益处必须与 CV 和骨骼风险相平衡,ATA 建议采用分层处理(图 15.1)[17]。ATA 建议采用持续风险分层的概念,对于治疗反应良好(影像学阴性和无法检测到抑制后的甲状腺球蛋白）的低危和中危患者，ATA 建议维持血清 TSH 水平在 0.5~2mU/L，而对于治疗反应良好的高危患者使用轻度的 TSH 抑制（TSH 水平在 0.1~0.5mU/L）。对于生化反应不完全的患者，也建议轻度抑制 TSH。对于有残余病灶或生化反应不完全的患者，如果患者年轻或 Exo SHyper 发生并发症的风险较低，建议使用更高强度的 TSH 抑制（即血清 TSH<0.1mU/L，但不一定需要抑制到无法检测的水平）。对患者的临床疾病状况以及危险因素的短期发展（如高龄、绝经后状态、骨质疏松和 / 或 CVD）进行动态评估，是适时停止治疗、防止患者病情恶化的关键，其比治疗疾病本身更重要。

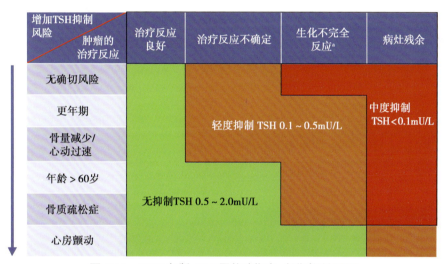

图 15.1　2015 年版 ATA 甲状腺指南：长期抑制 TSH

a 最初的 ATA 风险，甲状腺球蛋白（thyroglobulin，Tg）水平，随着时间推移的 Tg 趋势和抑制 TSH 的风险，导致生化不完全反应患者的 TSH 目标可能会有很大差异

（李　超　孙荣昊　周雨秋）

参考文献

1. McLeod DS. Thyrotropin in the development and management of differentiated thyroid cancer. Endocrinol Metab Clin North Am 2014;43:367–83.
2. Boelaert K, Horacek J, Holder RL, et al. Serum thyrotropin concentration as a novel predictor of malignancy in thyroid nodules investigated by fine-needle aspiration. J Clin Endocrinol Metab 2006;91:4295–301.
3. Haymart MR, Repplinger DJ, Leverson GE, et al. Higher serum thyroid stimulating hormone level in thyroid nodule patients is associated with greater risks of differ-

entiated thyroid cancer and advanced tumor stage. J Clin Endocrinol Metab 2008;93:809–14.
4. McLeod DS, Watters KF, Carpenter AD, et al. Thyrotropin and thyroid cancer diagnosis: a systematic review and dose-response meta-analysis. J Clin Endocrinol Metab 2012;97:2682–92.
5. McLeod DS, Cooper DS, Ladenson PW, et al. Prognosis of differentiated thyroid cancer in relation to serum thyrotropin and thyroglobulin antibody status at time of diagnosis. Thyroid 2014;24:35–42.
6. Suzuki H, Willingham MC, Cheng SY. Mice with a mutation in the thyroid hormone receptor beta gene spontaneously develop thyroid carcinoma: a mouse model of thyroid carcinogenesis. Thyroid 2002;12:963–9.
7. Franco AT, Malaguarnera R, Refetoff S, et al. Thyrotrophin receptor signaling dependence of Braf-induced thyroid tumor initiation in mice. Proc Natl Acad Sci U S A 2011;108:1615–20.
8. Xing M, Usadel H, Cohen Y, et al. Methylation of the thyroid-stimulating hormone receptor gene in epithelial thyroid tumors: a marker of malignancy and a cause of gene silencing. Cancer Res 2003;63:2316–21.
9. McGriff NJ, Csako G, Gourgiotis L, et al. Effects of thyroid hormone suppression therapy on adverse clinical outcomes in thyroid cancer. Ann Med 2002;34:554–664.
10. Ito Y, Masuoka H, Fukushima M, et al. Prognosis and prognostic factors of patients with papillary carcinoma showing distant metastasis at surgery (M1 patients) in Japan. Endocr J 2010;57:523–31.
11. Diessl S, Holzberger B, Mäder U, et al. Impact of moderate vs stringent TSH suppression on survival in advanced differentiated thyroid carcinoma. Clin Endocrinol (Oxf) 2012;76:586–92.
12. Cooper DS, Specker B, Ho M, et al. Thyrotropin suppression and disease progression in patients with differentiated thyroid cancer: results from the National Thyroid Cancer Treatment Cooperative Registry. Thyroid 1998;8:737–44.
13. Jonklaas J, Sarlis NJ, Litofsky D, et al. Outcomes of patients with differentiated thyroid carcinoma following initial therapy. Thyroid 2006;16:1229–42.
14. Carhill AA, Litofsky DR, Ross DS, et al. Long-term outcomes following therapy in differentiated thyroid carcinoma: NTCTCS Registry Analysis 1987-2012. J Clin Endocrinol Metab 2015;100:3270–9.
15. Hovens GC, Stokkel MP, Kievit J, et al. Associations of serum thyrotropin concentrations with recurrence and death in differentiated thyroid cancer. J Clin Endocrinol Metab 2007;92:2610–5.
16. Sugitani I, Fujimoto Y. Does postoperative thyrotropin suppression therapy truly decrease recurrence in papillary thyroid carcinoma? A randomized controlled trial. J Clin Endocrinol Metab 2010;95:4576–83.
17. Haugen BR, Alexander EK, Bible KC, et al. 2015 American Thyroid Association management guidelines for adult patients with thyroid nodules and differentiated thyroid cancer. Thyroid 2016;26:1–133.
18. Park S, Kim WG, Han M, et al. Thyrotropin suppressive therapy for low-risk small thyroid cancer: a propensity score-matched cohort study. Thyroid 2017;27:1164–70.
19. Biondi B, Cooper DS. Benefits of thyrotropin suppression versus the risks of adverse effects in differentiated thyroid cancer. Thyroid 2010;20:135–46.
20. Biondi B, Fazio S, Carella C, et al. Cardiac effects of long term thyrotropin-

suppressive therapy with levothyroxine. J Clin Endocrinol Metab 1993;77:334-8.
21. Jonklaas J, Davidson B, Bhagat S, et al. Triiodothyronine levels in athyreotic individuals during Levothyroxine therapy. JAMA 2008;299:769-77.
22. Gullo D, Latina A, Frasca F, et al. Levothyroxine monotherapy cannot guarantee euthyroidism in all athyreotic patients. PLoS One 2011;6:e2255.
23. Ito M, Miyauchi A, Morita S, et al. TSH-suppressive doses of levothyroxine are required to achieve preoperative native serum triiodothyronine levels in patients who have undergone total thyroidectomy. Eur J Endocrinol 2012;167:373-8.
24. Botella-Carretero JI, Galan JM, Caballero C, et al. Quality of life and psychometric functionality in patients with differentiated thyroid carcinoma. Endocr Relat Cancer 2003;10(4):601-10.
25. Eustatia-Rutten CF, Corssmit EP, Pereira AM, et al. Quality of life in long-term exogenous subclinical hyperthyroidism and the effects of restoration of euthyroidism, a randomized controlled trial. Clin Endocrinol 2006;64:284-91.
26. Hoftijzer HC, Heemstra KA, Corssmit EP, et al. Quality of life in cured patients with differentiated thyroid carcinoma. J Clin Endocrinol Metab 2008;93:200-3.
27. Tagay S, Herpertz S, Langkafel M, et al. Health-related quality of life, anxiety and depression in thyroid cancer patients under short-term hypothyroidism and TSH-suppressive levothyroxine treatment. Eur J Endocrinol 2005;153:755-63.
28. Vigario Pdos S, Chachamovitz DS, Cordeiro MF, et al. Effects of physical activity on body composition and fatigue perception in patients on thyrotropin-suppressive therapy for differentiated thyroid carcinoma. Thyroid 2011;21:695-700.
29. Ching G, Franklyn J, Stallard TJ, et al. Cardiac hypertrophy as a result of long-term thyroxine therapy and thyrotoxicosis. Heart 1996;75:363-8.
30. Gullu S, Altuntas F, Dincer İ, et al. Effects of TSH-suppressive therapy on cardiac morphology and function: beneficial effects of the addition of beta-blockade on diastolic dysfunction. Eur J Endocrinol 2004;150:655-61.
31. Abdulrahman RM, Delgado V, Hoftijzer HC, et al. Both exogenous subclinical hyperthyroidism and short-term overt hypothyroidism affect myocardial strain in patients with differentiated thyroid carcinoma. Thyroid 2011;21:471-6.
32. Fazio S, Biondi B, Carella C, et al. Diastolic dysfunction in patients on thyroid-stimulating hormone suppressive therapy with levothyroxine: beneficial effect of beta-blockade. J Clin Endocrinol Metab 1995;80:2222-6.
33. Abdulrahman RM, Delgado V, Ng A, et al. Abnormal cardiac contractility in long term exogenous subclinical hyperthyroid patients as demonstrated by two-dimensional echocardiography speckle tracking imaging. Eur J Endocrinol 2010;163:435-41.
34. Smit JW, Eustatia-Rutten CF, Corssmit EP, et al. Reversible diastolic dysfunction after long-term exogenous subclinical hyperthyroidism: a randomized, placebo-controlled study. J Clin Endocrinol Metab 2005;90:6041-7.
35. Shargorodsky M, Serov S, Gavish D, et al. Long-term thyrotropin-suppressive therapy with Levothyroxine impairs small and large artery elasticity and increases left ventricular mass in patients with thyroid carcinoma. Thyroid 2006;16:381-6.
36. Biondi B, Fazio S, Cuocolo A, et al. Impaired cardiac reserve and exercise capacity in patients receiving long-term thyrotropin suppressive therapy with Levothyroxine. J Clin Endocrinol Metab 1996;81:4224-8.
37. Mercuro G, Panzuto MG, Bina A, et al. Cardiac function, physical exercise capacity, and quality of life during long-term thyrotropin mild thyrotropin-suppressive

therapy with levothyroxine: effect of individual dose tailoring. J Clin Endocrinol Metab 2000;85:159–64.
38. Taillard V, Sardinoux M, Oudot C, et al. Early detection of isolated left ventricular diastolic dysfunction in high-risk differentiated thyroid carcinoma patients on TSH-suppressive therapy. Clin Endocrinol (Oxf) 2011;75:709–14.
39. Biondi B, Fazio S, Carella C, et al. Control of adrenergic overactivity by β-blockade improves the quality of life in patients receiving long term suppressive therapy with levothyroxine. J Clin Endocrinol Metab 1994;78:1028–33.
40. Pajamäki N, Metso S, Hakala T1, et al. Long-term cardiovascular morbidity and mortality in patients treated for differentiated thyroid cancer. Clin Endocrinol (Oxf) 2018;88:303–10.
41. Flynn RW, Bonellie SR, Jung RT, et al. Serum thyroid-stimulating hormone concentration and morbidity from cardiovascular disease and fractures in patients on long-term thyroxine therapy. J Clin Endocrinol Metab 2010;95:186–93.
42. Abonowara A, Quraishi A, Sapp JL, et al. Prevalence of atrial fibrillation in patients taking TSH suppression therapy for management of thyroid cancer. Clin Invest Med 2012;35:152–6.
43. Klein Hesselink EN, Lefrandt JD, Schuurmans EP, et al. Increased risk of atrial fibrillation after treatment for differentiated thyroid carcinoma. J Clin Endocrinol Metab 2015;100:4563–9.
44. Wang LY, Smith AW, Palmer FL, et al. Thyrotropin suppression increases the risk of osteoporosis without decreasing recurrence in ATA low-and intermediate-risk patients with differentiated thyroid carcinoma. Thyroid 2015;25:300–7.
45. Spitzweg C, Joba W, Eisenmenger W, et al. Analysis of human sodium iodide symporter gene expression in extrathyroidal tissues and cloning of its complementary deoxyribonucleic acids from salivary gland, mammary gland, and gastric mucosa. J Clin Endocrinol Metab 1998;83:1746–51.
46. Klein Hesselink EN, Klein Hesselink MS, de Bock GH, et al. Long-term cardiovascular mortality in patients with differentiated thyroid carcinoma: an observational study. J Clin Oncol 2013;31:4046–53.
47. Eustatia-Rutten CFA, Corssmit EPM, Biermasz NR, et al. Survival and death causes in differentiated thyroid carcinoma. J Clin Endocrinol Metab 2006;91:313–9.
48. Links TP, van Tol KM, Jager PL, et al. Life expectancy in differentiated thyroid cancer: a novel approach to survival analysis. Endocr Relat Cancer 2005;12:273–80.
49. Zoltek M, Andersson TML, Hedman C, et al. Cardiovascular mortality in 6900 patients with differentiated thyroid cancer: a Swedish population-based study. Clin Surg 2017;2:1–6.
50. Bassett JH, Williams GR. Role of thyroid hormones in skeletal development and bone maintenance. Endocr Rev 2016;37:135–87.
51. Abe E, Marians RC, Yu W, et al. TSH is a negative regulator of skeletal remodeling. Cell 2003;115:151–62.
52. Mazziotti G, Sorvillo F, Piscopo M, et al. Recombinant human TSH modulates in vivo C-telopeptides of type-1 collagen and bone alkaline phosphatase, but not osteoprotegerin production in postmenopausal women monitored for differentiated thyroid carcinoma. J Bone Miner Res 2005;20:480–6.
53. Quan ML, Pasieka JL, Rorstad O. Bone mineral density in well-differentiated thyroid cancer patients treated with suppressive thyroxine: a systematic overview of

the literature. J Surg Oncol 2002;79:62-9.
54. Heemstra KA, Hamdy NA, Romijn JA, et al. The effects of thyrotropin-suppressive therapy on bone metabolism in patients with well-differentiated thyroid carcinoma. Thyroid 2006;16:583-91.
55. Faber J, Galloc AM. Changes in bone mass during prolonged subclinical hyperthyroidism due to L-thyroxine treatment: a meta-analysis. Eur J Endocrinol 1994; 130:350-6.
56. Uzzan B, Campos J, Cucherat M, et al. Effect on bone mass of long term treatment with thyroid hormones: a meta analysis. J Clin Endocrinol Metab 1996;81: 4278-489.
57. Moon JH, Kim KM, Oh TJ, et al. The effect of TSH suppression on vertebral trabecular bone scores in patients with differentiated thyroid carcinoma. J Clin Endocrinol Metab 2017;102:78-85.
58. Tournis S, Antoniou JD, Liakou CG, et al. Volumetric bone mineral density and bone geometry assessed by peripheral quantitative computed tomography in women with differentiated thyroid cancer under TSH suppression. Clin Endocrinol (Oxf) 2015;82:197-204.
59. Kim K, Kim IJ, Pak K, et al. Evaluation of bone mineral density using DXA and central QCT in postmenopausal patients under thyrotropin suppressive therapy. Evaluation of bone mineral density using DXA and central QCT in postmenopausal patients under thyrotropin suppressive therapy. J Clin Endocrinol Metab 2018. https://doi.org/10.1210/jc.2017-02704.
60. Mazziotti G, Formenti AM, Frara S, et al. High prevalence of radiological vertebral fractures in women on thyroid-stimulating hormone-suppressive therapy for thyroid carcinoma. J Clin Endocrinol Metab 2018;103:956-64.
61. Sugitani I, Fujimoto Y. Effect of postoperative thyrotropin suppressive therapy on bone mineral density in patients with papillary thyroid carcinoma: a prospective controlled study. Surgery 2011;150:1250-7.
62. Turner MR, Camacho X, Fischer HD, et al. Levothyroxine dose and risk of fractures in older adults: nested case-control study. BMJ 2011;342:d2238.
63. Bauer DC, Ettinger B, Nevitt MC, et al, Study of Osteoporotic Fractures Research Group. Risk for fracture in women with low serum levels of thyroid-stimulating hormone. Ann Intern Med 2001;134:561-8.
64. Lee JS, Buzková P, Fink HA, et al. Subclinical thyroid dysfunction and incident hip fracture in older adults. Arch Intern Med 2010;170:1876-83.
65. Blum MR, Bauer DC, Collet TH, et al. Subclinical thyroid dysfunction and fracture risk: a meta-analysis. JAMA 2015;313:2055-65.
66. Wirth CD, Blum MR, da Costa BR, et al. Subclinical thyroid dysfunction and the risk for fractures: a systematic review and meta-analysis. Ann Intern Med 2014; 161:189-99.
67. Yan Z, Huang H, Li J, et al. Relationship between subclinical thyroid dysfunction and the risk of fracture: a meta-analysis of prospective cohort studies. Osteoporos Int 2016;27:115-25.
68. Yang R, Yao L, Fang Y, et al. The relationship between subclinical thyroid dysfunction and the risk of fracture or low bone mineral density: a systematic review and metaanalysis of cohort studies. J Bone Miner Metab 2018;36(2):209-20.
69. Biondi B, Cooper DS. Subclinical hyperthyroidism. N Engl J Med 2018;378: 2411-9.
70. Gammage MD, Parle JV, Holder RL, et al. Association between free thyroxine

concentration and atrial fibrillation. Arch Intern Med 2007;167:928–34.
71. Heeringa J, Hoogendoorn EH, van der Deure WM, et al. High normal thyroid function and risk of atrial fibrillation. Arch Intern Med 2008;168:2219–24.
72. Chaker L, Heeringa J, Dehghan A, et al. Normal thyroid function and the risk of atrial fibrillation: the Rotterdam Study. J Clin Endocrinol Metab 2015;100: 3718–24.
73. Yeap BB, Alfonso H, Hankey GJ, et al. Higher free thyroxine levels are associated with all-cause mortality in euthyroid older men: the Health In Men Study. Eur J Endocrinol 2013;169:401–8.
74. Aubert CE, Floriani C, Bauer DC, et al. Thyroid function tests in the reference range and fracture: individual participant analysis of prospective cohorts. J Clin Endocrinol Metab 2017;102:2719–28.
75. Panebianco P, Rosso D, Destro G, et al. Use of disphosphonates in the treatment of osteoporosis in thyroidectomized patients on levothyroxin replacement therapy. Arch Gerontol Geriatr 1997;25:219–25.
76. Sharma A, Einstein AJ, Vallakati A, et al. Risk of atrial fibrillation with use of oral and intravenous bisphosphonates. Am J Cardiol 2014;113:1815–21.

第16章
进展性放射性碘难治性甲状腺癌的新药治疗

Steven P. Weitzman, Steven I. Sherman

关键词

- 甲状腺肿瘤 • 丝裂原活化蛋白激酶 • 血管生成 • MEK 激酶
- TOR 丝氨酸-苏氨酸激酶 • 酪氨酸激酶受体 RET • 原癌基因蛋白 TRK
- 免疫治疗

要点

- 与摄碘性分化型甲状腺癌相比,碘难治性分化型甲状腺癌患者的预后较差。
- lenvatinib 与 sorafenib 是用于治疗进展性碘难治性分化型甲状腺癌的抗血管生成的多激酶抑制剂(aMKI)。
- 目前的药物并非治愈性,因此在治疗前应仔细评估治疗的风险和获益。
- 甲状腺癌新型治疗中有很多颇具前景的手段,如免疫治疗及针对 BRAF、TRK 和 RET 的靶向治疗。
- 体细胞基因变异检测对于辅助选择合适的治疗药物及发现潜在的新靶点至关重要。

引言

大多数分化型甲状腺癌(differentiated thyroid cancer, DTC)患者经过治疗后预后良好,据 SEER 数据库显示,甲状腺癌初诊后 5 年生存率高达

98.1%[1]，然而，对于出现远处转移的患者，其 5 年生存率从仅局限于甲状腺内的 99.9% 降至 55.5%。很多之前的文章已经对 DTC 的规范化诊疗进行了详细的阐述，然而仍有部分患者经过手术，促甲状腺激素（thyroid-stimulating hormone，TSH）抑制治疗及 RAI（radioiodine）治疗后出现病情进展，这类患者亟需新的治疗方法。

RAI 治疗长期以来一直是临床医生的主要治疗方法，RAI 难治性 DTC 因而成为临床挑战。出现以下任一情况即可考虑为碘难治性 DTC（radioiodine-refractory differentiated thyroid cancer，RAIR-DTC）[2-4]：①已知的转移性病灶（一处或多处病变）在初次治疗后显像或之后的诊断性显像中表现为不摄碘或失去摄碘能力；②在 RAI 治疗后短期（通常在 1 年内）即出现病情进展；③治疗累积放射性活度 ≥600mCi，这是由于随着剂量增加，辐射相关风险增加，而患者的潜在获益减少。累积放射性活度的增加与继发恶性肿瘤的风险升高密切相关，继发恶性肿瘤常见于血液系统、唾液腺和骨[5]。

据报道，存在持续性摄碘病灶的患者 10 年生存率为 29%，而初始即无摄碘的持续性病灶患者的 10 年生存率仅为 10%[2]。然而，许多病情持续的患者可能因病灶稳定、病灶较小、进展缓慢而没有症状；对于这部分患者而言，系统性治疗的毒性作用可能会大于获益。因此，评价病灶进展速度对判断患者是否获益至关重要。实体瘤反应评估标准（response evaluation criteria in solid tumor，RECIST）1.1 广泛用于评估临床试验中是否存在病情快速进展，也可直接应用于常规临床实践。进展性疾病定义为靶病灶直径总和增长 ≥20% 或出现明显的新病灶[6]。

当病灶迅速进展而无法行手术或放疗等局部治疗时，应考虑全身系统治疗。回顾之前的治疗手段，尽管美国食品药品管理局（US Food and Drug Administration，FDA）批准了阿霉素，但细胞毒性化疗的疗效令人失望[7,8]。因此，对肿瘤转移和进展至关重要的血管生成以及信号转导途径中的致癌基因变化引起了人们的广泛研发兴趣。正在研究及评估中的新疗法包括恢复甲状腺相关生物学过程以控制肿瘤生长，如肿瘤的诱导再分化以增敏 RAI 治疗，以及免疫疗法。

抗血管生成多激酶抑制剂

首先讨论的药物是抗血管生成多激酶抑制剂（antiangiogenic multikinase inhibitor，aMKI）。这是唯一一类获得包括美国 FDA 在内的许多机构批准的抗甲状腺癌药物。尽管它们以不同的效能阻断了不同靶点的多种激酶，但其共同的作用机制是抑制血管内皮生长因子(vascular endothelial growth factor, VEGF)及其同源 VEGF 受体(vascular endothelial growth factor receptor, VEGFR)之间的相互作用，从而干扰肿瘤形成、生长和转移所必需的血管生成[9]。

lenvatinib

lenvatinlb 是一种靶向 VEGFR1~VEGFR3, FGFR1~FGFR4, PDGFR, RET 和 cKIT 激酶的 aMKI。Ⅰ期试验在接受 lenvatinib 治疗的甲状腺癌患者中观察到疗效反应。Ⅱ期试验中，58 例进展性 RAIR-DTC 患者的客观缓解率为 50%，中位无进展生存时间(progression-free survival, PFS)为 12.6 个月[10]，中位缓解期为 12.7 个月。基于一项双盲、安慰剂对照、多中心Ⅲ期临床试验的结果，lenvatinib 随后在 2015 年被 FDA 批准用于进展性 RAIR-DTC 的患者。该试验即 lenvatinib(E7080)在 DTC 中的研究[Study of (E7080) Lenvatinib in Differentiated Cancer of the Thyroid, SELECT][11]。SELECT 试验根据 RECIST 标准招募了具有进展性碘难治性 DTC 的受试者，将其以 2∶1 的比例随机分配至接受 lenvatinib(起始剂量为每日 24mg)组或安慰剂组；主要研究终点是 PFS 的改善，定义为从随机分组到病情进展或死亡的时间。392 人被随机分组并达到试验主要终点，两组之间的 PFS 显著不同($P<0.001$)。lenvatinib 治疗组 PFS 为 18.3 个月，安慰剂组 PFS 为 3.6 个月(HR=0.21)。安慰剂组中的短 PFS 提示整个受试者队列中疾病进展迅速。不论之前是否接受过其他抗血管生成治疗，所有组织学亚型(乳头状、滤泡状、低分化及 Hürthle 细胞)的患者均可观察到 PFS 延长。此外，lenvatinib 组的客观缓解率为 64.8%，中位起效时间仅为 2 个月；其中 4 名受试者表现为完全缓解并持续至最后一次评估。由于方案允许安慰剂组的受试者在出现病情进展后交叉至治疗组，交叉后患者的中位 PFS 和客观缓解率分别为 10.1 个月和 52.3%。虽然 BRAF 野生型状态本身可能是疾病阴性预后指标，但是 *BRAF* 突变状态并未影响该药物的疗效[12]。可能是因为允许交叉入组这一设计的影响，lenvatinib 对队列总体生存期(overall survival, OS)改善呈阴性结果，但进一步的亚组分析显示 65 岁以上进展性 RAIR-DTC 患者存在良好的 OS 获益(HR 0.53, 95% CI 0.31~0.91, $P=0.020$)[13]。

两种治疗方案的不良反应都很常见。接受 lenvatinib 治疗的受试者中有 97.3% 出现了不良反应，而安慰剂组为 59.5%。lenvatinib 治疗最常见的不良反应包括高血压、腹泻、疲劳、食欲下降和体重减轻。值得注意的是，

lenvatinitb 组有 2.3% 的受试者出现被认为与治疗有关的致命性不良反应。这进一步强调了使用 lenvatinib 治疗时需要进行周密的患者选择和密切监测。除了与该药相关的风险异常增高的特定人群,由于使所有患者的 PFS 显著改善,65 岁以上患者的 OS 延长,与安慰剂相比较高的效价比,lenvatinib 被公认为进展性 RAIR-DTC 患者的一线治疗[14,15]。

sorafenib

sorafenib 是另一种靶向 VEGFR1~VEGFR3,RET,RET/PTC 和 BRAF 激酶的 aMKI。两项单中心 Ⅱ 期临床试验初步提示其对转移性 RAIR-DTC 患者有效,客观缓解率分别为 23% 和 15%[16,17]。基于一项随机、双盲、安慰剂对照、多中心 Ⅲ 期临床研究的结果,sorafenib 于 2013 年被美国 FDA 批准为局部复发或转移性、进展性 RAIR-DTC 患者的一线治疗药物[18]。这项 sorafenib 在局部晚期或转移性 RAIR-DTC 患者中的试验(DECISION),依据 RECIST 标准招募了未经治疗的进展性 RAIR-DTC 受试者,以 1∶1 的比例随机分配至接受 sorafenib(起始剂量为每日 2 次 400mg)组或安慰剂组,主要终点是 PFS 的改善。417 人被随机分组,两组之间的 PFS 显著不同($P<0.001$)。sorafenib 治疗组 PFS 为 10.8 个月,安慰剂组 PFS 为 5.8 个月(HR 0.59);sorafenib 组客观缓解率为 12.2%。两组 OS 无明显差异。与 SELECT 试验类似,sorafenib 的疗效不受 *BRAF* 突变状态的影响,两组(sorafenib 组与对照组)的 BRAF 野生型状态均与较短的 PFS 相关。sorafenib 组受试者中有 98.6% 出现了不良反应,而安慰剂组为 87.6%。最常见的不良反应包括手足皮肤反应、腹泻、脱发、皮疹和疲劳。两组各有 1 例受试者死亡,这 2 例死亡被认为与治疗有关。

虽然不能直接比较 SELECT 和 DECISION 试验,但在安慰剂组 PFS 较短的情况下,lenvatinib 对 PFS 的改善更为显著,且性价比优于 sorafenib;提示其应是首选的抗血管生成药物[14,15]。然而,对于那些可能对强效抗血管生成药物禁忌的患者,如有气管食管瘘或肠穿孔风险的患者,sorafenib 可能是更合理的初始治疗药物。

vandetanib

vandetanib 是一种靶向 RET,RET/PTC,VEGFR2,VEGFR3 和上皮生长因子受体(epithelial growth factor receptor,EGFR)激酶的 aMKI,于 2011 年被美国 FDA 批准用于治疗无法切除的局部晚期或转移性的症状性/进展性甲状腺髓样癌（medullary thyroid cancer, MTC）。考虑到 vandetanib 可以抑制一系列激酶，一项随机、双盲、安慰剂对照的多中心Ⅱ期试验招募了被认为不适合 RAI 治疗的局部晚期或转移性 DTC 受试者[19]。145 名受试者以 1∶1 的比例随机分配至 vandetanib 组（起始剂量为每日 300mg）或安慰剂组，主要终点是 PFS 的改善。试验达到了主要终点，vandetanib 组的 PFS 为 11.1 个月，而安慰剂组的 PFS 为 5.9 个月（HR=0.63）；vandetanib 治疗组的总缓解率仅为 8%，而安慰剂组为 5%，差异无统计学意义。

vandetanib 治疗最常见的不良反应包括腹泻、高血压、痤疮、乏力、食欲下降、皮疹、疲劳和 QTc 间期延长。实际上 3 级或更高级别的 QTc 间期延长可见于 14% 的安全人群[19]；因此，在开具 vandetanib 之前，处方者必须先进行风险评估及对症处理的相关培训。由于很多非抗肿瘤药物可延长 QT 间期，对用药前 QT 间期稍有延长的患者来说，vandetanib 治疗颇具挑战。

cabozantinib

cabozantinib 是一种靶向 VEGFR2、cMET 和 RET 激酶的 aMKI，已获得美国 FDA 批准用于治疗进展性转移 MTC。一项旨在评估潜在药物相互作用的开放标签Ⅰ期试验纳入了来自 2 个中心的 15 名存在转移性 RAIR 或不可切除病灶的 DTC 受试者[20]；次要终点包括总体缓解率和 OS 率。其中 8 位受试者（53%）可见部分缓解；6 位受试者（40%）可见病情稳定；而 1 人因瘘管形成死亡[20,21]。随后，一项多中心Ⅱ期试验招募了 25 名患有 RAIR-DTC 且进行了至少 1 年 VEGFR 靶向治疗后病情进展的受试者，cabozantinib 起始剂量为每日 60mg，主要终点为总缓解率[22]。在这些受试者中，40% 的患者部分缓解，52% 的患者疾病稳定，还有 8% 的患者无法评估（由于临床进展或难以耐受的不良反应）。中位 PFS 为 12.7 个月，中位 OS 为 34.7 个月。该试验是第一个在接受过 aMKI 治疗的受试者中显示出疗效的前瞻性试验。另有一项Ⅱ期试验初步报道了研究 cabozantinib 在一线治疗中的作用；起始剂量每日 60mg[23]。总体缓解率为 54%，中位缓解期为 40 周，中位 PFS 尚未获得。预期将进行Ⅲ期临床试验以评估 cabozantinib 在前期经抗血管生成治疗出现疾病进展的 DTC 患者中的疗效。

pazopanib

pazopanib 是另一种靶向 VEGFR1~VEGFR3、FGFR1~FGFR3、PDGFR 和 cKit 激酶的 aMKI。一项Ⅱ期试验招募了转移性、快速进展性 RAIR-DTC

的患者接受 pazopanib 治疗,起始剂量为每日 800mg,主要终点为客观缓解率[24]。在 37 名可评估的受试者中,客观缓解率为 49%,1 年 PFS 为 47%,1 年 OS 为 81%。该药物总体耐受性良好,最常见的不良反应为疲劳,皮肤和头发色素减少,腹泻和恶心。尽管 pazopanib 有希望用于治疗甲状腺癌,但尚缺乏进一步的试验证实其疗效。

sunitinib

sunitinib 是一种靶向 VEGFR、PDGFR 和 RET 激酶的 aMKI。目前已有两个 II 期试验评估 sunitinib 在 DTC 患者中的应用。第一项试验是单机构研究,评估了其在 ^{18}F-FDG-PET 显像上高摄取的转移灶、转移性 RAIR DTC 或 MTC 受试者中的潜在效用。在 28 名 DTC 受试者中,疾病控制率(定义为出现缓解或 3 个月内疾病稳定)为 78%[25]。最近的一项单中心、开放标签的非随机试验纳入了 23 位转移性 / 残留性 / 复发性或进展性 DTC 患者,其中 6 名受试者(26%)出现部分缓解[26]。

axitinib

axitinib 是一种可抑制 VEGFR 和 PDGFR 激酶的 aMKI。一项多中心、开放标签、单臂 II 期研究招募了 45 名存在 RAIR 或转移性或不可切除的局部晚期病灶的晚期甲状腺癌患者[27]。受试者中有 38% 出现部分缓解;29% 病情稳定。尽管 DTC 受试者并未进行亚组分析,但该试验仍显示出一定疗效。

安全使用抗血管生成的多激酶抑制剂

鉴于与使用 aMKI 有关的不良事件的发生率很高,对不良事件的精密监控和积极管理至关重要。最常见或最严重(但不常见)的不良反应包括高血压、疲劳、慢性体重减轻、腹泻、QT 间期延长、充血性心力衰竭、蛋白尿、肝损伤、骨髓抑制、出血、血栓形成、手足皮肤反应及皮疹等。有关此类药物的安全使用以及与药物相关的不良反应的管理,在相关指南中已作概述[28-30]。

肿瘤的精准治疗

鉴于通过丝裂原激活的蛋白激酶(mitogen-activated protein kinase,MAPK)和磷脂酰肌醇 3- 激酶 /AKT 途径激活的信号转导在 DTC 的发生和生物学行为中都非常重要，人们对使用更具选择性靶向于这些通路的激酶抑制剂产生了浓厚兴趣（见第 3 章）。特别是现已发现具有 *BRAF* 阳性突变的肿瘤通常更具侵袭性，且与分化功能（如对 RAI 治疗的反应）丧失有关。许多临床研究都致力于评估 BRAF 激酶抑制剂在抑制肿瘤生长或诱导再分化增敏 RAI 治疗中的效果。针对这些通路中其他激酶抑制剂的研究较少，但单一疗法或与其他药物联合使用仍是令人感兴趣的研究方向，包括可提高或恢复对 RAI 治疗反应的辅助手段。目前，最新的治疗主要针对与 DTC 发展相关的一些罕见融合突变，仍在早期临床试验阶段，且有鼓舞人心的初步结果。

BRAF——靶向治疗

两种目前被批准用于治疗突变型黑色素瘤的 BRAF 激酶抑制剂已被研究证实对 *BRAF* 突变的 DTC 有效：vemurafenib 和 dabrafenib[31]。两种药物均为与 *V600E* 突变型激酶优先结合的 ATP 竞争性 I 型抑制剂[32]，然而，它们也增强了野生型 BRAF 的异二聚作用并促进了 CRAF 的反式激活，这反而会促进 MAPK 通路信号转导，特别是在 *RAS* 突变的情况下。因此，其使用仅限于有明确 *BRAF* 突变的患者且特别禁忌于存在 *RAS* 突变者。

在 I 期试验中，研究者最初考虑将 vemurafenib 用于 *BRAF* 突变型 PTC，因为其对 *V6000E* 突变型激酶（IC_{50} 31nM）的选择性是野生型的 3 倍[33,34]。在 3 位存在 RAIR 转移灶、*BRAF* 突变阳性的受试者中，有 1 位出现肺转移灶缩小，达部分缓解。在随后的一项多中心 II 期试验中，vemuratenib 被用于两组进展性、转移性、*BRAF V600E* 突变阳性的 RAIR-PTC 患者，起始剂量为 960mg 每日 2 次[35]。在从未接受过抗血管生成多靶点激酶抑制剂治疗的 26 位受试者中，有 38.5% 的患者出现了部分缓解，中位缓解期为 16.5 个月，中位 PFS 为 18.2 个月。在第二组曾接受抗血管生成多靶点激酶抑制剂（包括 sorafenib）治疗的 25 位受试者中，有 27.3% 的人出现了部分缓解，中位缓解期为 7.4 个月，中位 PFS 为 8.9 个月。因此，vemuratenib 作为使用抗血管生成激酶抑制剂后的二线治疗手段的疗效可能不及其作为一线治疗。该试验报告的不良事件与其他研究相似，包括皮疹（69%）、疲劳（67%）、体重减轻（51%）、食欲下降（45%）、脱发（41%）和关节痛（41%）。约 1/3 的受试者出现血清肌酐升高，其中部分可达剂量限值。1/5 的受试者出现皮肤鳞状细胞癌，2 名受试者出现头或颈部的非皮肤鳞状细胞癌，这可能是甲状腺原发灶去分化的结果。在一项 vemurafenitb 真实世界研究中，15 例受试者（其中 12 例无激酶抑制剂治疗史)的部分缓解率为 47%,中位治疗失败时间为 13 个月[36]。这些研究表明 vemurafenib 可有效治疗 *BRAF V600E* 突变的 RAIR-PTC,尤其作为一线治疗。

鉴于 vemurafenib 在治疗进展性转移性疾病中的作用,最近完成的一项单中心试验探索了应用其缩小巨大颈部肿瘤的术前新辅助治疗作用[37]。尽管主要转化终点尚未报道,但次要研究终点显示,对于存在局部晚期病灶的 *BRAF* 突变阳性的 PTC 患者,术前 vemurafenib 治疗 8 周可使 2/3 以上的患者出现临床显著的肿瘤缩小,这可能会提高术后极少或无残留病灶的概率。

dabrafenib 是一种高效的 *BRAF V600E* 激活突变(*V600E* IC$_{50}$ 0.5nM)拮抗剂。在一项 I 期临床试验的初步报告中,接受治疗的 *BRAF* 突变阳性转移性 RAIR-PTC 的 9 名受试者中有 3 名出现部分缓解[38]。随后,一份来自该试验的 *BRAF* 突变阳性 PTC 患者扩展队列的完整报告称,14 名进展性 RAIR-PTC 患者,dabrafenib 剂量为 150mg 每日 2 次,其部分缓解率为 29%,中位 PFS 为 11.3 个月[39]。在患有甲状腺癌的受试者中,最常见的不良反应包括皮肤乳头状瘤、角化过度、脱发、关节痛和发热。

考虑到 dabrafenib 联合 MEK 拮抗剂 trametinib 在黑色素瘤中的疗效和耐受性,一项随机 II 期临床试验对比了 dabrafenib 单药治疗与 dabrafenib 和 trametinib 联合治疗[40]。53 名 *BRAF* 突变阳性的 RAIR-PTC 患者被随机分配至 dabrafenib 组(每日 2 次 150mg)或联合治疗组:dabrafenib(每日 2 次 150mg)和 trametinib(每日 2mg)。两组间客观缓解率无显著差异,其中单药治疗组的客观缓解率(定义为部分和次要缓解率)为 50%(中位缓解期 15.6 个月);联合治疗组客观缓解率为 54%(中位缓解期 13.3 个月)。两组的毒性反应也相似。为改善患者对联合用药的耐受性,联合治疗组患者曾接受剂量调整以延长患者在治疗中的稳定状态[41]。

dabrafenib 和 trametinib 联合治疗在 *BRAF* 突变阳性的甲状腺未分化癌中似乎特别有效,因此靶向 BRAF 激酶的治疗可能在更具侵袭性的分化型癌中意义更大[42]。例如,笔者最近收治了 1 例 *BRAF* 突变阳性且颈部转移灶迅速进展并伴有皮肤受累的低分化癌患者,我们将 dabrafenib 和 trametinib 作为肿瘤新辅助治疗方法,目的是使后续手术治疗成为可能,联合用药治疗 2 个月后患者出现影像学完全缓解,后因无明显病灶而推迟手术(图 16.1)。

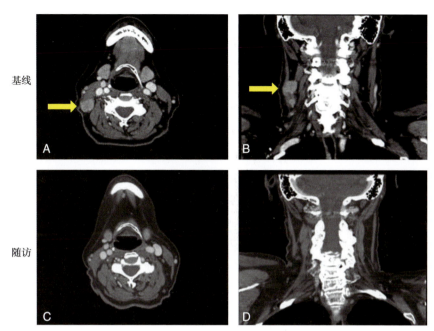

图 16.1 *BRAF V600E* 突变型低分化甲状腺癌患者治疗后颈部 CT 轴向和冠状增强图像。治疗前的基线图像(A,B)示右侧颈部转移灶明显强化伴皮下组织受累(箭头)。2 个月后随访图像(C,D)示上述病变已完全缓解,消退至无法检测到

MEK——靶向治疗

MEK 是 RAS 或 BRAF 激活信号的常见下游效应子,但除与 BRAF 激酶抑制剂组合外,尚无关于 MEK 拮抗剂在此病中的广泛研究。在一项关于 MEK 拮抗剂 selumetinib 的 Ⅱ 期临床试验中,39 名进展性 RAIR-PTC 的受试者里只有 1 位出现部分缓解,中位 PFS 为 32 周[43]。据报道,严重不良反应被认为限制了该药的长期耐受性,因此,未能在该人群中进行后续试验。尽管 MEK 拮抗剂 cobimetinib 在美国市售用于治疗黑色素瘤,但尚无与其相关的研究报道。

PI3K 通路——靶向治疗

三项近期的 Ⅱ 期研究评估了 PI3K 抑制剂 everolimus 在转移性 RAIR-DTC 患者中的作用。第一项研究纳入 28 例进展性疾病的患者,采用 everolimus 治疗,初始剂量每日 10mg;未观察到客观缓解,中位 PFS 和 OS 分别为 9 个月和 18 个月[44]。第二项研究中纳入了 33 名进展性 RAIR-DTC 受试者,初始剂量每日 10mg;作为主要终点,中位 PFS 为 12.9 个月;仅观察到 1 例部分缓解;预估 2 年 PFS 和 OS 率分别为 23.6% 和 73.5%[45]。尽管每个基因组特征的亚组受

试者人数都非常少，*BRAF V600E* 突变阳性的受试者获得了最长的 PFS。第三项试验中纳入 24 名具有转移灶 RAIR-DTC 的受试者，everolimus 初始剂量每日 10mg[46]，2 名受试者出现部分缓解，中位 PFS 为 43 周。在这三项研究中，常见的不良反应包括黏膜炎或口腔炎、贫血、咳嗽和高血糖症。

已有三项独立的Ⅱ期试验对 everolimus 及 temsirolimus 与 sorafenib 联用进行了研究。在一项纳入 36 名进展性 RAIR 甲状腺癌（包括 2 名未分化癌）受试者的试验中，temsirolimus 与 sorafenib 联用（起始剂量分别为每周 25mg 和每日 2 次 200mg），部分缓解率达到 22%[47]。1 年 PFS 率为 31%，中位 OS 为 24.6 个月。最常见的 3~5 级不良事件为高血糖、疲劳、贫血和口腔黏膜炎。在 28 名 RAIR-DTC 患者中试验了 everolimus 和 sorafenib 联用，初始剂量分别为每日 5mg 和每日 2 次 400mg；初步报告中部分缓解率达 61%，其中包含 9 名 Hürthle 细胞亚型受试者中的 7 名[48]。第三项试验中对 33 名已经接受 sorafenib 单药治疗且病情进展的 DTC 受试者中加用 everolimus 每日 10 mg；同时增加了 sorafenib 的剂量[49]。增大 sorafenib 剂量及加用 everolimus 后，中位 PFS 为 13.7 个月，仅 1 名出现部分缓解。

MAPK 靶向的诱导分化治疗

对 MAPK 信号通路高度激活的 DTC 摄碘能力下降这一现象的认识向我们提示，对该通路的抑制有可能恢复 DTC 病灶的 RAI 摄取。在强力霉素诱导的 *BRAF V600E* 突变转基因小鼠模型中，通过使用 BRAF 或 MEK 拮抗剂恢复了 RAI 摄取，使上述假说得到了完美的验证[50]。在随后的探索性试验中，20 名 RAIR-DTC 患者（未限制 *BRAF* 或 *RAS* 突变阳性受试者入组）接受了 4 周 MEK 拮抗剂 selumetinib 治疗[51]。^{124}I-PET 显像及剂量学研究提示其中 60% 的受试者病灶出现 RAI 摄取的显著恢复，其中 7 名受试者能够继续接受 RAI 治疗。在接受了初步治疗的 20 名受试者中，有 5 名出现部分缓解，表现为肿瘤显著减少，客观缓解率达 25%。无显著短期毒性，除了之前 1 名接受过近 1 000mCi RAI 及前列腺癌盆腔照射治疗的受试者在治疗后约 1 年出现骨髓增生异常综合征。在另一项试验中，10 位受试者接受了 BRAF 拮抗剂 dabrafenib 治疗，以判断治疗 25 日后病灶能否重获 RAI 摄取能力[52]。RAI 扫描示 6 名受试者出现明显摄取并随后接受了 RAI 治疗，2 名受试者出现部分缓解，总缓解率为 20%。

笔者最近回顾了 13 名在进行 BRAF 或 MEK 靶向治疗进展性转移性 RAIR-DTC 时常规行 RAI 扫描的患者[53]。其中 9 名患者因存在 *BRAF* 突变而行 BRAF 拮抗剂治疗，另外 4 名患者接受了 MEK 拮抗剂治疗。9 名激酶抑制剂治疗的受试者出现了 RAI 摄取的显著恢复,中位治疗时间为 14 个月,使患者后期得以进行 200mCi 的 RAI 治疗。随后停止激酶抑制剂治疗,在约 8 个月的中位随访时间中,7 名受试者无病情进展。尽管应用了 RAI 剂量测定,仍有 2 名受试者出现短暂性放射性肺炎,这可能是提示激酶抑制剂治疗促进 RAI 摄取及滞留的进一步证据。

许多新研究正在探索增敏 RAI 疗法的临床作用,这反映了此方法在该领域引发的广泛兴趣。目前正在招募中的两项多中心研究正在尝试扩增先前初步观察到的对 RAI 治疗有反应的转移性疾病的受试者队列,其中包括一项安慰剂对照试验[54,55]。在另一项不同的治疗方案中,ASTRA 试验被用于评估以下假设:初次手术后,在中高复发风险的受试者中,与安慰剂组相比,在 RAI 治疗前先行 5 周 selumetinib 治疗能明显提高受试者 18 个月的完全缓解率[56]。但最近有报道提示该研究未能达到主要终点[57]。

基因重排——靶向治疗

除了点突变外,导致新型嵌合激酶异常表达及功能变化的基因重排也是甲状腺癌中具有治疗意义的致瘤性基因改变[58]。RET 激酶融合重排最先在甲状腺乳头状癌中发现,最近被认为是包括非小细胞肺癌在内近 2% 的实体恶性肿瘤中可被干预的突变[59]。由于存在多种可能接受 RET 靶向治疗的肿瘤类型,人们的兴趣集中于开发比现有药物更具选择性的 RET 拮抗剂来降低药物不良反应,而现有药物如 lenvatinib 或 sorafenib 的毒性作用主要归因于其抗血管生成特性。目前,Ⅰ期试验中有三种此类药物的初步疗效和安全性数据:RXDX-105,BLU-667 和 LOXO-292,每种药物野生型 RET 激酶的 IC_{50} 均明显低于 VEGFR,且不论实体肿瘤类型如何,其均有广泛的临床疗效[60-62]。LOXO-292 治疗中,在 *RET* 融合阳性转移性 PTC 组 (5/6) 部分缓解率为 83%,在非小细胞肺癌中为 65%[63]。BLU-667 治疗时,在 1 名可评估的 *RET/PTC1*(*CCDC6*)融合重排阳性的 PTC 患者中,肿瘤缩小近 80%,在非小细胞肺癌中的缓解率达 50%[64]。

一些乳头状癌以及许多其他实体瘤中也发现了导致激酶活化的 *NTRK* 基因重排,这促进了选择性 TRK 拮抗剂的发展。larotrectinib 在纳摩尔浓度下能够作为全部三种 TRK 蛋白共同的拮抗剂[65]。在一份总结了几项Ⅰ期试验中接受治疗的受试者的报告中,具有 *TRK* 基因重排的 DTC 患者的总缓解率为 100%(4 例部分缓解,1 例完全缓解),而在样本量更大的实体瘤受试者中,总体缓解率约为 75%[66,67]。这些研究中最常见的不良反应是肝功能异常、疲劳、呕吐、头晕和恶心。进行中的 larotrectinib 和 entrectinib(也抑制 ROS1

和 ALK 重排的激酶)篮子试验正在积极招募 *NTRK* 异常的甲状腺癌患者。larotrectinib 最近已获得美国 FDA 批准用于任何需要系统治疗的 *NTRK* 突变阳性的实体瘤。已有报道称 BRTC、ALK 和 ROS1 等其他激酶重排可能是 DTC 的致癌性基因改变,但相关靶向治疗尚未见报道。

转录因子配对盒 8(transcription factor paired box 8,PAXB)和过氧化物酶体增殖物活化受体 γ(peroxisome proliferator-activated receptor gamma,PPARγ)的基因融合产物是 DTC 罕见的驱动因素,尤其可见于滤泡样组织学亚型。临床前期数据提示 PPARγ 激动剂 piogitazone 可显著缩小此类基因融合阳性的转移性甲状腺癌,报道称 1 名受试者在 piogitazone 治疗后出现滤泡状癌骨转移灶显著缩小及症状缓解[68]。目前拟行一项多中心试验以评估在相似人群中的疗效,但尚未确定是否有已知的其他基因重排参与。从这项充满挑战的研究中所获的经验,以及从其他靶向重排基因治疗的 I 期试验中汲取的教训,提示我们应将大规模并行测序方法如全转录组测序(RNA-Seq)应用到或可接受该治疗的患者评估体系中[58]。

免疫治疗

鉴于针对 T 细胞相关的免疫检查点(抑制 T 细胞抗癌免疫反应)的新型疗法的成功,人们产生了对将新的免疫疗法应用于转移性 DTC 的兴趣[69]。较低的非同源突变的发生率和 DTC 中发现的新抗原可能提示 CTLA-4,PD-1 或 PD-L1 不是拮抗剂单药治疗的合适靶点[70]。事实上,PD-1 拮抗剂 pembrolizumab 的篮子试验的初步报告证实了这一假设[71]。在 22 位经 pembrolizumab 治疗的 RAIR-DTC 受试者中,尽管每个受试者至少有 1% 的肿瘤细胞存在 PD-L1 表达,但经初始剂量为每 2 周 10mg/kg 的治疗后,部分缓解率仅为 9.1%。与其他探索有关 PD-1 拮抗剂的试验一致,常见的不良反应包括腹泻、疲劳,以及 1 例大肠菌病。

尽管为免疫冷状态,但已显示某些癌症在与其他增加检查点蛋白自身表达的治疗方法结合时会产生对检查点抑制剂的反应,这亦可能适用于 DTC[69]。遵循这种方法,目前正在进行一项多中心试验评估 lenvatinib 与 pembrolizumab 联合使用后的反应,试验招募了单用 lenvatinib 后病情进展的受试者或直接作为一线联合治疗(NCT02973997)的受试者。一项 CTLA-4 拮抗剂 ipilimumab 联合立体定向消融放疗治疗肺、肝或肾上腺转移瘤(NCT02239900)的研究招募了转移性甲状腺癌(包括 RAIR-DTC)的扩大亚组,以进一步研究单纯放疗后的伴随远隔效应[72]。

初始治疗的选择

目前,只有两种美国 FDA 批准的有效药物可用于治疗进展性转移性 RAIR-DTC 的患者:lenvatinib 和 sorafenib。尚无对这两种获批药物进行比较的随机试验。实际上,除了单用 dabrafenib 与 dabrafenib 和 trametinib 联用的研究,还没有随机试验比较任何两种或可成为 RAIR-DTC 患者初始选择的药物或方案[14]。因此,有关选择这些治疗方法的决策均基于主观判断而非确定的数据。此外,选择适合于靶向特定致癌改变(例如 *BRAF* 突变或 *TRK* 重排)的精准肿瘤治疗的患者时,要检测特定的体细胞基因异常,而这并非目前的常规临床诊疗步骤。

在作者所在的医疗机构,lenvatinib 基于其已被证明的显著改善 PFS、明显缩小肿瘤和改善 OS(至少在老年患者中如此)的功效被认为是首选药物。但进行该初始系统治疗的选择前,患者应进行接受抗血管生成治疗的风险评估。肿瘤体细胞突变谱分析可用于评估患者是否适合采取某种特定的肿瘤精准治疗,如商品化的 BRAF 拮抗剂或临床试验药物。如果有效,可进一步评估其是否可能诱导再分化增敏进一步的 RAI 治疗。以上各种因素的综合考量如图 16.2 所示。

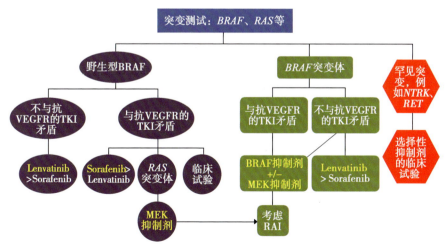

图 16.2 一种确定进展性转移性 RAIR-DTC 的初始治疗选择的算法
TKI,酪氨酸激酶抑制剂

(孙 迪 林岩松)

参考文献

1. Noone A, Howlader N, Krapcho M, et al. SEER cancer statistics review, 1975-2015. Bethesda (MD): National Cancer Institute; 2018. Available at: https://seer.cancer.gov/csr/1975_2015/. Based on November 2017 SEER data submission. Accessed September 1, 2018.
2. Durante C, Haddy N, Baudin E, et al. Long-term outcome of 444 patients with distant metastases from papillary and follicular thyroid carcinoma: benefits and limits of radioiodine therapy. J Clin Endocrinol Metab 2006;91(8):2892–9.
3. Schlumberger M, Brose M, Elisei R, et al. Definition and management of radioactive iodine-refractory differentiated thyroid cancer. Lancet Diabetes Endocrinol 2014;2(5):356–8.
4. Haugen BR, Alexander EK, Bible KC, et al. 2015 American Thyroid Association Management Guidelines for Adult Patients with Thyroid Nodules and Differentiated Thyroid Cancer: the American Thyroid Association Guidelines Task Force on Thyroid Nodules and Differentiated Thyroid Cancer. Thyroid 2016;26(1):1–133.
5. Endo M, Liu JB, Dougan M, et al. Incidence of second malignancy in patients with papillary thyroid cancer from surveillance, epidemiology, and end results 13 dataset. J Thyroid Res 2018;2018:8765369.
6. Eisenhauer EA, Therasse P, Bogaerts J, et al. New response evaluation criteria in solid tumours: revised RECIST guideline (version 1.1). Eur J Cancer 2009;45(2):228–47.
7. Shimaoka K, Schoenfeld DA, DeWys WD, et al. A randomized trial of doxorubicin versus doxorubicin plus cisplatin in patients with advanced thyroid carcinoma. Cancer 1985;56(9):2155–60.
8. Sherman SI. Cytotoxic chemotherapy for differentiated thyroid carcinoma. Clin Oncol (R Coll Radiol) 2010;22:464–8.
9. Lin JD, Chao TC. Vascular endothelial growth factor in thyroid cancers. Cancer Biother Radiopharm 2005;20(6):648–61.
10. Cabanillas ME, Schlumberger M, Jarzab B, et al. A phase 2 trial of lenvatinib (E7080) in advanced, progressive, radioiodine-refractory, differentiated thyroid cancer: a clinical outcomes and biomarker assessment. Cancer 2015;121(16):2749–56.
11. Schlumberger M, Tahara M, Wirth LJ, et al. Lenvatinib versus placebo in radioiodine-refractory thyroid cancer. N Engl J Med 2015;372(7):621–30.
12. Tahara M, Schlumberger M, Elisei R, et al. Exploratory analysis of biomarkers associated with clinical outcomes from the study of lenvatinib in differentiated cancer of the thyroid. Eur J Cancer 2017;75:213–21.
13. Brose MS, Worden FP, Newbold KL, et al. Effect of age on the efficacy and safety of lenvatinib in radioiodine-refractory differentiated thyroid cancer in the phase III select trial. J Clin Oncol 2017;35(23):2692–9.
14. Rao SN, Cabanillas ME. Navigating systemic therapy in advanced thyroid carcinoma: from standard of care to personalized therapy and beyond. J Endocr Soc 2018;2(10):1109–30.
15. Wilson L, Huang W, Chen L, et al. Cost effectiveness of lenvatinib, sorafenib and

placebo in treatment of radioiodine-refractory differentiated thyroid cancer. Thyroid 2017;27(8):1043–52.
16. Kloos RT, Ringel MD, Knopp MV, et al. Phase II trial of sorafenib in metastatic thyroid cancer. J Clin Oncol 2009;27(10):1675–84.
17. Gupta-Abramson V, Troxel AB, Nellore A, et al. Phase II trial of sorafenib in advanced thyroid cancer. J Clin Oncol 2008;26(29):4714–9.
18. Brose MS, Nutting CM, Jarzab B, et al. Sorafenib in radioactive iodine-refractory, locally advanced or metastatic differentiated thyroid cancer: a randomised, double-blind, phase 3 trial. Lancet 2014;384(9940):319–28.
19. Leboulleux S, Bastholt L, Krause T, et al. Vandetanib in locally advanced or metastatic differentiated thyroid cancer: a randomised, double-blind, phase 2 trial. Lancet Oncol 2012;13(9):897–905.
20. Cabanillas ME, Brose MS, Holland J, et al. A phase I study of cabozantinib (XL184) in patients with differentiated thyroid cancer. Thyroid 2014;24(10):1508–14.
21. Blevins DP, Dadu R, Hu M, et al. Aerodigestive fistula formation as a rare side effect of antiangiogenic tyrosine kinase inhibitor therapy for thyroid cancer. Thyroid 2014;24(5):918–22.
22. Cabanillas ME, de Souza JA, Geyer S, et al. Cabozantinib as salvage therapy for patients with tyrosine kinase inhibitor-refractory differentiated thyroid cancer: results of a multicenter phase II international thyroid oncology group trial. J Clin Oncol 2017;35(29):3315–21.
23. Brose MS, Shenoy S, Bhat N, et al. A phase II trial of cabozantinib (CABO) for the treatment of radioiodine (RAI)-refractory differentiated thyroid carcinoma (DTC) in the first-line setting. J Clin Oncol 2018;36(15_suppl):6088.
24. Bible KC, Suman VJ, Molina JR, et al. Efficacy of pazopanib in progressive, radioiodine-refractory, metastatic differentiated thyroid cancers: results of a phase 2 consortium study. Lancet Oncol 2010;11(10):962–72.
25. Carr LL, Mankoff DA, Goulart BH, et al. Phase II study of daily sunitinib in FDG-PET-positive, iodine-refractory differentiated thyroid cancer and metastatic medullary carcinoma of the thyroid with functional imaging correlation. Clin Cancer Res 2010;16(21):5260–8.
26. Bikas A, Kundra P, Desale S, et al. Phase 2 clinical trial of sunitinib as adjunctive treatment in patients with advanced differentiated thyroid cancer. Eur J Endocrinol 2016;174(3):373–80.
27. Locati LD, Licitra L, Agate L, et al. Treatment of advanced thyroid cancer with axitinib: phase 2 study with pharmacokinetic/pharmacodynamic and quality-of-life assessments. Cancer 2014;120(17):2694–703.
28. Carhill AA, Cabanillas ME, Jimenez C, et al. The noninvestigational use of tyrosine kinase inhibitors in thyroid cancer: establishing a standard for patient safety and monitoring. J Clin Endocrinol Metab 2013;98(1):31–42.
29. Resteghini C, Cavalieri S, Galbiati D, et al. Management of tyrosine kinase inhibitors (TKI) side effects in differentiated and medullary thyroid cancer patients. Best Pract Res Clin Endocrinol Metab 2017;31(3):349–61.
30. Lacouture ME. Management of dermatologic toxicities. J Natl Compr Canc Netw 2015;13(5 Suppl):686–9.
31. Cabanillas ME, Patel A, Danysh BP, et al. BRAF inhibitors: experience in thyroid cancer and general review of toxicity. Horm Cancer 2015;6(1):21–36.
32. Holderfield M, Deuker MM, McCormick F, et al. Targeting RAF kinases for cancer

therapy: BRAF-mutated melanoma and beyond. Nat Rev Cancer 2014;14(7): 455–67.
33. Kim KB, Cabanillas ME, Lazar AJ, et al. Clinical responses to vemurafenib in patients with metastatic papillary thyroid cancer harboring BRAF(V600E) mutation. Thyroid 2013;23(10):1277–83.
34. Sala E, Mologni L, Truffa S, et al. BRAF silencing by short hairpin RNA or chemical blockade by PLX4032 leads to different responses in melanoma and thyroid carcinoma cells. Mol Cancer Res 2008;6(5):751–9.
35. Brose MS, Cabanillas ME, Cohen EE, et al. Vemurafenib in patients with BRAF(V600E)-positive metastatic or unresectable papillary thyroid cancer refractory to radioactive iodine: a non-randomised, multicentre, open-label, phase 2 trial. Lancet Oncol 2016;17(9):1272–82.
36. Dadu R, Shah K, Busaidy NL, et al. Efficacy and tolerability of vemurafenib in patients with BRAF(V600E) -positive papillary thyroid cancer: M.D. Anderson Cancer Center off label experience. J Clin Endocrinol Metab 2015;100(1):E77–81.
37. Cabanillas ME, Busaidy NL, Zafereo M, et al. Neoadjuvant vemurafenib in patients with locally advanced papillary thyroid cancer (PTC). Eur Thyroid J 2017; 6(Suppl 1):38.
38. Falchook GS, Long GV, Kurzrock R, et al. Dabrafenib in patients with melanoma, untreated brain metastases, and other solid tumours: a phase 1 dose-escalation trial. Lancet 2012;379(9829):1893–901.
39. Falchook GS, Millward M, Hong D, et al. BRAF inhibitor dabrafenib in patients with metastatic BRAF-mutant thyroid cancer. Thyroid 2015;25(1):71–7.
40. Shah MH, Wei L, Wirth LJ, et al. Results of randomized phase II trial of dabrafenib versus dabrafenib plus trametinib in BRAF-mutated papillary thyroid carcinoma. J Clin Oncol 2017;35(15_suppl):6022.
41. White PS, Pudusseri A, Lee SL, et al. Intermittent dosing of dabrafenib and trametinib in metastatic BRAFV600E mutated papillary thyroid cancer: two case reports. Thyroid 2017;27(9):1201–5.
42. Subbiah V, Kreitman RJ, Wainberg ZA, et al. Dabrafenib and trametinib treatment in patients with locally advanced or metastatic BRAF V600-mutant anaplastic thyroid cancer. J Clin Oncol 2018;36(1):7–13.
43. Hayes DN, Lucas AS, Tanvetyanon T, et al. Phase II efficacy and pharmacogenomic study of selumetinib (AZD6244; ARRY-142886) in iodine-131 refractory papillary thyroid carcinoma (IRPTC) with or without follicular elements. Clin Cancer Res 2012;18(7):2056–65.
44. Schneider TC, de Wit D, Links TP, et al. Everolimus in patients with advanced follicular-derived thyroid cancer: results of a phase II clinical trial. J Clin Endocrinol Metab 2017;102(2):698–707.
45. Hanna GJ, Busaidy NL, Chau NG, et al. Genomic correlates of response to everolimus in aggressive radioiodine-refractory thyroid cancer: a phase II study. Clin Cancer Res 2018;24(7):1546–53.
46. Lim SM, Chang H, Yoon MJ, et al. A multicenter, phase II trial of everolimus in locally advanced or metastatic thyroid cancer of all histologic subtypes. Ann Oncol 2013;24(12):3089–94.
47. Sherman EJ, Dunn LA, Ho AL, et al. Phase 2 study evaluating the combination of sorafenib and temsirolimus in the treatment of radioactive iodine-refractory thyroid cancer. Cancer 2017;123(21):4114–21.

48. Sherman EJ, Ho AL, Fury MG, et al. Combination of everolimus and sorafenib in the treatment of thyroid cancer: update on phase II study. J Clin Oncol 2015; 33(15suppl):6069.
49. Brose MS, Troxel AB, Yarchoan M, et al. A phase II study of everolimus (E) and sorafenib (S) in patients (PTS) with metastatic differentiated thyroid cancer who have progressed on sorafenib alone. J Clin Oncol 2015;33(15suppl):6072.
50. Chakravarty D, Santos E, Ryder M, et al. Small-molecule MAPK inhibitors restore radioiodine incorporation in mouse thyroid cancers with conditional BRAF activation. J Clin Invest 2011;121(12):4700–11.
51. Ho AL, Grewal RK, Leboeuf R, et al. Selumetinib-enhanced radioiodine uptake in advanced thyroid cancer. N Engl J Med 2013;368(7):623–32.
52. Rothenberg SM, McFadden DG, Palmer EL, et al. Redifferentiation of iodine-refractory BRAF V600E-mutant metastatic papillary thyroid cancer with dabrafenib. Clin Cancer Res 2015;21(5):1028–35.
53. Jaber T, Waguespack SG, Cabanillas ME, et al. Targeted therapy in advanced thyroid cancer to resensitize tumors to radioactive iodine. J Clin Endocrinol Metab 2018;103(10):3698–705.
54. Iodine I-131 with or without selumetinib in treating patients with recurrent or metastatic thyroid cancer. 2018. Available at: https://clinicaltrials.gov/ct2/show/NCT02393690?term=selumetinib&cond=Thyroid+Cancer&rank=3. Accessed September 3, 2018.
55. Wadsley J, Gregory R, Flux G, et al. SELIMETRY-a multicentre I-131 dosimetry trial: a clinical perspective. Br J Radiol 2017;90(1073):20160637.
56. Ho A, Keating K, Skolnik J, et al. The ASTRA study: adjuvant selumetinib for differentiated thyroid cancer (DTC); remission after radioiodine. Paper presented at: World Congress on Thyroid Cancer. Boston, MA, July 2013.
57. Soriot P, Frederickson D, Mallon M, et al. H1 2018 results. 2018. Available at: https://www.astrazeneca.com/content/dam/az/PDF/2018/h1-2018/H1%202018%20Results%20Presentation.pdf. Accessed September 3, 2018.
58. Yakushina VD, Lerner LV, Lavrov AV. Gene fusions in thyroid cancer. Thyroid 2018; 28(2):158–67.
59. Kato S, Subbiah V, Marchlik E, et al. RET aberrations in diverse cancers: next-generation sequencing of 4,871 patients. Clin Cancer Res 2017;23(8):1988–97.
60. Subbiah V, Velcheti V, Tuch BB, et al. Selective RET kinase inhibition for patients with RET-altered cancers. Ann Oncol 2018;29(8):1869–76.
61. Li GG, Somwar R, Joseph J, et al. Antitumor activity of RXDX-105 in multiple cancer types with RET rearrangements or mutations. Clin Cancer Res 2017;23(12): 2981–90.
62. Rahal R, Evans EK, Hu W, et al. The development of potent, selective RET inhibitors that target both wild-type RET and prospectively identified resistance mutations to multi-kinase inhibitors. Cancer Res 2016;76(14 Supplement):2641.
63. Drilon AE, Subbiah V, Oxnard GR, et al. A phase 1 study of LOXO-292, a potent and highly selective RET inhibitor, in patients with RET-altered cancers. J Clin Oncol 2018;36(15_suppl):102.
64. Subbiah V, Taylor M, Lin J, et al. Highly potent and selective RET inhibitor, BLU-667, achieves proof of concept in a phase I study of advanced, RET-altered solid tumors. Cancer Res 2018;78(13 Supplement):CT043.
65. Khotskaya YB, Holla VR, Farago AF, et al. Targeting TRK family proteins in cancer. Pharmacol Ther 2017;173:58–66.

66. Wirth L, Drilon A, Albert C, et al. Larotrectinib is highly active in patients with advanced recurrent TRK fusion thyroid (TC) and salivary gland cancers (SGC). Int J Radiat Oncol Biol Phys 2018;100(5):1318.
67. Drilon A, Laetsch TW, Kummar S, et al. Efficacy of larotrectinib in TRK fusion-positive cancers in adults and children. N Engl J Med 2018;378(8):731–9.
68. Giordano TJ, Haugen BR, Sherman SI, et al. Pioglitazone therapy of PAX8-PPARgamma fusion protein thyroid carcinoma. J Clin Endocrinol Metab 2018; 103(4):1277–81.
69. French JD, Bible K, Spitzweg C, et al. Leveraging the immune system to treat advanced thyroid cancers. Lancet Diabetes Endocrinol 2017;5(6):469–81.
70. Colli LM, Machiela MJ, Myers TA, et al. Burden of nonsynonymous mutations among TCGA cancers and candidate immune checkpoint inhibitor responses. Cancer Res 2016;76(13):3767–72.
71. Mehnert JM, Varga A, Brose M, et al. Pembrolizumab for advanced papillary or follicular thyroid cancer: preliminary results from the phase 1b KEYNOTE-028 study. J Clin Oncol 2016;34(15_suppl):6091.
72. Welsh JW, Tang C, de Groot P, et al. Phase 2 5-arm trial of ipilimumab plus lung or liver stereotactic radiation for patients with advanced malignancies. Int J Radiat Oncol Biol Phys 2017;99(5):1315–U1337.

第17章
分化型甲状腺癌复发的监测

Prasanna Santhanam, Paul W. Ladenson

关键词

- 分化型甲状腺癌 ● 肿瘤复发 ● 血清甲状腺球蛋白测定
- 甲状腺癌影像学

要点

- 血清甲状腺球蛋白测定以及解剖学和功能学影像检查在分化型甲状腺癌的初始治疗后的监测中发挥着主导作用。
- 对于依据疾病分期需要进行甲状腺残余物消融治疗或怀疑有转移病灶的患者,术后数月进行的诊断性放射性碘全身扫描是重要的检查手段。
- 复发风险中低危的患者,颈部超声(和甲状腺激素替代治疗下的血清甲状腺球蛋白测定)是首选的评估手段,通常也是唯一必要的检查。
- 对怀疑有远处转移病灶的患者,如果CT、MRI和 ^{18}F-FDG-PET 显像应用得当,都可以对残余病灶的定位、监测病灶的进展和对治疗的反应作出重要的判断。

引言

分化型甲状腺癌的复发很常见,根据ATA(American Thyroid Association)指南的复发危险分层,低危患者的复发率为3%~13%,中危患者的复发率为21%~36%,高危患者的复发率高达68%[1,2]。对几乎所有复发的患者来说,复发是由初始治疗时没有被发现也没有进行外科治疗的残留病灶引起,或者是由于没有进行术后的放射性碘治疗所致。血清甲状腺球蛋白监测对怀疑可能存在的复发病灶有警示作用,当有正常甲状腺组织残留时,甲状腺球蛋白就缺乏特异性,也不能提示少数的低分化甲状腺癌的残留,只能根据甲状腺球蛋白的水平来大致提供残余肿瘤位置的线索[3-5]。因此,解剖学和功能学影像技术对甲状腺癌患者的肿瘤复发的监测、定位、治疗决策和疗效评估等方面具有重要作用。本章涉及的解剖学影像技术包括超声、CT(computed tomography)和MRI,功能学影像技术有放射性碘显像和PET扫描。

采用高敏感的方法对治疗后的甲状腺癌患者进行监测,也有很大的局限性。甲状腺球蛋白作为肿瘤标志物,很少能鉴别与临床不相关的残留的正常甲状腺组织或肿瘤组织。在手术治疗后有可检测的血清甲状腺球蛋白的患者中,大约2/3的患者可能没有局部结构性病灶的存在,也没有可能或必要的治疗,并且这些患者的预后通常较好。一项研究显示,接受甲状腺手术和放射性碘消除残余物治疗6个月后,左甲状腺素钠抑制治疗下的甲状腺球蛋白水平为1~5ng/ml的患者,在没有进一步治疗的情况下,最终有54%的患者的血清甲状腺球蛋白水平低于1ng/ml[6]。另一项对生化不完全反应的患者(如可检测到甲状腺球蛋白)进行的研究,发现34%的患者的肿瘤自发缓解,仅有20%的患者的残余肿瘤出现临床表现[1,2,7]。

影像学检查同样也会有许多假阳性的结果。超声常通过不确定的特征来判断良性颈部淋巴结肿大,诸如圆形或淋巴门消失。CT会经常显示肺、肝或骨内与原发病变无关的意外影像。甚至放射性碘的诊断性扫描和治疗后的显像也可能产生影像结果的误导,这是由于乳腺和胸腺的生理性摄取、组织炎症(如支气管炎和结节病)、皮肤污染和异常结构(如食管和气管憩室)的放射性滞留所致[8,9]。

因此,应仔细考虑联合应用甲状腺球蛋白和影像学手段,尤其应时刻牢记,基于患者的年龄和术后肿瘤的病理学发现,患者存在肿瘤残留的可能性。在此,我们对目前用于发现残余病变的技术进行回顾,并提出了一种有效而又经济的策略对残余肿瘤进行定位诊断。

血清甲状腺球蛋白在甲状腺癌监测中的作用和局限性

甲状腺球蛋白是甲状腺来源的特异的循环蛋白质,它是甲状腺癌初始治疗后甲状腺组织残留的高度特异和敏感的标志物[10]。1973年,Van Herle及其同事[11]描述了最早用于检测人血清甲状腺球蛋白的特异而又可重复的双抗体免疫分析法,这种方法测定甲状腺球蛋白的分析敏感性为 1.6ng/ml。同一团队随后发现,未进行治疗的分化型甲状腺癌患者的血清甲状腺球蛋白的平均水平为 144ng/ml,治疗后平均值下降到 6ng/ml;但有转移灶的患者,血清甲状腺球蛋白持续升高,平均值达到 465ng/ml[12]。Spencer 及其同事[13]通过整合残留的良性甲状腺和/或肿瘤组织的体积、TSH(thyroid-stimulating hormone)受体的刺激程度,以及肿瘤组织合成和释放甲状腺球蛋白的能力,将甲状腺球蛋白恰当地描述为一种循环标志物。

在正常甲状腺组织和肿瘤组织中可以看到甲状腺球蛋白对 TSH 刺激的反应,这就意味着对血清甲状腺球蛋白水平的解释要考虑 TSH 的刺激作用。由于给予重组 TSH 后,短期集中的 TSH 刺激可增加血清甲状腺球蛋白检测的敏感性,此时通常也要进行放射性碘扫描。已经证实,肌肉注射重组 TSH,0.9ng/d,连用 2 日,用甲状腺球蛋白测定来检测残余甲状腺和肿瘤组织的准确性与停用甲状腺激素的准确性相当;在给予第 2 次重组 TSH 后的 72 小时,血清甲状腺球蛋白达到最高水平[14]。分化型甲状腺癌患者给予重组 TSH 后,血清甲状腺球蛋白升高近 10 倍,而低分化甲状腺癌患者的血清甲状腺球蛋白增加不超过 3 倍[13]。甲状腺球蛋白测定方法的检测极限为 1~2ng/ml 或更高时,重组 TSH 刺激试验最有助于甲状腺球蛋白的测定[15,16]。一篇选择性的文献综述发现,在给予重组 TSH 后,甲状腺球蛋白测定的截断值为 1ng/ml 时,不能发现 36% 的残余病灶;而以 2ng/ml 作为甲状腺球蛋白检测的截断值,则可以发现 91% 的残余肿瘤[3]。然而,高敏的甲状腺球蛋白检测方法的问世,使检测极限可低达 0.1ng/ml,减少了重组 TSH 在甲状腺球蛋白检测前的应用[17]。

甲状腺球蛋白监测的一个重要局限性存在于 20% 的分化型甲状腺癌患者中,由于这些患者体内有循环甲状腺球蛋白抗体,抗体干扰了应用最广泛的免疫分析法(三明治法)对甲状腺球蛋白的测定,错误地降低了甲状腺球蛋白的测定结果[13,18]。双抗体免疫分析法和液相色谱串联质谱法都可以克服抗体的干扰,是两种可替换免疫分析法的甲状腺球蛋白测定方法[19-21]。用同一种检测方法连续测定甲状腺球蛋白抗体阳性患者的甲状腺球蛋白抗体水平,常常也能提供残余病灶,以及病灶进展和对治疗反应的信息[22-24]。

2015 年 ATA 临床实践指南用术后 3~4 周测定的最低甲状腺球蛋白水平对患者进行:①初始治疗反应分类;②指导甲状腺癌患者预后的判断;③推荐监测方案[7,25-27](表 17.1)。TSH 抑制或 TSH 刺激下的甲状腺球蛋白低于 1ng/ml,也并不完全排除在随后的 ^{131}I 治疗后的扫描中发现疾病的可能性,但发现病灶的可能性极低,除非是肿瘤分期高的患者。复发(残余病灶的出现)的风险随术后的甲状腺球蛋白水平升高达到 5~10ng/ml 而增加[7]。

表 17.1
甲状腺癌初始治疗后的疗效分类

分类	特点	预后
完全缓解	影像学阴性 抑制下的 Tg[a]<0.2(和无 Tg 抗体干扰)或 刺激下的 Tg<1	1%~4% 的复发率 <1% 的死亡风险
生化不完全反应	影像学阴性 抑制下的 Tg≥1 或 刺激下的 Tg≥10 或 Tg 抗体水平升高	30% 的患者自然缓解 20% 的患者需要其他的治疗获得完全缓解 20% 的患者进展出现结构性病灶 死亡风险<1%
结构不完全反应	有结构性病灶,不论 Tg 水平如何	病灶持续的发生率 50%~85% 局部转移的死亡风险为 11% 远处转移的死亡风险为 50%
不确定反应	非特异的影像学发现 抑制下的 Tg<1 刺激下的 Tg<10 Tg 抗体水平稳定或下降	15%~20% 会表现出复发,其余会自发缓解 <1% 的死亡风险

[a] 甲状腺球蛋白(简称 Tg)的单位为 ng/ml

Adapted from Haugen BR, Alexander EK, Bible KC, et al. 2015 American Thyroid Association Management guidelines for adult patients with thyroid nodules and differentiated thyroid cancer: the American Thyroid Association guidelines task force on thyroid nodules and differentiated thyroid cancer. Thyroid 2016;26(1):48;with permission.

甲状腺癌患者在初始手术和可能的放射性碘治疗后的随访过程中,连续监测血清甲状腺球蛋白有助于以下几种情形的判断。第一,对大多数临床分期低且复发风险极低的患者,血清甲状腺球蛋白检测不到或处于非常低的水平,可以提供对非特异性影像检查需求更少的保证。第二,可以反驳或证实可能代表残留病灶的放射学影像的意义。第三,指定血清甲状腺球蛋白水平升高的患者定期进行影像学检查以定位病灶。第四,当怀疑颈部淋巴结复发,而细胞学检查为阴性时,测定细针穿刺抽吸物的甲状腺球蛋白水平有时能揭示疾病[28]。第五，对已知存在局部或远处肿瘤转移的患者，血清甲状腺球蛋白水平的连续变化可作为治疗反应的标志物，有助于决定何时开始或重复 ^{131}I 治疗和/或化疗。最后，血清甲状腺球蛋白水平与影像学已知的肿瘤负荷的比例，可以判断肿瘤的分化程度以及对 ^{131}I 治疗和其他治疗方法产生反应的可能性。

检测残余病变的传统影像学方法
颈部超声

超声是发现甲状腺癌在颈部淋巴结或软组织残留的高度敏感的手段[29,30]。欧洲指南推荐至少使用 12MHz 的超声探头对甲状腺床及双侧颈部 Ⅱ~Ⅵ 区的淋巴结进行灰阶超声成像，采用多普勒进行血流评估[31]。ATA 指南推荐使用频率为 10MHz 的超声来评估颈部淋巴结的转移[7]。高频换能器（>10MHz或以上）对浅表淋巴结的分辨率较好，但对深部组织的穿透性差；而低频率超声（5MHz）对深部组织的穿透性好，但分辨率低[32]。超声检查发现颈部残余肿瘤的灵敏度可高达 94%，而 TSH 刺激后的甲状腺球蛋白和诊断性碘扫描发现残余病变的灵敏度接近 50%[30]。

然而，颈部超声检查也存在假阳性，尤其是 ATA 危险分层的中低危患者[33]。双侧甲状腺切除术后，甲状腺床通常是一个平坦的倒三角形，被纤维脂肪组织填充[34]。甲状腺床的小结节（<5mm）很常见，有 60% 或更多的结节在初次超声评估时表现出可疑恶性的特征，包括低回声、纵横比>1、微钙化、边缘不规则和/或血流增加等，但在 5 年的随访中，仅有不到 10% 的结节体积增大[35]。超声能发现良性颈部淋巴结和瘢痕组织，但意义通常不明。甲状腺床内或与甲状腺床相邻的正常组织也可能被误认为是残留的病变，包括残余的小块甲状腺组织、环状软骨和甲状腺软骨、颈部的胸腺、交感神经节、胸导管末端、颈椎横突和神经根[36]。慢性肉芽肿病变、手术瘢痕、咽食管憩室（有时伴钙化）、甲状旁腺瘤和甲状舌管囊肿的影像也可能产生误诊。此外，在颈侧区也可以看到创伤性神经瘤、神经鞘瘤和副神经节瘤等[36]。

当颈部淋巴结出现以下 1 个或多个超声影像特征时应怀疑转移，包括淋巴门消失、出现囊性区域、淋巴结内点状的高回声病变、周围型血流增加[37]；然而，用这些标准来诊断或排除恶性肿瘤并不完美[7]。淋巴结淋巴门消失的灵敏度最高可达 100%，而特异度仅有 29%[38]。淋巴结内微钙化的特异度最高可达 100%，但灵敏度较差[37]。周围型血流特征的灵敏度和特异度分别为

86% 和 82%[7]。淋巴结长轴与短轴的比<2 和短轴的直径>8mm 都是怀疑淋巴结转移的特征[31,39]。

2015 年 ATA 指南推荐,根据复发危险分层和血清甲状腺球蛋白水平,应间隔 6~12 个月进行中央区和颈侧区的超声评估[7]。我们推荐放射性碘治疗后 6 个月进行颈部超声检查,在随后的 1~3 年内,特别是对复发风险高危的患者应间隔 6~12 个月进行 1 次超声检查[31]。在随后的几年中,推荐复发风险高危的患者每年进行 1 次超声检查。对于复发风险低的患者,应根据临床发现和血清甲状腺球蛋白水平来判断是否行超声检查。不应该常规对以下的患者作进一步的超声评估,包括:根据手术发现判断为复发风险低危和极低危的患者;术后 2 年的超声检查再次确认颈部淋巴结为阴性;接受放射性碘治疗后检测不到血清甲状腺球蛋白,或未进行甲状腺消融治疗但血清甲状腺球蛋白水平长期稳定并低于 2ng/ml 以下的患者。对这些患者来说,不确定的超声检查发现更有可能是假阳性结果,而不足真阳性结果。然而,对于血清甲状腺球蛋白预示有肿瘤残留的中高危患者,间隔 6~12 个月连续进行超声检查是恰当的,超声影像检查最有可能确定复发肿瘤的位置。

颈部、胸部和其他部位的 CT 扫描

CT 在甲状腺癌中有许多方面的应用,包括术前分期、监测、再分期、定位转移病灶、连续扫描监测肿瘤的进展和对治疗的反应等。从颅底到气管分叉处的 CT 平扫及静脉使用对比剂的增强扫描,可以对颈部淋巴结残留或复发病灶的超声定位进行补充,尤其是定位术前中央区和术后胸骨后方及颈侧方转移淋巴结[8-40]。如果 CT 影像发现肿大的颈部淋巴结出现囊性成分、钙化和 / 或强化,则怀疑淋巴结转移。有时,转移病灶中也可能出现反映出血性或高蛋白含量的高密度 CT 影像[40]。

CT 扫描对确定残余甲状腺肿瘤的范围和侵袭性甲状腺恶性肿瘤的解剖关系也很关键,包括导致或威胁喉或气管浸润、呼吸道梗阻,或椎旁或肌肉浸润的侵袭性甲状腺恶性肿瘤[41]。2015 年版 ATA 指南推荐,对血清甲状腺球蛋白水平高而颈部超声检查阴性的患者行 CT 扫描[7],尤其是血清甲状腺球蛋白>10ng/ml 和 / 或用左甲状腺素钠进行 TSH 抑制治疗时血清甲状腺球蛋白升高的患者[42,43]。甲状腺癌也会导致罕见的恶性胸腔积液,CT 也是可选用的检查手段[44]。

虽然 CT 扫描并不是所有甲状腺癌患者术后常规推荐的监测手段,但在未被超声充分揭示的残留或复发病变的定位中起着关键作用。CT 检查需要

使用碘增强剂来显示颈部包块,因此,必须协调好增强 CT 的使用与计划中的 ^{131}I 扫描和治疗的关系[45]。

MRI 的作用

MRI 在甲状腺癌的术前分期、监测、术后再分期、转移病灶定位,以及连续监测疾病进展和对治疗反应中的具体应用有限。MRI 检查包括轴位和冠状位 T_1 加权像、脂肪饱和 T_2 加权像,还有就是增强后的轴位和冠状位 T_1 加权像[40]。无论是手术前还是手术后,MRI 检查发现脂肪组织完全消失则预示着喉返神经受累(准确性为 88%,敏感性为 94%,特异性为 82%,n=32)[46]。联合气管软骨出现软组织信号、气管腔内出现包块和/或肿瘤包绕气管 180° 的周径来预测甲状腺癌浸润气管的准确性为 90%[47]。相似地,有时 MRI 也能发现食管浸润[48]。MRI 有助于术前发现受累的淋巴结和术后复发的淋巴结,但 MRI 鉴别转移淋巴结和良性反应性淋巴结的特异性不如放射性碘全身扫描[49]。与传统 CT 扫描相比,MRI 和 ^{18}F-FDG-PET/CT 发现骨转移的敏感性更好,尤其在肿瘤累及脊柱时[50]。

新的磁共振弥散加权成像的原理是基于水分子在细胞丰富的组织中有较低的弥散系数,目前正在评价这种成像技术用于检测甲状腺癌的特异特征的能力。对甲状腺癌患者的小队列研究发现,发生甲状腺外浸润的甲状腺乳头状癌的弥散系数显著低于发生转移而无甲状腺外浸润的肿瘤[51]。

检测残余病变的功能性成像方法

放射性碘平面成像和单光子发射计算机断层成像术/计算断层扫描(SPECT/CT)

放射性碘显像应用甲状腺细胞固有的碘浓集能力,可以用于:①为潜在的后续 ^{131}I 消融治疗发现残余的正常甲状腺组织,或持续性循环甲状腺球蛋白的鉴别诊断;②分化型甲状腺癌的摄碘转移灶的鉴别、定位,以及监测转移灶的进展或对治疗的反应。常用的放射性碘的同位素有三种(表 17.2)。依据临床病理分期判定术后放射性碘治疗是合理的患者,通常在术后 2~12 周进行放射性碘的全身扫描[7]。在大多数情况下,^{123}I 是首选的放射性碘同位素,这是由于它的放射线适合平面成像和 SPECT/CT 显像;且它不会产生"顿抑",也就是说甲状腺细胞的损伤轻微,并不影响甲状腺细胞对后续治疗剂量的 ^{131}I 的浓集能力[52,53]。^{131}I 治疗后的全身扫描发现转移肿瘤的敏感性更高,这是由于治疗用的放射性碘剂量较高,且 ^{131}I 有更长的物理半衰期,从而可以在放射性背景活性消失后更晚的时间进行显像[54]。示踪剂量的 ^{131}I 也常用于治疗剂量的计算,由于它的衰变较慢,从而允许在给予 ^{131}I 后 5~10 日或更长的时间来定量预测摄碘转移灶和放射线敏感的正常组织(如骨髓和肺)对进入体内的放射剂量的摄取率。

表 17.2
用于分化型甲状腺癌显像的放射性同位素

同位素	放射线	物理半衰期 $t_{1/2}$	经典的扫描剂量	特征	用途
^{131}I	β 粒子（606keV）能级跃迁释放伽马射线（364keV）	8.02 日	2~3mCi（诊断性扫描）30~200mCi（治疗后扫描）	正常摄取：鼻区、口咽和唾液腺、胃和肠道 甲状腺床残余摄取：可能是残余的甲状腺或残留的肿瘤组织	给予示踪剂量后的 48 小时进行诊断性全身显像 治疗后的 5~7 日进行治疗后的全身显像
^{123}I	伽马射线（159keV）	13.2 小时	1.5~2.0mCi	正常摄取：鼻区、口咽和唾液腺、胃和肠道 甲状腺床可能见到残余摄取,但难以辨别是残余甲状腺组织还是残留的病变	甲状腺切除术后的诊断性扫描 9~12 个月后的随访期诊断性显像,用于发现嗜 RAI 的残余病灶
^{124}I	多种射线、高能量光子、伽马射线、正电子	4.18 日	1.5~1.7mCi	如同上述,但高能量光子增加了分辨率	研究阶段,包括 3D 全身扫描和基于病灶的剂量学研究

mCi,毫居里;RAI,放射性碘
数据来自参考文献[82-84]

放射性碘扫描需要 TSH 刺激残余的正常甲状腺组织和甲状腺癌组织摄取碘。传统上是通过术后不给予或停用甲状腺激素治疗 4 周左右的时间使内源性 TSH 升高。这种方法对大多数患者有效,但也存在许多缺点。第一,这种方法会导致几乎所有的患者出现导致生活质量(躯体和精神)下降的严重的临床甲状腺功能减退症[55]。第二,持久而频繁的 TSH 刺激,偶尔也会刺激肿瘤生长而导致严重的后果,尤其是当转移肿瘤位于关键部位时。第三,少数患者可能无法实现内源性 TSH 升高,包括合并垂体或下丘脑疾病的患者,以及部分老年患者[56]。重组 TSH(rTSH,促甲状腺激素-α,thyrogen)也可获得同样准确的放射性碘扫描和甲状腺球蛋白刺激试验的结果,同时又可以避免临床甲状腺功能减退[14,57]。然而,给予重组 TSH 也很少与转移病灶迅速增大导致的上呼吸道梗阻、骨折和神经系统并发症有关。

当患者循环血液中的碘水平较低时,放射性碘显像的结果更准确,这是由于循环血液中的碘与诊断性和治疗性应用的放射性碘竞争摄碘性甲状腺组织。因此,在进行放射性碘显像和潜在的放射性碘治疗之前,患者常被安排 1 周的低碘饮食(https://www.thyrogen.com/patients/Low-Iodine-Diet.aspx)[58]。患者在计划行放射性碘扫描前的 6~8 周接受了含碘的放射对比剂或含碘药物,对他们进行尿碘水平测定有助于确认体内的碘已被清除。

诊断性 ^{123}I 扫描对揭示病变的范围的敏感性不如 ^{131}I 治疗后的显像。两种同位素对诊断甲状腺床复发和骨转移的敏感性有较高的一致性,但诊断淋巴结转移和肺转移的一致性较差,分别为 60% 和 40%[59]。

对甲状腺癌患者来说,无论是诊断性 ^{123}I 扫描还是 ^{131}I 治疗后的全身扫描,阳性扫描结果的特异性并不完美。假阳性的放射性浓集灶可能由于皮肤污染、非对称的唾液腺活动和乳腺的摄取、气管和食管憩室、肺的炎症性疾病(如支气管炎和肺结节)、阑尾腔内的胃肠道内容物滞留、子宫内膜异位症、卵巢皮样囊肿、骨折愈合、精液囊肿、肾肉芽肿和囊肿、皮下脂肪瘤等引起[60-63]。

联合放射性碘扫描与 CT 扫描(SPECT/CT),可以对 1/4 的患者在平面成像时表现为模糊影像的微量碘浓集灶进行更准确的定位[64]。因此,SPECT/CT 显像有助于确认前面描述的造成假阳性结果的放射性活动点。额外病灶的发现、TNM 分期的改变和疾病预后的改善都与 SPECT/CT 显像的应用有关,尤其是放射性碘治疗后的显像[65,66]。

在实际工作中,根据疾病分期可能需要后续 ^{131}I 治疗的患者进行术后 ^{123}I 诊断性全身扫描,^{131}I 治疗也通常在诊断性扫描后的数日内进行。通常推荐在 ^{131}I 治疗后的 9~12 个月进行第二次 ^{123}I 全身显像,以确认甲状腺残余组织和任何摄碘残余病灶是否被清除。一旦第二次诊断性扫描为阴性结果,则放射性碘扫描对大多数患者的监测就不再有意义[67]。有摄碘转移灶的甲状腺滤泡状癌和乳头状癌的患者属于少见的例外情况,这些患者就需要进行额外数次的 ^{131}I 治疗。

[^{18}F]- 氟代脱氧葡萄糖(^{18}F-FDG)-PET/CT 扫描

^{18}F-FDG-PET 成像是基于正电子和电子相互湮灭后,以相反方向释放出 2 个 511keV 的高能光子的原理。高代谢的肿瘤组织对葡萄糖的摄取增强,特别是与 CT 联合应用时,可以对多种空间分辨率高的肿瘤进行定位[68]。根据患者的复发高风险的临床病理分期、血清甲状腺球蛋白浓度或临床发现,怀疑有额外但尚未确认的转移灶时,^{18}F-FDG-PET/CT 成像就成为定位转移灶的二线检查手段。如果这些可疑的病变逃脱了 ^{123}I 或 ^{131}I 的放射性碘扫描、超声检查和 CT 扫描,有不同的报道认为,^{18}F-FDG-PET/CT 检查可以发现 45%~100% 的患者的额外病灶,并且可以改变多达 50% 的患者的管理[69]。在 PET/CT 显像前应用重组 TSH 的刺激,可以提高成像方法的敏感性和特异性[70]。

一项纳入 515 例患者的 meta 分析发现,^{18}F-FDG-PET/CT 检查发现分化型甲状腺癌残留的总敏感度为 0.84(95% CI 1.77~0.89),总特异度为 0.78(95% CI 0.67~0.86)[71]。随着血清甲状腺球蛋白水平的增加,^{18}F-FDG-PET/CT 发现残余肿瘤的敏感性增加,且血清甲状腺球蛋白可以反映残余肿瘤的体积。一项研究显示,当血清甲状腺球蛋白水平高于 4.6ng/ml 时,^{18}F-FDG-PET/CT 诊断残余肿瘤的敏感性可达 90% 以上[72]。血清甲状腺球蛋白水平在 12~32ng/ml 时,^{18}F-FDG-PET/CT 的诊断敏感性和特异性均最高[73]。如果联合 ^{18}F-FDG-PET/CT 和 ^{131}I 扫描,则 PET 可以发现 14% 的分化型甲状腺癌患者存在额外的病灶[74,75]。

定量 ^{18}F-FDG-PET/CT 检查也被用来评估甲状腺癌的复发。第 90 分钟的标准摄取值>2.75,且第 60 分钟和第 90 分钟的最大标准摄取值变化>−1.1%,对 1cm 以下转移淋巴结诊断的灵敏度、特异度和准确率分别为 81%、90% 和 83%[76]。与野生型甲状腺乳头状癌相比,*BRAF V600E* 突变的甲状腺乳头状癌具有更高的 ^{18}F-FDG-PET/CT 亲和可能性,并且与更高的标准摄取值相关[77]。最后,^{18}F-FDG-PET/CT 发现的病灶与预后不良有关,也可能与较低的化疗反应有关[78]。一项研究联合应用 ^{18}F-FDG-PET/CT 和 MRI,由于提供了关于疾病范围的额外信息,改变了将近一半的分化型甲状腺癌的患者的治疗策略[79]。

同样也可以用正电子发射同位素 ^{124}I 进行全身扫描和病灶剂量学研究(表 17.2)[80,81],但目前这种方法正处于研究阶段。

总结

血清甲状腺球蛋白测定以及解剖学和功能学影像检查在分化型甲状腺

癌的初始治疗后的监测中发挥着主导作用。对于依据疾病分期需要进行甲状腺残余物的放射性碘消融治疗或怀疑有转移病灶的患者，放射性碘的诊断性全身扫描是术后数月内进行的重要检查手段。颈部淋巴结或软组织是中低危患者最常见的复发部位，超声是首选的最佳评估手段，通常也是唯一必要的检查。对怀疑有多处远处转移病灶的患者，CT、MRI 和 ^{18}F-FDG-PET/CT 显像都可以对残余病灶的定位、监测病灶进展和对治疗的反应作出重要的判断。

（苏艳军　程若川）

参考文献

1. Vaisman F, Momesso D, Bulzico DA, et al. Spontaneous remission in thyroid cancer patients after biochemical incomplete response to initial therapy. Clin Endocrinol 2012;77(1):132-8.
2. Tuttle RM, Tala H, Shah J, et al. Estimating risk of recurrence in differentiated thyroid cancer after total thyroidectomy and radioactive iodine remnant ablation: using response to therapy variables to modify the initial risk estimates predicted by the new American Thyroid Association staging system. Thyroid 2010;20(12):1341-9.
3. Mazzaferri EL, Robbins RJ, Spencer CA, et al. A consensus report of the role of serum thyroglobulin as a monitoring method for low-risk patients with papillary thyroid carcinoma. J Clin Endocrinol Metab 2003;88(4):1433-41.
4. Torlontano M, Crocetti U, Augello G, et al. Comparative evaluation of recombinant human thyrotropin-stimulated thyroglobulin levels, 131I whole-body scintigraphy, and neck ultrasonography in the follow-up of patients with papillary thyroid microcarcinoma who have not undergone radioiodine therapy. J Clin Endocrinol Metab 2006;91(1):60-3.
5. Robbins RJ, Srivastava S, Shaha A, et al. Factors influencing the basal and recombinant human thyrotropin-stimulated serum thyroglobulin in patients with metastatic thyroid carcinoma. J Clin Endocrinol Metab 2004;89(12):6010-6.
6. Padovani RP, Robenshtok E, Brokhin M, et al. Even without additional therapy, serum thyroglobulin concentrations often decline for years after total thyroidectomy and radioactive remnant ablation in patients with differentiated thyroid cancer. Thyroid 2012;22(8):778-83.
7. Haugen BR, Alexander EK, Bible KC, et al. 2015 American Thyroid Association Management guidelines for adult patients with thyroid nodules and differentiated thyroid cancer: the American Thyroid Association guidelines task force on thyroid nodules and differentiated thyroid cancer. Thyroid 2016;26(1):1-133.
8. Chudgar AV, Shah JC. Pictorial review of false-positive results on radioiodine scintigrams of patients with differentiated thyroid cancer. Radiographics 2017;37(1):298-315.

9. Yang SP, Bach AM, Tuttle RM, et al. Serial neck ultrasound is more likely to identify false-positive abnormalities than clinically significant disease in low-risk papillary thyroid cancer patients. Endocr Pract 2015;21(12):1372–9.
10. Refetoff S, Lever EG. The value of serum thyroglobulin measurement in clinical practice. JAMA 1983;250(17):2352–7.
11. Van Herle AJ, Uller RP, Matthews NI, et al. Radioimmunoassay for measurement of thyroglobulin in human serum. J Clin Invest 1973;52(6):1320–7.
12. Herle AJ, Uller RP. Elevated serum thyroglobulin. A marker of metastases in differentiated thyroid carcinomas. J Clin Invest 1975;56(2):272–7.
13. Spencer CA, LoPresti JS, Fatemi S, et al. Detection of residual and recurrent differentiated thyroid carcinoma by serum thyroglobulin measurement. Thyroid 1999;9(5):435–41.
14. Haugen BR, Pacini F, Reiners C, et al. A comparison of recombinant human thyrotropin and thyroid hormone withdrawal for the detection of thyroid remnant or cancer. J Clin Endocrinol Metab 1999;84(11):3877–85.
15. Torrens JI, Burch HB. Serum thyroglobulin measurement. Utility in clinical practice. Endocrinol Metab Clin North Am 2001;30(2):429–67.
16. Woodmansee WW, Haugen BR. Uses for recombinant human TSH in patients with thyroid cancer and nodular goiter. Clin Endocrinol 2004;61(2):163–73.
17. Giovanella L, Clark PM, Chiovato L, et al. Thyroglobulin measurement using highly sensitive assays in patients with differentiated thyroid cancer: a clinical position paper. Eur J Endocrinol 2014;171(2):R33–46.
18. Spencer CA, Takeuchi M, Kazarosyan M, et al. Serum thyroglobulin autoantibodies: prevalence, influence on serum thyroglobulin measurement, and prognostic significance in patients with differentiated thyroid carcinoma. J Clin Endocrinol Metab 1998;83(4):1121–7.
19. Kushnir MM, Rockwood AL, Straseski JA, et al. Comparison of LC-MS/MS to immunoassay for measurement of thyroglobulin in fine-needle aspiration samples. Clin Chem 2014;60(11):1452–3.
20. Netzel BC, Grebe SK, Algeciras-Schimnich A. Usefulness of a thyroglobulin liquid chromatography-tandem mass spectrometry assay for evaluation of suspected heterophile interference. Clin Chem 2014;60(7):1016–8.
21. Netzel BC, Grebe SK, Carranza Leon BG, et al. Thyroglobulin (Tg) testing revisited: Tg assays, TgAb assays, and correlation of results with clinical outcomes. J Clin Endocrinol Metab 2015;100(8):E1074–83.
22. Spencer CA. Clinical review: clinical utility of thyroglobulin antibody (TgAb) measurements for patients with differentiated thyroid cancers (DTC). J Clin Endocrinol Metab 2011;96(12):3615–27.
23. Gianoukakis AG. Thyroglobulin antibody status and differentiated thyroid cancer: what does it mean for prognosis and surveillance? Curr Opin Oncol 2015;27(1):26–32.
24. Spencer C, Fatemi S. Thyroglobulin antibody (TgAb) methods—strengths, pitfalls and clinical utility for monitoring TgAb-positive patients with differentiated thyroid cancer. Best Pract Res Clin Endocrinol Metab 2013;27(5):701–12.
25. Piccardo A, Arecco F, Puntoni M, et al. Focus on high-risk DTC patients: high postoperative serum thyroglobulin level is a strong predictor of disease persistence and is associated to progression-free survival and overall survival. Clin Nucl Med 2013;38(1):18–24.

26. Giovanella L, Ceriani L, Ghelfo A, et al. Thyroglobulin assay 4 weeks after thyroidectomy predicts outcome in low-risk papillary thyroid carcinoma. Clin Chem Lab Med 2005;43(8):843–7.
27. Polachek A, Hirsch D, Tzvetov G, et al. Prognostic value of post-thyroidectomy thyroglobulin levels in patients with differentiated thyroid cancer. J Endocrinol Invest 2011;34(11):855–60.
28. Torres MR, Nobrega Neto SH, Rosas RJ, et al. Thyroglobulin in the washout fluid of lymph-node biopsy: what is its role in the follow-up of differentiated thyroid carcinoma? Thyroid 2014;24(1):7–18.
29. Matrone A, Gambale C, Piaggi P, et al. Postoperative thyroglobulin and neck ultrasound in the risk restratification and decision to perform 131I ablation. J Clin Endocrinol Metab 2017;102(3):893–902.
30. Frasoldati A, Pesenti M, Gallo M, et al. Diagnosis of neck recurrences in patients with differentiated thyroid carcinoma. Cancer 2003;97(1):90–6.
31. Leenhardt L, Erdogan MF, Hegedus L, et al. 2013 European Thyroid Association guidelines for cervical ultrasound scan and ultrasound-guided techniques in the postoperative management of patients with thyroid cancer. Eur Thyroid J 2013; 2(3):147–59.
32. Ying M, Ahuja A. Sonography of neck lymph nodes. Part I: normal lymph nodes. Clin Radiol 2003;58(5):351–8.
33. Peiling Yang S, Bach AM, Tuttle RM, et al. Frequent screening with serial neck ultrasound is more likely to identify false-positive abnormalities than clinically significant disease in the surveillance of intermediate risk papillary thyroid cancer patients without suspicious findings on follow-up ultrasound evaluation. J Clin Endocrinol Metab 2015;100(4):1561–7.
34. Shin JH, Han BK, Ko EY, et al. Sonographic findings in the surgical bed after thyroidectomy: comparison of recurrent tumors and nonrecurrent lesions. J Ultrasound Med 2007;26(10):1359–66.
35. Rondeau G, Fish S, Hann LE, et al. Ultrasonographically detected small thyroid bed nodules identified after total thyroidectomy for differentiated thyroid cancer seldom show clinically significant structural progression. Thyroid 2011;21(8): 845–53.
36. Chua WY, Langer JE, Jones LP. Surveillance neck sonography after thyroidectomy for papillary thyroid carcinoma: pitfalls in the diagnosis of locally recurrent and metastatic disease. J Ultrasound Med 2017;36(7):1511–30.
37. Leboulleux S, Girard E, Rose M, et al. Ultrasound criteria of malignancy for cervical lymph nodes in patients followed up for differentiated thyroid cancer. J Clin Endocrinol Metab 2007;92(9):3590–4.
38. Kuna SK, Bracic I, Tesic V, et al. Ultrasonographic differentiation of benign from malignant neck lymphadenopathy in thyroid cancer. J Ultrasound Med 2006; 25(12):1531–7 [quiz: 1538–40].
39. Steinkamp HJ, Cornehl M, Hosten N, et al. Cervical lymphadenopathy: ratio of long- to short-axis diameter as a predictor of malignancy. Br J Radiol 1995; 68(807):266–70.
40. Hoang JK, Branstetter BF, Gafton AR, et al. Imaging of thyroid carcinoma with CT and MRI: approaches to common scenarios. Cancer Imaging 2013;13:128–39.
41. Ahmed M, Saleem M, Al-Arifi A, et al. Obstructive endotracheal lesions of thyroid cancer. J Laryngol Otol 2002;116(8):613–21.
42. Moneke I, Kaifi JT, Kloeser R, et al. Pulmonary metastasectomy for thyroid cancer

as salvage therapy for radioactive iodine-refractory metastases. Eur J Cardiothorac Surg 2018;53(3):625–30.
43. Wang R, Zhang Y, Tan J, et al. Analysis of radioiodine therapy and prognostic factors of differentiated thyroid cancer patients with pulmonary metastasis: an 8-year retrospective study. Medicine 2017;96(19):e6809.
44. Liu M, Shen Y, Ruan M, et al. Notable decrease of malignant pleural effusion after treatment with sorafenib in radioiodine-refractory follicular thyroid carcinoma. Thyroid 2014;24(7):1179–83.
45. Loevner LA, Kaplan SL, Cunnane ME, et al. Cross-sectional imaging of the thyroid gland. Neuroimaging Clin N Am 2008;18(3):445–61, vii.
46. Takashima S, Takayama F, Wang J, et al. Using MR imaging to predict invasion of the recurrent laryngeal nerve by thyroid carcinoma. AJR Am J Roentgenol 2003; 180(3):837–42.
47. Wang JC, Takashima S, Takayama F, et al. Tracheal invasion by thyroid carcinoma: prediction using MR imaging. AJR Am J Roentgenol 2001;177(4):929–36.
48. Wang J, Takashima S, Matsushita T, et al. Esophageal invasion by thyroid carcinomas: prediction using magnetic resonance imaging. J Comput Assist Tomogr 2003;27(1):18–25.
49. Mihailovic J, Prvulovic M, Ivkovic M, et al. MRI versus (1)(3)(1)I whole-body scintigraphy for the detection of lymph node recurrences in differentiated thyroid carcinoma. AJR Am J Roentgenol 2010;195(5):1197–203.
50. Lange MB, Nielsen ML, Andersen JD, et al. Diagnostic accuracy of imaging methods for the diagnosis of skeletal malignancies: a retrospective analysis against a pathology-proven reference. Eur J Radiol 2016;85(1):61–7.
51. Lu Y, Moreira AL, Hatzoglou V, et al. Using diffusion-weighted MRI to predict aggressive histological features in papillary thyroid carcinoma: a novel tool for pre-operative risk stratification in thyroid cancer. Thyroid 2015;25(6):672–80.
52. Kao CH, Yen TC. Stunning effects after a diagnostic dose of iodine-131. Nuklearmedizin 1998;37(1):30–2.
53. Urhan M, Dadparvar S, Mavi A, et al. Iodine-123 as a diagnostic imaging agent in differentiated thyroid carcinoma: a comparison with iodine-131 post-treatment scanning and serum thyroglobulin measurement. Eur J Nucl Med Mol Imaging 2007;34(7):1012–7.
54. Chong A, Song HC, Min JJ, et al. Improved detection of lung or bone metastases with an I-131 whole body scan on the 7th day after high-dose I-131 therapy in patients with thyroid cancer. Nucl Med Mol Imaging 2010;44(4):273–81.
55. Ladenson PW, Braverman LE, Mazzaferri EL, et al. Comparison of administration of recombinant human thyrotropin with withdrawal of thyroid hormone for radioactive iodine scanning in patients with thyroid carcinoma. N Engl J Med 1997; 337(13):888–96.
56. Ringel MD, Ladenson PW. Diagnostic accuracy of 131I scanning with recombinant human thyrotropin versus thyroid hormone withdrawal in a patient with metastatic thyroid carcinoma and hypopituitarism. J Clin Endocrinol Metab 1996; 81(5):1724–5.
57. Schroeder PR, Haugen BR, Pacini F, et al. A comparison of short-term changes in health-related quality of life in thyroid carcinoma patients undergoing diagnostic evaluation with recombinant human thyrotropin compared with thyroid hormone withdrawal. J Clin Endocrinol Metab 2006;91(3):878–84.
58. Lee M, Lee YK, Jeon TJ, et al. Low iodine diet for one week is sufficient for

adequate preparation of high dose radioactive iodine ablation therapy of differentiated thyroid cancer patients in iodine-rich areas. Thyroid 2014;24(8):1289-96.
59. Iwano S, Kato K, Nihashi T, et al. Comparisons of I-123 diagnostic and I-131 post-treatment scans for detecting residual thyroid tissue and metastases of differentiated thyroid cancer. Ann Nucl Med 2009;23(9):777-82.
60. Triggiani V, Giagulli VA, Iovino M, et al. False positive diagnosis on (131)iodine whole-body scintigraphy of differentiated thyroid cancers. Endocrine 2016; 53(3):626-35.
61. Hannoush ZC, Palacios JD, Kuker RA, et al. False positive findings on I-131 WBS and SPECT/CT in patients with history of thyroid cancer: case series. Case Rep Endocrinol 2017;2017:8568347.
62. Campenni A, Giovinazzo S, Tuccari G, et al. Abnormal radioiodine uptake on post-therapy whole body scan and sodium/iodine symporter expression in a dermoid cyst of the ovary: report of a case and review of the literature. Arch Endocrinol Metab 2015;59(4):351-4.
63. Mi YX, Sui X, Huang JM, et al. Incidentally polycystic kidney disease identified by SPECT/CT with post-therapy radioiodine scintigraphy in a patient with differentiated thyroid carcinoma: a case report. Medicine 2017;96(43):e8348.
64. Zilioli V, Peli A, Panarotto MB, et al. Differentiated thyroid carcinoma: incremental diagnostic value of (131)I SPECT/CT over planar whole body scan after radioiodine therapy. Endocrine 2017;56(3):551-9.
65. Kohlfuerst S, Igerc I, Lobnig M, et al. Posttherapeutic (131)I SPECT-CT offers high diagnostic accuracy when the findings on conventional planar imaging are inconclusive and allows a tailored patient treatment regimen. Eur J Nucl Med Mol Imaging 2009;36(6):886-93.
66. Ciappuccini R, Heutte N, Trzepla G, et al. Postablation (131)I scintigraphy with neck and thorax SPECT-CT and stimulated serum thyroglobulin level predict the outcome of patients with differentiated thyroid cancer. Eur J Endocrinol 2011; 164(6):961-9.
67. Gonzalez Carvalho JM, Gorlich D, Schober O, et al. Evaluation of (131)I scintigraphy and stimulated thyroglobulin levels in the follow up of patients with DTC: a retrospective analysis of 1420 patients. Eur J Nucl Med Mol Imaging 2017;44(5): 744-56.
68. Farwell MD, Pryma DA, Mankoff DA. PET/CT imaging in cancer: current applications and future directions. Cancer 2014;120(22):3433-45.
69. Leboulleux S, Schroeder PR, Schlumberger M, et al. The role of PET in follow-up of patients treated for differentiated epithelial thyroid cancers. Nat Clin Pract Endocrinol Metab 2007;3(2):112-21.
70. Chin BB, Patel P, Cohade C, et al. Recombinant human thyrotropin stimulation of fluoro-D-glucose positron emission tomography uptake in well-differentiated thyroid carcinoma. J Clin Endocrinol Metab 2004;89(1):91-5.
71. Kim SJ, Lee SW, Pak K, et al. Diagnostic performance of PET in thyroid cancer with elevated anti-Tg Ab. Endocr Relat Cancer 2018;25(6):643-52.
72. Giovanella L, Ceriani L, De Palma D, et al. Relationship between serum thyroglobulin and 18FDG-PET/CT in 131I-negative differentiated thyroid carcinomas. Head Neck 2012;34(5):626-31.
73. Santhanam P, Solnes LB, Rowe SP. Molecular imaging of advanced thyroid cancer: iodinated radiotracers and beyond. Med Oncol 2017;34(12):189.

74. Lee JW, Lee SM, Lee DH, et al. Clinical utility of 18F-FDG PET/CT concurrent with 131I therapy in intermediate-to-high-risk patients with differentiated thyroid cancer: dual-center experience with 286 patients. J Nucl Med 2013;54(8):1230–6.
75. Kaneko K, Abe K, Baba S, et al. Detection of residual lymph node metastases in high-risk papillary thyroid cancer patients receiving adjuvant I-131 therapy: the usefulness of F-18 FDG PET/CT. Clin Nucl Med 2010;35(1):6–11.
76. Kunawudhi A, Pak-art R, Keelawat S, et al. Detection of subcentimeter metastatic cervical lymph node by 18F-FDG PET/CT in patients with well-differentiated thyroid carcinoma and high serum thyroglobulin but negative 131I whole-body scan. Clin Nucl Med 2012;37(6):561–7.
77. Santhanam P, Khthir R, Solnes LB, et al. The relationship of BRAF(V600E) mutation status to FDG PET/CT avidity in thyroid cancer: a review and meta-analysis. Endocr Pract 2018;24(1):21–6.
78. Gaertner FC, Okamoto S, Shiga T, et al. FDG PET performed at thyroid remnant ablation has a higher predictive value for long-term survival of high-risk patients with well-differentiated thyroid cancer than radioiodine uptake. Clin Nucl Med 2015;40(5):378–83.
79. Seiboth L, Van Nostrand D, Wartofsky L, et al. Utility of PET/neck MRI digital fusion images in the management of recurrent or persistent thyroid cancer. Thyroid 2008;18(2):103–11.
80. Sgouros G, Hobbs RF, Atkins FB, et al. Three-dimensional radiobiological dosimetry (3D-RD) with 124I PET for 131I therapy of thyroid cancer. Eur J Nucl Med Mol Imaging 2011;38(Suppl 1):S41–7.
81. Santhanam P, Taieb D, Solnes L, et al. Utility of I-124 PET/CT in identifying radioiodine avid lesions in differentiated thyroid cancer: a systematic review and meta-analysis. Clin Endocrinol 2017;86(5):645–51.
82. Rault E, Vandenberghe S, Van Holen R, et al. Comparison of image quality of different iodine isotopes (I-123, I-124, and I-131). Cancer Biother Radiopharm 2007;22(3):423–30.
83. Ziessman HA, O'Malley JP, Thrall JH, et al. Nuclear Medicine: The Requisites. Philadelphia: Elsevier Saunders; 2014.
84. Kuker R, Sztejnberg M, Gulec S. I-124 imaging and dosimetry. Mol Imaging Radionucl Ther 2017;26(Suppl 1):66–73.

第18章
甲状腺未分化癌的诊断与治疗

Ashish V. Chintakuntlawar, Robert L. Foote, Jan L. Kasperbauer,
Keith C. Bible

关键词

- 甲状腺未分化癌 • 放化疗 • 多学科治疗 • 系统治疗

要点

- 甲状腺未分化癌预后极差,总死亡率接近100%。
- 放化疗联合手术治疗或单纯放化疗是局部进展期甲状腺未分化癌的首选治疗。
- 包括BRAF与MEK拮抗剂在内的新型靶向治疗药物,有可能为转移性未分化癌提供新的治疗手段。

引言

甲状腺未分化癌(anaplastic thyroid cancer, ATC)占所有甲状腺癌的1%~2%,是一种恶性程度极高且罕见的甲状腺癌[1]。近年来,由于甲状腺微小乳头状癌的诊出数量越来越多,分化型甲状腺癌(differentiated thyroid cancer, DTC)的发病率也越来越高;但在过去的几十年中,甲状腺未分化癌的发病率似乎一直很稳定,死亡率在多年间也几乎保持一致,其死亡人数占了甲状腺癌患者死亡总数的20%~50%[2]。根据众多大规模基于人群研究的结果,甲状腺未分化癌的中位生存期在3~6个月,而且在最近几十年都没有得到改善[3,4]。

因此，直到 2018 年，甲状腺未分化癌仍然是一种令人望而生畏的癌症。然而，随着我们对这种癌症的病理生理学的认识逐渐加深、新的治疗技术不断发展、众多富有启发性并与治疗相关的临床试验的不断出现，一线希望的曙光出现了。本章将聚焦甲状腺未分化癌，并根据肿瘤的不同分期阐释目前对甲状腺未分化癌的治疗手段。

临床表现

甲状腺未分化癌常常表现为迅速增大的颈部肿块，可能伴有表面皮肤红肿以及压迫邻近器官（如颈部血管、食管和气管）的症状。它可以侵犯邻近的喉返神经并导致单侧声带麻痹[5]，表现为声音嘶哑、发声障碍；还能侵犯或压迫气管，导致通气功能障碍并产生喘鸣音。甲状腺未分化癌患者还可能有吞咽困难、呼吸困难、咳嗽、疼痛，以及远处转移或脑转移导致的相应症状[6]，少数患者会表现为咯血。有时，在分化型甲状腺癌患者的病理标本中会意外发现甲状腺未分化癌细胞[7,8]，偶尔在分化型甲状腺癌的远处转移灶中，会发现一些失分化的癌成分[9]。

甲状腺未分化癌的好发年龄是 50~70 岁，偶尔见于年轻患者，但与分化型甲状腺癌不同，甲状腺未分化癌几乎不会在小于二三十岁的人群中出现。甲状腺未分化癌多见于女性患者[10]；大约一半的甲状腺未分化癌患者有分化型甲状腺癌的病史。与原发于甲状腺的淋巴瘤不同，桥本氏甲状腺炎病史和甲状腺未分化癌并不相关[5]。

鉴别诊断与病理诊断

甲状腺未分化癌需要与其他导致颈部肿块迅速增大的疾病相鉴别，比如低分化甲状腺癌、原发性甲状腺淋巴瘤、肉瘤，以及罕见的甲状腺原发鳞状细胞癌。上消化道、上呼吸道的转移性低分化恶性肿瘤也可能出现迅速增大的颈部肿块。由于后续治疗方法截然不同，迅速鉴别并排除诊断变得非常重要，而诊断的关键在于有效的病理活检。所以在初诊阶段，病理科医生迅速作出鉴别诊断变得非常重要。

甲状腺癌包括较多的病理组织学类型，其范围包括从惰性的肿瘤（如微小乳头状癌）到高度侵袭性的肿瘤（如未分化癌）。鉴别 ATC 与分化差的甲状腺癌是非常重要的，然而这些肿瘤的病理学特征有时候差别非常细微，需要有经验的病理科医生仔细读片才能鉴别出来。常用的诊断方式包括细针穿刺，但细针穿刺通常只能取出部分肿瘤细胞，标本中的细胞形态可能存在较大差异，且混杂着中性粒细胞等急性炎症细胞。大约 20%~50% 的甲状腺未分化癌会与分化型甲状腺癌共存，所以分化型甲状腺癌的细胞可能混杂在未分化癌的穿刺标本中[5]。甲状腺未分化癌有多种组织学亚型，包括肉瘤样、鳞状上皮样亚型、破骨细胞样亚型、寡细胞亚型、横纹肌样亚型和癌肉瘤样亚型。尽管存在不同种类的组织学亚型，但在治疗手段上并无区别。部分亚型不能单靠细针穿刺诊断，需要提供更多的活检组织或至少需要空心针穿刺活检才能诊断。甲状腺未分化癌的病理标本常常表现为细胞坏死和细胞碎片，伴有分裂像增加。免疫组织化学染色下，角蛋白（keratin）常表现为局部阳性。波形蛋白（vimentin）也多为阳性，尤其是在梭形细胞中。甲状腺转录因子 -1、甲状腺球蛋白和降钙素呈阴性，而 PAX8 及 P53 在组织中广泛表达[11]。除了寡细胞亚型，大多数甲状腺未分化癌都存在炎症细胞重度浸润，包括肿瘤相关巨噬细胞及 T 细胞[12,13]。甲状腺未分化癌同时存在着 PD-L1 高表达[14]。空心针穿刺在诊断上有非常高的敏感性和阳性预测值，免去了诊断性手术的必要[15]。

尽管甲状腺未分化癌和其他所有低分化癌在形态学表现上几乎一致，两者之间仍然存在鉴别点。最重要的是甲状腺未分化癌 PAX8 免疫组化染色阳性，以及可能与其他类型的甲状腺癌共存，这两个明显的特征有助于更快地明确甲状腺未分化癌的诊断。

病理生理学

大约一半的甲状腺未分化癌患者都有分化型甲状腺癌病史，这意味着相当一部分甲状腺未分化癌经历了分化型甲状腺癌逐渐去分化、侵袭性增加的过程。除此之外，分化型甲状腺癌和甲状腺未分化癌之间基因组的对比发现，两者之间既有许多共同的部分，但又有一些额外的变异，而这些变异常见于（但不仅见于）DTC-PDTC-ATC 这一转化途径，这也暗示了一系列连续的获得性基因突变最终导致了甲状腺未分化癌的产生。值得注意的是，甲状腺未分化癌比分化型甲状腺癌更常出现 *TP53* 突变，及并存 *BRAF* 与 *TERT* 基因突变，而且甲状腺未分化癌突变负荷也更大。Landa 等人[16]和 Kunstman 等人[17]首次发表了一项关于甲状腺未分化癌的大规模队列研究，发现它频繁携带 *BRAF*、*P53* 和 *RAS* 突变。Landa 等人[15]还发现了其 *TERT* 启动子序列的突变率很高。事实上，甲状腺未分化癌的体细胞突变负荷非常高，其中既包括了分化型甲状腺癌常见的 BRAF 和 RAS 突变，还包括了 P53、TERT 启动子这些高致病性的突变。上述结论已经得到了后续更大规模研究的证实[18-20]。一项纳入了中国和美国患者的队列研究显示，TERT 启动子突变与 BRAF 突变、年龄大和远处转移相关[21]。实际上，上述基因组的突变导致了增生和凋亡通路的激活[22]。表 18.1 列出了部分常见基因的突变频率，表中同一个基因在不同研究中的突变率差异可能是由研究方法以及人群差异导致的。这些研究都支持一个结论：带有驱动基因突变的 DTC 可能进一步突变成高致病性的亚型，比如低分化甲状腺癌或甲状腺未分化癌[19,23]。

除此之外，还有其他潜在因素导致这些肿瘤侵袭性增加，例如其他基因突变，其中包括 PI3-激酶通路中的基因（PTEN、PIK3CA、mTOR），转录因子（EIF1AX、NF1），细胞周期调控因子（CDKN1B），受体酪氨酸激酶（FLT1），以及组蛋白甲基化转移酶（KMT）。基因复制数改变和基因融合（ALK）也可能导致肿瘤恶性程度增加[16]。

表 18.1
甲状腺未分化癌中主要基因的突变频率

临床研究	病例数	P53/%	TERT/%	BRAF/%	RAS(N-,H-,K)/%
Kunstman 等[17], 2015	22	29	—	20	32
Landa 等[16], 2016	33	73	73	45	24
Bonhomme 等[18], 2017	144	54	54	14	42
Tiedje 等[20], 2017	118	55	73	11	19
Pozdeyev 等[19], 2018	196	65	65	41	27

图 18.1 列出了主要的可为甲状腺未分化癌提供潜在治疗靶点的信号转导通路。最近，越来越多的研究结果阐明了这些基因突变导致甲状腺未分化癌发生的机制。这些激酶活性改变不单导致经典通路的活化，还导致 TERT 激活[24]和细胞周期检查点激酶活性失调[25,26]。尽管遗传学研究并未发现 ATC 中涉及 shh 通路（sonic hedgehog pathway）的激活，但该通路和其他参与了甲状腺未分化癌发生的信号通路互相作用[27]，使肿瘤细胞保持类似干细胞的特性[28]以及耐药性。表观遗传机制如甲基化[29]也逐渐被发现参与了甲状腺未分化癌的发生，有望成为潜在的临床治疗方法[30]。另一方面，小 RNA（micro-RNA）在发病过程中所扮演的角色也开始受到关注，尽管它在短期内离

临床应用还相当遥远[31,32]，但这也让我们认识到甲状腺未分化癌的发生机制涉及多个环节，相当复杂。

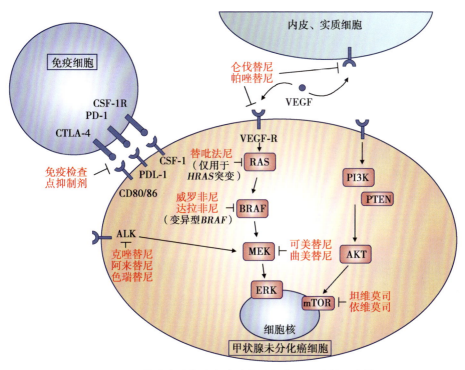

图 18.1 甲状腺未分化癌中主动免疫与信号通路的示意简图

在甲状腺未分化癌的发生过程中，需要重点考虑的因素还包括：经典的信号通路并不孤立地发挥作用，而是相互影响。使用药物抑制其中一条通路会激活其他通路，导致耐药性的产生[33]，有时甚至会导致癌细胞微环境中产生免疫抑制[34,35]。甲状腺未分化癌有非常多看似可调控的免疫逃逸机制，这使得免疫治疗成为了非常有潜力的治疗手段[36,37]。甲状腺未分化癌富含中性粒细胞、T 细胞和肿瘤相关巨噬细胞[13]，伴有 PD-L1 高表达[12,14]，这些特性都与预后不良相关，同时也暗示了肿瘤细胞处于一个免疫力强但疲惫的微环境中[14]。针对这些通路（CSF-1/CSF-1R、CTLA4、PD-1/PD-L1）和其他免疫调节因子（OX-40、4-1BB、GITR、NK 细胞等）的靶向治疗药物已经得到了美国食品药品管理局（US Food and Drug Administration，FDA）的批准上市或处于研发阶段。对甲状腺未分化癌患者单独或联合应用 CTLA4、PD-1 单抗的临床试验目前正在进行中，其与激酶抑制剂都有望在未来成为新的治疗手段。

诊断试验与影像学表现

不同于分化型甲状腺癌可以用甲状腺球蛋白作为有效的肿瘤标志物,甲状腺未分化癌并没有特异性的肿瘤标志物。如果甲状腺未分化癌中没有混杂分化型甲状腺癌的成分,甲状腺球蛋白染色通常是阴性结果。尽管如此,甲状腺未分化癌患者仍然需要进行基本的实验室检查,以评估骨髓及其他器官功能情况。

颈部原发灶的超声检查有助于提示恶性病变,通常表现为低回声的不规则结构伴局部浸润;也有助于发现颈部淋巴结转移。如果计划行手术治疗,则还需要增加其他检查,比如颈部增强 CT。如果要评估远处转移情况,笔者推荐行 FDG-PET-CT 检查[38]。如果没有条件行 PET-CT,可以用颈、胸、腹、盆 CT 评估肿瘤分期。除此之外,甲状腺未分化癌脑转移风险高,因此建议在初次判定分期时通过脑部 MRI 排除颅内转移[39]。

尽管仍缺少相关的前瞻性研究,但回顾性研究的结果显示,PET-CT 对于监测甲状腺未分化癌治疗效果更加敏感和高效[40]。患者经放化疗后颈部肿块常常持续存在,直到数个月后才能达到最大的治疗效果。回顾性分析显示,放化疗后病灶仍持续摄取 FDG 的患者的预后往往更差,但目前没有前瞻性研究证实这一结论[40]。

第 8 版 AJCC 分期中[41],T 和 N 的分类标准有轻微改变,然而,ⅣA、ⅣB、ⅣC 这一预后分期基本没有变化。局限于甲状腺内的未分化癌为ⅣA 期;病灶超出甲状腺以外,或累及颈部淋巴结者属于ⅣB 期;有远处转移的属ⅣC 期。然而临床上常常会遇到可能与分化型甲状腺癌相关的 1cm 以下的肺部结节以及远处转移病灶,这些情况下肿瘤分期的难度会增加,因此,应该结合临床背景以及患者个人的治疗目标,谨慎地作出评估。

治疗方法

考虑到甲状腺未分化癌进展迅速,如不及时处理,可能快速累及气道和食管,在数日内危及生命,故应当将它作为肿瘤科急症来处理。全面、迅速进行评估和诊断对于患者的治疗至关重要,而这项工作应该由一支经验丰富、协调合作的多学科团队完成。团队须涵盖内分泌专长的病理科医生、头颈外科医生、肿瘤内科医生、放疗科医生和内分泌科医生,理想情况下,最好再包括一名姑息治疗医生。由于甲状腺未分化癌整体上预后非常差,患者及其家属应该得到充分彻底的知情同意,内容包括这一疾病的自然病程、治疗目标、治疗不良反应,以及不同治疗方案可能带来的结果[42]。

一直以来甲状腺未分化癌的预后都非常差,这也导致了对它的治疗一度非常混乱,甚至被忽略而不行治疗。如果颈部病灶没有得到妥善治疗,几乎所有患者都会死于窒息。哪怕是对ⅣC期(远处转移)患者而言,颈部病灶都是危害生命最常见的主要因素。因此,必须把颈部病灶(甲状腺及淋巴结)的处理作为治疗的首要任务。

在开始进行ATC的多学科综合治疗之前的报告显示,2/3的患者死于窒息[43]。一项加拿大的基于人群的研究显示,在13位未经多学科会诊的患者中,11位在1个月内死亡,中位生存期只有6天,欧洲一项队列研究也得出了类似的结果,提示甲状腺未分化癌预后极差[44]。

初诊时应该进行详细的问诊、症状评估、体格检查,其中包括内镜下对喉、声门下和气管的评估,还有影像学检查以便分期。最重要的是,必须进行多学科会诊,全面地讨论患者的临床状况以及合适、有效的治疗手段。在每一位患者诊治的过程中,必须始终和患者及其家属保持紧密沟通,告知其疾病凶险的自然病程、预后以及治疗目标。另一方面,建立个体化的治疗目标对于治疗决策和计划是必不可少的,因为ATC中的所有治疗决策都需要在疾病风险和治疗风险之间进行认真权衡。图18.2展示了甲状腺未分化癌患者的初始诊治流程。

最佳支持治疗或临终关怀

首先,我们必须分清两个概念。一是对症治疗(palliative care),指专门用于缓解症状的治疗,不论甲状腺未分化癌患者选择哪种治疗方案,都应当接受对症治疗。二是最佳支持治疗或临终关怀(best supportive care or hospice),其唯一目标就是控制症状,而不行抗肿瘤治疗。临终关怀适合不愿意行积极多学科治疗的患者,以及基础条件较差、难以耐受抗肿瘤治疗的患者。尽管如此,临终关怀的应用必须要非常慎重,因为多数患有此病的患者在弥留之际都非常痛苦[43]。气管切开术作为临终关怀的手段仍然是有争议的,但对于那些气道阻塞进行性加重的患者,行气管切开有利于缓解症状,因此确为适应证。除此之外,在疾病诊断和分期阶段,行气管切开有助于缓解急性症状,为后续商讨治疗手段提供更宽裕的条件。尽管如此,气管切开本身对生活质量和生理功能有无法忽略的负面影响,需要对气管套管、伤口和分泌物进行妥善的护理。其他支持治疗手段,比如止痛药、针对缺氧的阿片类药物、缓解呼吸困难的氧疗以及类固醇激素,都能作为气管切开的替代治疗方式。选择临终关怀的患者的生存期几乎都一样,短以日计[44]。

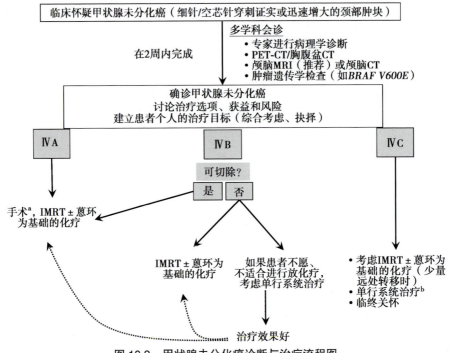

图 18.2　甲状腺未分化癌诊断与治疗流程图

a 目标是 R_0 或 R_1 切除而不是减瘤手术。尽量避免会推迟放化疗开始的手术,如部分咽切除术、部分食管切除术、气管切除术和喉切除术等
b 系统治疗包括达拉非尼和曲美替尼(*BRAF V600E* 基因突变阳性)、加入临床试验、化疗等

多学科治疗

表18.2 总结了目前发现的甲状腺未分化癌预后独立影响因素,包括年龄、患病时间(包括未出现远处转移的时间)、原发灶和颈部淋巴结放疗剂量以及多学科治疗情况[3,4,6,8,10]。基于这些研究和一些单中心的诊疗经验,笔者认为如果条件允许,对于病灶局限于颈部,尤其是仅发生在甲状腺的患者(ⅣA和ⅣB期),除非患者自愿选择临终关怀,否则应该接受手术以及后续放化疗,即调强放疗(intensity-modulated radiotherapy,IMRT)联合以紫杉类药物为基础的化疗。尽管如此,这种多学科联合治疗方法毒性大,不良反应明显,其利弊必须告知患者及其家属,进行充分评估后再取舍,因为对于大多数ⅣB(和

ⅣC)期患者而言,无论采取什么治疗方法,最终生存期都不超过1年。

Wallgren 和 Norin[45]发表了首项联合放化疗疗效研究的结果,后续的研究发现:包括手术、化疗、放疗在内的多学科治疗和传统上与温和的疗法相比,更有助于局部肿瘤控制[43]。瑞典和法国的研究人员早前针对不同化疗方案、分割放疗以及多学科序贯治疗进行了探索,发现经治疗后虽然局部肿瘤控制较好,但总体生存率较差,这主要是由于对远处转移灶的控制不足所致(表18.3)[46-48]。

近年来,多学科治疗在初治甲状腺未分化癌治疗中的地位持续上升,已经成为了目前治疗方案中的基石,越来越多的研究结果证明联合应用细胞毒性化疗和外放射治疗(尤其是IMRT)能取得更好的疗效。表18.3展示了数个单中心研究关于甲状腺未分化癌中位总生存期、局部肿瘤控制、远处转移灶控制率的结果。这些结果与此前的其他研究相比[49,50],都表明妥善控制原发灶与总生存期改善相关。对于ⅣB期,尤其是ⅣA期患者而言,生存期的改善尤为显著。对于ⅣB期患者而言,接受姑息治疗的患者的预后非常差,而接受较积极的多学科治疗的患者的生存期更长(4个月 vs. 22.4个月,HR=0.12,P=0.000 1)[50]。尽管如此,所有研究都未能控制远处转移灶。目前,迫切需要一种更有效的方法来治疗初诊时似乎已经普遍存在的隐匿性远处转移灶。

目前仍未发现能成为标准治疗的用于甲状腺未分化癌的放疗增敏剂。最早的时候,欧洲的研究大部分都采取联用细胞毒性药物的化疗方案[46,51]。后来,Kim 和 Leeper 等[52]发展出以多柔比星为基础的化疗方案[53,54]。最近几十年,蒽环类药物方案也被证实对甲状腺未分化癌有效[50,55,56]。尽管还没有随机对照的研究数据,但肿瘤放射治疗组(Radiation Therapy Oncology Group 0912)的研究结果显示,全身性的系统治疗可能对甲状腺未分化癌更有效[25]。在临床实践中,我们倾向于同期行放化疗,具体可以选择多西他赛+多柔比星或卡铂+紫杉醇,并同期每周行IMRT[50]。

近年来,放射治疗和计划的方式发生了非常大变化。超分割或加速放疗曾试用于甲状腺未分化癌的治疗,这些放疗方式尽管会增加放疗毒性[57,58],但是显著改善了原发灶的控制情况[47]。近年来,基于人群的研究和单中心研究都显示,40~45Gy是治疗甲状腺未分化癌的最佳剂量[4,8,59,60]。随着IMRT以及其他适形放射治疗方法的出现,在实现肿瘤区域的完整覆盖、提高局部放疗剂量的同时减少放疗毒性成为了可能[61]。对于甲状腺未分化癌患者,尤其是ⅣA和ⅣB期患者(R_1切除、R_2切除或不可切除),笔者所在的中心常规行6.5~7周IMRT,总剂量是66~70Gy/33~35次。这实际上是在用根治性的剂量来治疗不可切除的病灶[62]。对于体积较小的病灶，可以选择 66Gy/30 次的剂量；对于 R_0 切除的病例，我们会采用 60Gy/30 次的剂量，6 周完成。

表 18.2
甲状腺未分化癌的预后因素

作者，年份	研究类型	病例总数	女性患者/男性患者	年龄	中位生存期/月	改善预后因素
Goutsouliak 等[3], 2005	注册登记研究	75	51/24	74	5.1	放疗
Kebebew 等[10], 2005	注册登记研究	516	345/171	71	3	年龄、肿瘤局限、无远处转移、手术+放疗
Sugitani 等[8], 2012	多中心研究	547	339/208	约 70	—	年龄、急性症状、白细胞增多、肿瘤大小、无远处转移、手术切除、放化疗
Wendler 等[6], 2016	多中心研究	100	52/48	70	5.7	年龄、无远处转移、手术切除、放疗剂量>40Gy、化疗
Pezzi 等[4], 2017	注册登记研究	1 288	769/519	70	2.2	年龄、无共患病、无远处转移、手术、化疗、放疗剂量>45Gy

由于可切除性仍无定义、切除范围尚无定论，而且缺乏相关的前瞻性研究数据，手术切除对于治疗甲状腺未分化癌的作用目前还无法明确。然而，多项基于人群的研究均显示，手术是改善甲状腺未分化癌患者生存期的独立预后因素[4,10,63]，最近一项涵盖 40 多个研究的系统回顾也证实了这一结论[64]。值得注意的是，接受手术的ⅣA 和ⅣB 期患者的总生存期改善尤其显著[8,65]。减瘤手术对改善预后很可能并没有帮助，为了尽可能实现 R_0 或 R_1 切除，应当避免这种手术[57]。除此之外，还应当尽量避免单独行气管切开术[39]，况且大部分患者的肿瘤都在气管的表面，操作较为困难[66]。对于已经有远处转移，或者原发灶确定无法切除的患者，我们建议要非常慎重地决定是否行手术治疗。一些会导致术后放化疗延迟的手术，实际上没有足够证据证明能使患者获益，比如部分咽切除术、气管切除术、食管切除术和喉切除术。因为其很可能延误放化疗，增加远处转移的机会。

表 18.3 关于甲状腺未分化癌多学科治疗的重要研究

研究	年份	病例总数	女性患者/男性患者	年龄	手术率/%	放疗剂量/Gy	化疗方案	中位生存期/月	局部控制率/%	远处转移控制率/%
Werner	1975—1980	19	14/5	68~72	63	30~40	博来霉素+环磷酰胺+5-氟尿嘧啶	7~12	—	16
Kim	1979—1987	19	13/6	60	53	56	多柔比星	12	68	21
Schulumberger	1981—1990	20	11/9	—	60	52	米托蒽醌或多柔比星+顺铂	2~6	75	35
Tennvall	1984—1999	55	38/17	76	73	46	多柔比星	2~4.5	60	22
Crevoisier	1999—2000	30	18/12	59	24	40	多柔比星+顺铂	10	47	37
Sherman	1984—2007	37	20/17	63	51	58	多柔比星	6	50	—
Prasongsook	2003—2015	30	8/22	60	90	66	多柔比星+多西他赛	21	93	22

基于前述的多项研究结果,笔者提出了一套基于甲状腺未分化癌临床分期的诊治流程,如图 18.2 所示。在迅速完成初始评估后,我们认为大多数ⅣA 和ⅣB 期患者应该进行手术切除(可能的话),然后接受辅助放化疗。然而这种治疗方法仅仅适用于本人愿意、基本情况允许进行积极治疗,能耐受治疗不良反应的患者。在我们的临床实践中,对ⅣA 期患者应用这种治疗方案普遍让患者取得了良好的长期生存率,因此我们强烈建议ⅣA 期患者考虑这种治疗。不仅如此,我们发现ⅣB 期患者接受这种治疗后总生存期也得到了改善,尽管改善幅度不如ⅣA 期患者,但我们认为ⅣB 期患者也应接受这种疗法。

另外,我们建议原发灶无法切除的ⅣB 期患者应该接受同期化疗和放疗(最好是 IMRT)。这类患者也可以在新辅助治疗后行手术治疗[67]。然而,这一治疗方案并没有得到广泛验证,而且如果患者对系统治疗无效的话,会有窒息的危险。所以对我们的团队而言,只要有一线希望,我们都不愿意一开始就行全身性系统治疗而放弃切除颈部原发灶。

另一方面,对于全身广泛转移或ⅣC 期患者,应该根据患者个人的意愿接受对症治疗或临终关怀。对于极少数只有寡转移灶的甲状腺未分化癌患者,仍然应当考虑行多学科治疗,并对远处转移灶加做局部治疗(如立体定向放疗、立体定向放射外科治疗、射频消融、冷冻消融等)。然而,这种治疗方案似乎只有利于局部控制病情进展,对总生存期的改善并不明确[50]。

系统治疗(包括靶向和免疫治疗)

甲状腺未分化癌的系统治疗近年来有了显著变化。基于蒽环类或多柔比星的化疗成为了放化疗方案主要组成,被广泛应用。然而,对于远处转移的患者,单独使用这些化疗方案有效率低,有效时间较短[55,56,68]。此外,40%~50% 的甲状腺未分化癌携带 *BRAF V600E* 体突变。由于甲状腺未分化癌可以由分化程度较高的乳头状癌演变而来,也因此继承了在乳头状癌中常见的驱动因素 *BRAF V600E* 突变[16]。受这些研究启发,Subbiah 等人[69]最近对 16 位甲状腺未分化癌患者进行了一项研究,这些患者接受了 BRAF 拮抗剂达拉菲尼(darafenib)和 MEK 拮抗剂曲美替尼(trametinib)治疗后,有相当多患者获得了很好的治疗效果。目前,这项研究仍未达到中位总生存期,1 年生存率据报达到 80%。基于这项研究以及此前在恶性黑色素瘤上取得的成功,美国 FDA 批准了联合达拉菲尼 + 曲美替尼可用于局部治疗效果不佳的甲状腺未分化癌患者。在我们的临床实践中,也发现 *BRAF V600E* 靶向治疗对甲状腺未分化癌患者治疗效果非常好。然而,我们发现疗效持续时间只有短短几个月。其他激酶抑制剂,比如仑伐替尼[70](lenvatinib)和帕唑帕尼[71](pazopanib)对甲状腺未分化癌也有一定效果,可以作为 *BRAF* 突变阴性或达拉非尼+曲美替尼治疗失败患者的挽救治疗,然而它们的有效时间同样很短。任何能使转移性 ATC 受益的疗法都代表着治疗手段的进步,而我们迫切需要这些新进展。

免疫治疗很早就在细胞和动物试验中证实了对甲状腺未分化癌有效[35,72],但直到最近,人们开始越来越需要有效、可耐受的免疫治疗,这些研究成果才得到重视。甲状腺未分化癌的免疫研究结果令人鼓舞,但目前数量有限[67]。因此,在临床试验范围之外,尚未将这些药物并入甲状腺未分化癌的治疗方案。基于临床前研究[12,14]、病例报道[73]和 Wirth 等人[74]一项前瞻性研究的早期结果(抗 PD-1 单克隆抗体斯巴达丽珠 spartalizumab 的 Ⅰ 期和 Ⅱ 期临床试验),在没有适合患者的临床试验、免疫治疗没有禁忌证、患者没有严重的经济负担时,可以考虑对甲状腺未分化癌患者使用 PD-1 拮抗剂。

目前,PPARγ 激动剂 efatutazone(NCT02152137)[75]、复合免疫药物(NCT03122496、NCT03181100)以及 mTOR 拮抗剂(NCT02244463)等多种新药正在招募甲状腺未分化癌患者进行临床试验,部分患者也获得了一定的疗效。我们热切期待这些研究结果的出炉,同时希望能有更多类似的临床试验出现,早日找到针对进展期甲状腺未分化癌的有效的治疗手段。

总结

甲状腺未分化癌是一种罕见而高度致命的癌症。尽管如此,近来的研究发现早期采用积极的多学科治疗可以改善总生存期,尤其是对 ⅣA 和 ⅣB 期患者。然而,这种疗法的毒副作用较大,而且不能保证对所有患者都有效。因此,在选择这样激进的治疗前,医患双方必须结合患者本人个体化的治疗目标,认真权衡治疗的潜在获益、有效性和风险。经美国 FDA 批准可用于治疗甲状腺未分化癌的药物,除此前的多柔比星之外,最近还新增了达拉非尼+曲美替尼联合疗法,这一疗法适用于 *BRAF V600E* 突变的患者。对于转移性的 ⅣC 期患者而言,尽管最新研究出现了进展,但无论采用什么治疗方法,预后仍然非常差。尽管甲状腺未分化癌一直以来都被认为是非常致命、难治的,但通过将生物靶向药物和免疫治疗药物纳入多学科治疗方案,进一步设计新治疗方法和临床试验,我们面前出现了一线希望的曙光。笔者希望通过加强全球性多中心的协作,最终取得更多进展,为甲状腺未分化癌患者提供最佳的治疗方案。

致谢

笔者对无私参与文中各项临床研究的甲状腺未分化癌患者,为他们为其他患者改善预后作出的努力,致以最崇高的敬意。受篇幅所限,很多令人尊敬的同行所做的工作无法尽纳,我们深感歉意。

(陈颖乐　杨安奎)

参考文献

1. Mao Y, Xing M. Recent incidences and differential trends of thyroid cancer in the USA. Endocr Relat Cancer 2016;23(4):313–22.
2. Lim H, Devesa SS, Sosa JA, et al. Trends in thyroid cancer incidence and mortality in the United States, 1974-2013. JAMA 2017;317(13):1338 48.
3. Goutsouliak V, Hay JH. Anaplastic thyroid cancer in British Columbia 1985-1999: a population-based study. Clin Oncol 2005;17(2):75–8.
4. Pezzi TA, Mohamed ASR, Sheu T, et al. Radiation therapy dose is associated with improved survival for unresected anaplastic thyroid carcinoma: outcomes from the National Cancer Data Base. Cancer 2017;123(9):1653–61.
5. Nel CJ, van Heerden JA, Goellner JR, et al. Anaplastic carcinoma of the thyroid: a clinicopathologic study of 82 cases. Mayo Clin Proc 1985;60(1):51–8.
6. Wendler J, Kroiss M, Gast K, et al. Clinical presentation, treatment and outcome of anaplastic thyroid carcinoma: results of a multicenter study in Germany. Eur J Endocrinol 2016;175(6):521–9.
7. Yoshida A, Sugino K, Sugitani I, et al. Anaplastic thyroid carcinomas incidentally found on postoperative pathological examination. World J Surg 2014;38(9):2311–6.
8. Sugitani I, Miyauchi A, Sugino K, et al. Prognostic factors and treatment outcomes for anaplastic thyroid carcinoma: ATC Research Consortium of Japan cohort study of 677 patients. World J Surg 2012;36(6):1247–54.
9. Iniguez Ariza NM, Ryder M, Morris JC, et al. EXTRA-Thyroidal anaplastic thyroid cancer: a single institution experience, in 87th Annual Meeting of the American Thyroid Association. Victoria, British Columbia, Canada, October 18–22, 2007.
10. Kebebew E, Greenspan FS, Clark OH, et al. Anaplastic thyroid carcinoma. Treatment outcome and prognostic factors. Cancer 2005;103(7):1330–5.
11. Talbott I, Wakely PE Jr. Undifferentiated (anaplastic) thyroid carcinoma: practical immunohistochemistry and cytologic look-alikes. Semin Diagn Pathol 2015;32(4):305–10.
12. Bastman JJ, Serracino HS, Zhu Y, et al. Tumor-infiltrating T Cells and the PD-1 checkpoint pathway in advanced differentiated and anaplastic thyroid cancer.

J Clin Endocrinol Metab 2016;101(7):2863-73.
13. Ryder M, Ghossein RA, Ricarte-Filho JC, et al. Increased density of tumor-associated macrophages is associated with decreased survival in advanced thyroid cancer. Endocr Relat Cancer 2008;15(4):1069-74.
14. Chintakuntlawar AV, Rumilla KM, Smith CY, et al. Expression of PD-1 and PD-L1 in anaplastic thyroid cancer patients treated with multimodal therapy: results from a Retrospective Study. J Clin Endocrinol Metab 2017;102(6):1943-50.
15. Ha EJ, Baek JH, Lee JH, et al. Core needle biopsy could reduce diagnostic surgery in patients with anaplastic thyroid cancer or thyroid lymphoma. Eur Radiol 2016;26(4):1031-6.
16. Landa I, Ibrahimpasic T, Boucai L, et al. Genomic and transcriptomic hallmarks of poorly differentiated and anaplastic thyroid cancers. J Clin Invest 2016;126(3):1052-66.
17. Kunstman JW, Juhlin CC, Goh G, et al. Characterization of the mutational landscape of anaplastic thyroid cancer via whole-exome sequencing. Hum Mol Genet 2015;24(8):2318-29.
18. Bonhomme B, Godbert Y, Perot G, et al. Molecular pathology of anaplastic thyroid carcinomas: a retrospective study of 144 cases. Thyroid 2017;27(5):682-92.
19. Pozdeyev N, Gay LM, Sokol ES, et al. Genetic analysis of 779 advanced differentiated and anaplastic thyroid cancers. Clin Cancer Res 2018;24(13):3059-68.
20. Tiedje V, Ting S, Herold T, et al. NGS based identification of mutational hotspots for targeted therapy in anaplastic thyroid carcinoma. Oncotarget 2017;8(26):42613-20.
21. Shi X, Liu R, Qu S, et al. Association of TERT promoter mutation 1,295,228 C>T with BRAF V600E mutation, older patient age, and distant metastasis in anaplastic thyroid cancer. J Clin Endocrinol Metab 2015;100(4):E632-7.
22. Liu Z, Hou P, Ji M, et al. Highly prevalent genetic alterations in receptor tyrosine kinases and phosphatidylinositol 3-kinase/akt and mitogen-activated protein kinase pathways in anaplastic and follicular thyroid cancers. J Clin Endocrinol Mctab 2008;93(8):3106-16.
23. Bible KC, Smallridge RC, Morris JC, et al. Development of a multidisciplinary, multicampus subspecialty practice in endocrine cancers. J Oncol Pract 2012;8(3 Suppl):e1s-5s.
24. Liu R, Zhang T, Zhu G, et al. Regulation of mutant TERT by BRAF V600E/MAP kinase pathway through FOS/GABP in human cancer. Nat Commun 2018;9(1):579.
25. Isham CR, Bossou AR, Negron V, et al. Pazopanib enhances paclitaxel-induced mitotic catastrophe in anaplastic thyroid cancer. Sci Transl Med 2013;5(166):166ra3.
26. Marlow LA, von Roemeling CA, Cooper SJ, et al. Foxo3a drives proliferation in anaplastic thyroid carcinoma through transcriptional regulation of cyclin A1: a paradigm shift that impacts current therapeutic strategies. J Cell Sci 2012;125(Pt 18):4253-63.
27. Parascandolo A, Laukkanen MO, De Rosa N, et al. A dual mechanism of activation of the Sonic Hedgehog pathway in anaplastic thyroid cancer: crosstalk with RAS-BRAF-MEK pathway and ligand secretion by tumor stroma. Oncotarget 2018;9(4):4496-510.
28. Williamson AJ, Doscas ME, Ye J, et al. The sonic hedgehog signaling pathway

stimulates anaplastic thyroid cancer cell motility and invasiveness by activating Akt and c-Met. Oncotarget 2016;7(9):10472–85.
29. Hou P, Ji M, Xing M. Association of PTEN gene methylation with genetic alterations in the phosphatidylinositol 3-kinase/AKT signaling pathway in thyroid tumors. Cancer 2008;113(9):2440–7.
30. Zhang L, Zhang Y, Mehta A, et al. Dual inhibition of HDAC and EGFR signaling with CUDC-101 induces potent suppression of tumor growth and metastasis in anaplastic thyroid cancer. Oncotarget 2015;6(11):9073–85.
31. Boufraqech M, Nilubol N, Zhang L, et al. miR30a inhibits LOX expression and anaplastic thyroid cancer progression. Cancer Res 2015;75(2):367–77.
32. Xiong Y, Zhang L, Kebebew E. MiR-20a is upregulated in anaplastic thyroid cancer and targets LIMK1. PLoS One 2014;9(5):e96103.
33. Byeon HK, Na HJ, Yang YJ, et al. Acquired resistance to BRAF inhibition induces epithelial-to-mesenchymal transition in BRAF (V600E) mutant thyroid cancer by c-Met-mediated AKT activation. Oncotarget 2017;8(1):596–609.
34. Ryder M, Gild M, Hohl TM, et al. Genetic and pharmacological targeting of CSF-1/CSF-1R inhibits tumor-associated macrophages and impairs BRAF-induced thyroid cancer progression. PLoS One 2013;8(1):e54302.
35. Brauner E, Gunda V, Vanden Borre P, et al. Combining BRAF inhibitor and anti PD-L1 antibody dramatically improves tumor regression and anti tumor immunity in an immunocompetent murine model of anaplastic thyroid cancer. Oncotarget 2016;7(13):17194–211.
36. French JD, Bible K, Spitzweg C, et al. Leveraging the immune system to treat advanced thyroid cancers. Lancet Diabetes Endocrinol 2017;5(6):469–81.
37. French JD. Revisiting immune-based therapies for aggressive follicular cell-derived thyroid cancers. Thyroid 2013;23(5):529–42.
38. Bogsrud TV, Karantanis D, Nathan MA, et al. 18F-FDG PET in the management of patients with anaplastic thyroid carcinoma. Thyroid 2008;18(7):713–9.
39. Smallridge RC, Ain KB, Asa SL, et al. American Thyroid Association guidelines for management of patients with anaplastic thyroid cancer. Thyroid 2012;22(11):1104–39.
40. Poisson T, Deandreis D, Leboulleux S, et al. 18F-fluorodeoxyglucose positron emission tomography and computed tomography in anaplastic thyroid cancer. Eur J Nucl Med Mol Imaging 2010;37(12):2277–85.
41. Amin MB, Edge SB, Greene FL, et al, editors. AJCC Cancer Staging Manual. 8th edition. New York: Springer; 2017.
42. Cabanillas ME, Williams MD, Gunn GB, et al. Facilitating anaplastic thyroid cancer specialized treatment: a model for improving access to multidisciplinary care for patients with anaplastic thyroid cancer. Head Neck 2017;39(7):1291–5.
43. Tallroth E, Wallin G, Lundell G, et al. Multimodality treatment in anaplastic giant cell thyroid carcinoma. Cancer 1987;60(7):1428–31.
44. Besic N, Auersperg M, Us-Krasovec M, et al. Effect of primary treatment on survival in anaplastic thyroid carcinoma. Eur J Surg Oncol 2001;27(3):260–4.
45. Wallgren A, Norin T. Combined chemotherapy and radiation therapy in spindle and giant cell carcinoma of the thyroid gland. Report of a case. Acta Radiol Ther Phys Biol 1973;12(1):17–20.
46. Werner B, Abele J, Alveryd A, et al. Multimodal therapy in anaplastic giant cell thyroid carcinoma. World J Surg 1984;8(1):64–70.

47. Tennvall J, Lundell G, Wahlberg P, et al. Anaplastic thyroid carcinoma: three protocols combining doxorubicin, hyperfractionated radiotherapy and surgery. Br J Cancer 2002;86(12):1848–53.
48. Schlumberger M, Parmentier C. Phase II evaluation of mitoxantrone in advanced non anaplastic thyroid cancer. Bull Cancer 1989;76(4):403–6.
49. Foote RL, Molina JR, Kasperbauer JL, et al. Enhanced survival in locoregionally confined anaplastic thyroid carcinoma: a single-institution experience using aggressive multimodal therapy. Thyroid 2011;21(1):25–30.
50. Prasongsook N, Kumar A, Chintakuntlawar AV, et al. Survival in response to multimodal therapy in anaplastic thyroid cancer. J Clin Endocrinol Metab 2017;102(12):4506–14.
51. Tennvall J, Andersson T, Aspegren K, et al. Undifferentiated giant and spindle cell carcinoma of the thyroid. Report on two combined treatment modalities. Acta Radiol Oncol Radiat Phys Biol 1979;18(5):408–16.
52. Kim JH, Leeper RD. Treatment of locally advanced thyroid carcinoma with combination doxorubicin and radiation therapy. Cancer 1987;60(10):2372–5.
53. Tennvall J, Lundell G, Hallquist A, et al. Combined doxorubicin, hyperfractionated radiotherapy, and surgery in anaplastic thyroid carcinoma. Report on two protocols. The Swedish Anaplastic Thyroid Cancer Group. Cancer 1994;74(4):1348–54.
54. Schlumberger M, Parmentier C, Delisle MJ, et al. Combination therapy for anaplastic giant cell thyroid carcinoma. Cancer 1991;67(3):564–6.
55. Ain KB, Egorin MJ, DeSimone PA. Treatment of anaplastic thyroid carcinoma with paclitaxel: phase 2 trial using ninety-six-hour infusion. Collaborative Anaplastic Thyroid Cancer Health Intervention Trials (CATCHIT) Group. Thyroid 2000;10(7):587–94.
56. Onoda N, Sugitani I, Higashiyama T, et al. Concept and design of a nationwide prospective feasibility/efficacy/safety study of weekly paclitaxel for patients with pathologically confirmed anaplastic thyroid cancer (ATCCJ-PTX-P2). BMC Cancer 2015;15:475.
57. Dandekar P, Harmer C, Barbachano Y, et al. Hyperfractionated Accelerated Radiotherapy (HART) for anaplastic thyroid carcinoma: toxicity and survival analysis. Int J Radiat Oncol Biol Phys 2009;74(2):518–21.
58. Mitchell G, Huddart R, Harmer C. Phase II evaluation of high dose accelerated radiotherapy for anaplastic thyroid carcinoma. Radiother Oncol 1999;50(1):33–8.
59. Swaak-Kragten AT, de Wilt JH, Schmitz PI, et al. Multimodality treatment for anaplastic thyroid carcinoma–treatment outcome in 75 patients. Radiother Oncol 2009;92(1):100–4.
60. Pierie JP, Muzikansky A, Gaz RD, et al. The effect of surgery and radiotherapy on outcome of anaplastic thyroid carcinoma. Ann Surg Oncol 2002;9(1):57–64.
61. Bhatia A, Rao A, Ang KK, et al. Anaplastic thyroid cancer: clinical outcomes with conformal radiotherapy. Head Neck 2010;32(7):829–36.
62. Venkatesh YS, Ordonez NG, Schultz PN, et al. Anaplastic carcinoma of the thyroid. A clinicopathologic study of 121 cases. Cancer 1990;66(2):321–30.
63. Chen J, Tward JD, Shrieve DC, et al. Surgery and radiotherapy improves survival in patients with anaplastic thyroid carcinoma: analysis of the surveillance, epidemiology, and end results 1983-2002. Am J Clin Oncol 2008;31(5):460–4.
64. Hu S, Helman SN, Hanly E, et al. The role of surgery in anaplastic thyroid cancer: a systematic review. Am J Otolaryngol 2017;38(3):337–50.

65. Haigh PI, Ituarte PH, Wu HS, et al. Completely resected anaplastic thyroid carcinoma combined with adjuvant chemotherapy and irradiation is associated with prolonged survival. Cancer 2001;91(12):2335–42.
66. Shaha AR, Ferlito A, Owen RP, et al. Airway issues in anaplastic thyroid carcinoma. Eur Arch Otorhinolaryngol 2013;270(10):2579–83.
67. Cabanillas ME, Ferrarotto R, Garden AS, et al. Neoadjuvant BRAF- and immune-directed therapy for anaplastic thyroid carcinoma. Thyroid 2018;28(7):945–51.
68. Shimaoka K, Schoenfeld DA, DeWys WD, et al. A randomized trial of doxorubicin versus doxorubicin plus cisplatin in patients with advanced thyroid carcinoma. Cancer 1985;56(9):2155–60.
69. Subbiah V, Kreitman RJ, Wainberg ZA, et al. Dabrafenib and trametinib treatment in patients with locally advanced or metastatic BRAF V600-mutant anaplastic thyroid cancer. J Clin Oncol 2018;36(1):7–13.
70. Takahashi S, K N, Yamazaki T, et al. Phase II study of lenvatinib in patients with differentiated, medullary, and anaplastic thyroid cancer: final analysis results. in 2016 ASCO Annual Meeting. Chicago, IL, 2016: J Clin Oncol.
71. Bible KC, Suman VJ, Menefee ME, et al. A multiinstitutional phase 2 trial of pazopanib monotherapy in advanced anaplastic thyroid cancer. J Clin Endocrinol Metab 2012;97(9):3179–84.
72. Casterline PF, Jaques DA, Blom H, et al. Anaplastic giant and spindle-cell carcinoma of the thyroid: a different therapeutic approach. Cancer 1980;45(7):1689–92.
73. Kollipara R, Schneider B, Radovich M, et al. Exceptional response with immunotherapy in a patient with anaplastic thyroid cancer. Oncologist 2017;22(10):1149–51.
74. Wirth LJ, Eigendorff E, Capdevila J, et al. Phase I/II study of spartalizumab (PDR001), an anti-PD1 mAb, in patients with anaplastic thyroid cancer. J Clin Oncol 2018;36(15 Suppl):6024.
75. Smallridge RC, Copland JA, Brose MS, et al. Efatutazone, an oral PPAR-gamma agonist, in combination with paclitaxel in anaplastic thyroid cancer: results of a multicenter phase 1 trial. J Clin Endocrinol Metab 2013;98(6):2392–400.

第19章
甲状腺髓样癌的管理

David Viola, Rossella Elisei

关键词

- 甲状腺髓样癌 ● 降钙素 ● CEA ● *RET* ● MEN

要点

- 甲状腺髓样癌（medullary thyroid cancer, MTC）是甲状腺肿瘤中的少见类型，但发现时多为晚期。
- MTC 分为散发型和家族型，各占 75% 和 25%。筛查 *RET* 致癌基因可以区别这两种类型。
- 降钙素是 MTC 特异的血清标志物，它的倍增时间是最重要的肿瘤预测因子之一，时间越短，预后越差。
- 新的一些靶向治疗能够阻止或延缓肿瘤的发展。

引言

甲状腺髓样癌（medullary thyroid cancer, MTC）是甲状腺癌中发病率第三的肿瘤。它发生于甲状腺滤泡旁细胞，或者分泌降钙素的 C 细胞，且肿瘤细胞保留了这些内分泌细胞的特性[1,2]。

MTC 确切的发病率并不清楚，但是在所有甲状腺恶性肿瘤中的发病率为 3%~5%，在甲状腺结节中的发病率为 0.4%~1.4%。各个年龄段均可发病，但高峰集中在 40~50 岁，发病率在男女之间并没有性别差异[3]。MTC 分为散发型和家族型,各占 75% 和 25%。家族型常合并其他的内分泌疾病,如嗜铬细胞瘤(pheocromocytoma,PHEO)、甲状旁腺腺瘤 / 甲状旁腺增生引起的甲状旁腺亢进(hyperparathyroidism,HPTH)[4]。

尚未发现环境因素或者种族因素对 MTC 的发生有影响,它的发病机理主要与 RET 致癌基因突变有关[5,6]。大约 98% 的家族遗传病例中存在 RET 基因的种系突变。然而在散发型病例中,有大约 50% RET 基因体细胞突变,20% RAS 基因体细胞突变,20%~30% 仍是孤立的任意驱动癌基因突变[7]。进行 RET 基因筛查可以用来鉴别家族型和散发型。

MTC 的预后较差,10 年生存率大约为 50%。早期诊断以及早期的手术治疗能够影响肿瘤的治愈率和生存率[8,9]。

临床表现

大部分 MTC 是在甲状腺结节中发现的,不伴有其他的临床症状,结节可以为单发或者在结节性甲状腺肿中发现。少数一些患者可表现为顽固性腹泻和 / 或面部潮红(图 19.1),且发现时多已出现肿瘤晚期转移。所以必须详细调查家族史,因为在其他 MTC 患者中也有可能出现这些表现,同时也提示了可能是家族性或遗传性。这种猜想同样适用于嗜铬细胞瘤或者甲状旁腺亢进的患者。

遗传综合征不仅包含了 MTC (100%),同时也包含了多发性内分泌及非内分泌器官的紊乱,并据此分为:多发性内分泌腺瘤 2A 型(multiple endocrine neoplasia,MEN2A),临床表现为嗜铬细胞瘤(50%),甲状旁腺功能亢进(25%);多发性内分泌腺瘤 2B 型(multiple endocrine neoplasia,MEN2B),此型除了合并有嗜铬细胞瘤(50%),还表现为家族性的 MTC(familial MTC,FMTC),这是和散发型 MTC 最常见也是最主要的区别。MEN2A 最典型的特征是合并皮肤苔藓淀粉样变性(cutaneous lichen amyloidosis,CLA)(15%~20%)

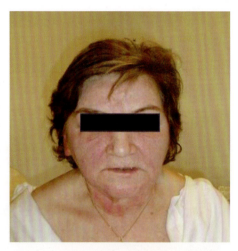

图 19.1　由于血清降钙素水平升高引起的典型的面部潮红:患者可表现为明显的阵发性面部潮红,尤其在肿瘤晚期发生转移的患者中多见

(图 19.2)。MEN2B 的临床特点主要是皮肤/黏膜神经瘤(100%)、巨结肠(100%),以及合并马方体型(100%)(图 19.3)[10]。

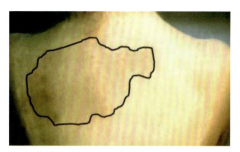

图 19.2　MEN2A 患者典型的 CLA:肩胛间区可见一红褐色的过度角化的伴有瘙痒的丘疹。病理改变是因为在特定区域内淀粉样蛋白在细胞外的过度沉积,有 *Cys634* 基因突变的患者容易合并有 CLA

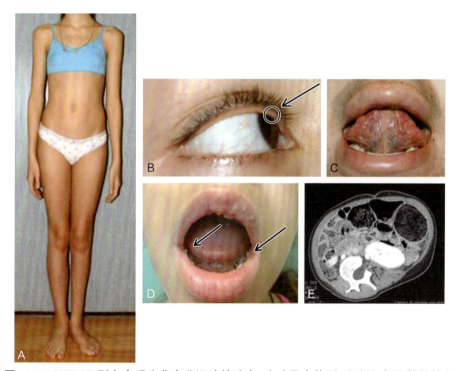

图 19.3　MEN2B 型多表现为非内分泌腺的改变。(A)马方体型:和躯干相比较长的上肢和下肢。(B)箭头所指的是眼结膜神经瘤。(C)凹凸不平的嘴唇,以及舌部的神经瘤。(D)箭头所指的是口腔黏膜两侧的神经瘤。(E)腹部 CT 可见由于横结肠的扩张引起的巨结肠,这种扩张是继发于 MEN2B 典型的节细胞性神经瘤病引起的

MTC 的临床表现主要分为三种综合征：进展较快且预后较差的 MEN2B 型；FMTC 多表现为惰性发展；MEN2A 肿瘤的严重程度介于两者之间。正因如此，出现上述临床表现，尤其是 MEN2 型特有的，需要被早期识别出来进行早期的诊断和治疗。

诊断

散发型

正如前面所描述的，散发型甲状腺髓样癌主要在甲状腺结节中发现。鉴于此，详细的体格检查、颈部超声以及超声引导下的甲状腺穿刺病理检查是诊断 MTC 最主要的手段。

MTC 的细胞涂片可见孤立、椭圆形的以及大的多边或者是纺锤样细胞。虽然这种细胞形态比较典型，但仍存在较高的概率在术前无法作出正确的诊断[11-13]。

与之不同的是当基础血清降钙素水平升高，尤其是 >100pg/ml 时[14]，对于 MTC 具有很好的诊断价值。对甲状腺结节患者常规检测血清降钙素有利于早期诊断意外发现的散发型 MTC[15-18]。降钙素的筛查可以及时发现 MTC，尤其是当肿瘤处于早期阶段，有利于及早进行外科治疗提高患者的治愈率。通过筛查降钙素诊断出来的甲状腺癌比通过细胞学或者组织学筛查出的甲状腺癌有更好的预后[17]。在其他一些情况下也会发生基础降钙素水平的升高[19-25]，可以通过钙刺激试验进行区别[26]。在 MTC 合并基础血清降钙素水平升高的患者中，钙刺激试验可以使血清降钙素水平 5~10 倍的升高，而其他疾病降钙素水平升高不明显或者不升高。

另外一种诊断 MTC 的方法是检测甲状腺结节穿刺后的穿刺针洗脱液中的降钙素水平，尤其是当血清降钙素水平升高不到 100pg/ml 时更有意义[27]。这种方法对于明确颈部超声检查发现的可疑的颈部淋巴结的性质尤其重要，有利于指导选择合适的外科治疗。

降钙素有着比较高的敏感性和特异性，从而成为比较可靠的肿瘤标志物。同时恶性转化 C 细胞分泌的其他一些多肽类物质也可以成为肿瘤标志物。例如，晚期发生转移的甲状腺癌患者中，血清 CEA（carcino embryonic antigen）会升高[28]。最近研究证实，在 MTC 的一种亚群中，血清 CA19.9 会升高，这一亚群预后更差，短期内死亡风险更高。像其他的一些神经内分泌肿瘤一样，MTC 患者可能会有血清嗜铬粒蛋白、生长激素抑制素、胃泌素释放蛋白、血管活性肠肽、神经元特异性烯醇酶,以及其他的一些神经内分泌物质的异常分泌,但是这些物质对诊断没有太多价值[28]。此外,MTC 分泌的一些多肽类物质可能会引起比较明显的临床症状,如:血管活性肠肽、5-羟色胺和前列腺素会引起面部潮红、腹泻。大约 1% 的 MTC 可能会出现 ACTH 相关的异位库欣综合征的表现[29]。

当 MTC 明确诊断后需要进行 RET 基因的分析以明确是散发型还是家族型[30]。如果突变存在于明显的散发型或者家族遗传型甲状腺癌患者中,那么对指导远期诊断和治疗策略有着极为重要的作用。不同的 RET 基因突变可能会产生不同的生物学行为,从而指导进一步检查。所有发现的完整的以及最新的 RET 基因种系突变和相应的临床表型数据可以在网上进行查阅(http://www.arup.utah.edu/database/MEN2/MEN2-welcome.php)。

家族型

MTC 遗传的特征多基于阳性的家族史或合并其他内分泌(如嗜铬细胞瘤和/或甲状旁腺功能亢进)或非内分泌紊乱,例如黏膜或皮肤的神经瘤、马方体型、MEN2B(图 19.3)中的巨结肠,以及 MEN2A 中的 CLA(图 19.2)。然而 7%~15% 明显的散发型 MTC 也发现有家族遗传病例[30-32]。

通常,嗜铬细胞瘤多在 MTC 发生和诊断以后发现,发病的中位年龄为 30~40 岁,24 小时尿中的 3-甲基肾上腺素升高是诊断无症状嗜铬细胞瘤最敏感和最特异的指标。一旦怀疑嗜铬细胞瘤,需要进行腹部超声探查肾上腺占位,必要时还可能需要进行腹部 CT 和/或 MRI 检查[28]。何时对嗜铬细胞瘤进行筛查,需要根据 RET 基因突变类型决定。因为早在 8 岁、12 岁和 19 岁诊断该病的患者就或多或少具有侵袭性 RET 基因突变[28]。

甲状旁腺病变只在 MEN2A 中出现,不管是腺瘤还是增生都可能引起甲状旁腺激素分泌的升高,从而引起高血钙以及高尿钙[33]。和 MEN1 型相比,甲状旁腺功能亢进多为轻度的且多数没有症状。MEN2A 中甲状旁腺功能亢进诊断的中位年龄为 30 岁,几乎所有的专家都建议在具有或多或少侵袭性 RET 基因突变的患者中筛查甲状旁腺功能亢进的时间分别不要早于 11 岁和 16 岁。在 MEN2A 家族中,先天性巨结肠可能和 MTC 或者其他的内分泌腺瘤有关,这种关系是比较独特的,因为先天性巨结肠的发病机理是因为 RET 基因功能缺失的突变,然而 MEN2 综合征的基因突变是功能获得性突变[34]。因为只有 4 个 RET 密码子控制着功能缺失突变或者功能获得突变(图 19.4),所以被称为 Janus 突变[34]。

被确诊为遗传性患者的所有一级亲属应该检测是否携带相同的 *RET* 种系突变。基因筛查能够将可能发展为综合征风险的基因携带者和没有携带这种基因且不需要进行密切随访的患者区别开来。与之不同的是基因携带者需要立刻收住院进行生物化学评估，明确是否已经存在了综合征中的某种临床表现。对基因携带者中还没有表现出 MEN2A 综合征中的任何一种临床表型的，需要密切随访。很多 *RET* 种系突变已经被识别出来并且发现和一些特定的临床表型有关[35]，根据不同的 *RET* 基因突变以及相关的表型，美国甲状腺协会（American Thyroid Association, ATA）根据发展为 MTC 的风险高低将 *RET* 突变分为三个等级：最高风险（highest, ATA-HST），高风险（high, ATA-H）和中风险（moderate, ATA-MOD）（图 19.4）。这种分级联合血清降钙素水平[36]，更有利于制订合适的筛查和治疗策略[28]。

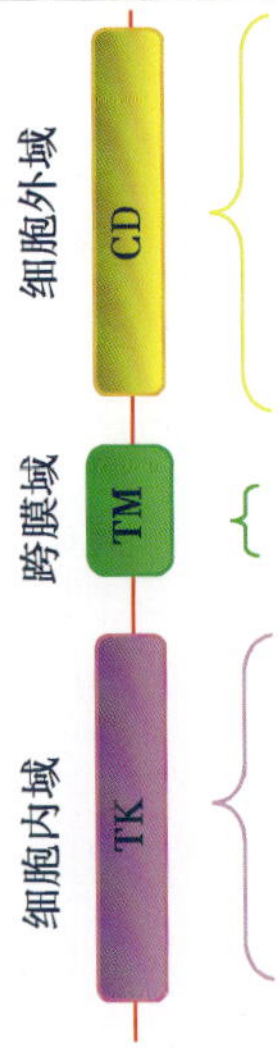

RET 受体	密码子	外显子	ATA 风险	HPTH	PHEO	CLA	HD	MH/MG/MN/BL
细胞外域 CD	533	8	MOD	−	+	A	A	A
	609	10	MOD	+	+/++	A	P	A
	611	10	MOD	+	+/++	A	P	A
	618	10	MOD	+	+/++	A	P	A
	620	10	MOD	+	+/++	A	P	A
	630	11	MOD	+	+/++	A	A	A
	631	11	MOD	−	+++	A	A	A
	634	11	H	++	+++	P	A	A
跨膜域 TM	666	11	MOD	−	+	A	A	A
细胞内域 TK	768	13	MOD	−	−	A	A	A
	790	13	MOD	−	+	A	A	A
	804	14	MOD	+	+	P	A	A
	883	15	H	−	+++	A	A	A
	891	15	MOD	+	+	A	A	A
	912	16	MOD	−	−	A	A	A
	918	16	HST	−	+++	A	A	P

图 19.4 基因型 - 表型的相关性和发展为内分泌新生物和其他非内分泌疾病相关 MTC 的风险水平（根据 ATA 分类）

+, 10%; ++, 20%~30%; +++, 50%; A, 缺乏; BL, 凹凸不平的嘴唇; CD, 富含半胱氨酸的区域; H, 高危; HD, Hirschsprung 病; HST, 最高危; MG, 巨结肠; MH, 马方体型; MN, 黏膜神经瘤; MOD, 中度发展风险（2015 年版 ATA 指南）; P, 具有; TK, 酪氨酸激酶区域

治疗及随访

初始治疗

MTC 治疗的基础是在疾病早期手术切除病灶。无论是散发型 MTC 还是遗传性 MTC,标准手术方式是甲状腺全切或近全切除术。而之所以需要全甲状腺切除,是因为大多数遗传性 MTC 和约 6% 的散发型 MTC 均存在多灶病变,并累及双侧甲状腺[37]。另外,约 7%~15% 的散发型 MTC 实际上是遗传性的,存在 C 细胞增生以及多灶病变[30-32]。

MTC 发生中央区淋巴结(central compartment lymph node,CCLND)转移的概率为 50%~75%,而这种转移概率与肿瘤直径无关,无论是直径<1cm 还是>4cm 的 MTC 病灶均具有相同的转移概率。因此,无论肿瘤大小,也无论术前有无淋巴结受累的证据,许多临床医生建议首次手术包括中央区淋巴结(CCLND)清扫。

近期的研究显示 MTC 患者术前降钙素水平可以决定淋巴结清扫的范围。当术前降钙素水平<20pg/ml 时(参考值<10pg/ml),几乎没有淋巴结转移的风险[38]。此时不应开展预防性 CCLND,从而避免术后并发症,尤其是永久性甲状旁腺功能减低症的发生。术前降钙素>20pg/ml、50pg/ml、200pg/ml、500pg/ml 时,分别与同侧中央组和同侧外侧组、对侧中央组、对侧外侧组、上纵隔淋巴结转移相关[38]。血清降钙素的最高值可以评估是否出现了转移病灶,然而一旦出现了转移病灶,预防性 CCLND 可能无法控制疾病的进展。在这样的情况下,手术范围应该局限于超声发现的转移淋巴结。

手术年龄显著影响 MTC 患者的复发与死亡情况,这在婴儿患者中尤为明显。在这种情况下,最大的问题来自年轻 RET 基因携带者手术后的甲状旁腺功能减退症,因为一旦发生,则需终身接受钙剂和维生素 D 替代治疗。根据 ATA 指南,预防性甲状腺切除术在 MEN2B 患者中,需在出生后 1 个月或 1 年内进行,MEN2A(ATA-HST)患者需在 5 岁前进行,MEN2A(ATA-MOD)患者在降钙素水平升高时或父母不希望患儿面对长程的评估时 5 岁前进行。然而,由于不同家系以及同一家系不同个体 MTC 发病年龄具有很大的差异,临床医生也可以根据基础和激发后降钙素水平为患者制订个性化的手术治疗方式。这主要出于如下两点考虑:即使对于经验丰富的外科医生而言,术中定位儿童和婴儿甲状旁腺的技术难度也很大;此外,一部分儿科医生认为甲状腺激素替代治疗不充分可能对患儿的大脑发育和生长产生不利影响。因此,1 岁以内进行预防性甲状腺切除术和 CCLND 只适用于 MEN2B 患者。不管是在成人还是儿童，CCLND 都与术后甲状旁腺功能减退的发生密切相关，因此，ATA 指南建议对于降钙素值<40pg/ml 且超声未显示淋巴结转移的 MEN2 儿童，仅进行甲状腺全切术而不进行 CCLND [28,36,39]。

对于遗传性以及尚未明确是否真正为散发的 MTC 患者，不管年龄与症状如何，都必须进行嗜铬细胞瘤（PHEO）和甲状旁腺功能亢进症（HPTH）的筛查。如果患者存在 PHEO，必须在甲状腺手术前治疗 PHEO，并在术前进行充分的准备确保不会出现高血压危象。HPTH 的筛查也很重要，如果延迟诊断，会导致同一部位反复多次手术，增加术后并发症的发生风险。

患者术后应该立即接受左旋甲状腺素（L-thyroxine，LT_4）替代治疗。与分化型甲状腺癌不同，滤泡旁细胞和 MTC 的生长均不依赖于 TSH，因而不需要"LT_4"抑制治疗，只需要将 TSH 维持在正常水平即可。

对于局部侵袭性 MTC，手术无法全部切除病灶，可以考虑体外放射疗法（external beam radiotherapy，EBRT）。但由于缺乏前瞻性的随机对照研究，EBRT 的实际治疗作用仍存在争议。最近的 SEER 分析显示，EBRT 不会给淋巴结转移的 MTC 患者带来生存获益[40]。因此，应综合评估 EBRT 的治疗获益以及 EBRT 的急慢性毒副作用。EBRT 增加了后续手术难度，患者更易发生严重并发症，因此，此类患者接受再次颈部手术时应谨慎考虑。

持续性和复发性 MTC 的随访与诊断

术后 3 个月应进行体格检查以及颈部超声、血清 TSH、基础降钙素、CEA 的评估，比较手术前后的差异。血清降钙素和 CEA 半衰期较长，因此术前水平较高的患者术后不宜过早复查。术后基础降钙素水平低于检测下限的患者视为临床缓解，MTC 复发率约 10%[41]。钙激发降钙素水平仍低于检测下限的患者，复发率可低至 3%[42]。当降钙素水平低于检测下限时，无须进行 CEA 检测。

术后降钙素水平<150pg/ml 的患者，可能会出现远处转移，但多数情况下持续性/复发性 MTC 病灶仅限于颈部淋巴结。对于这部分患者，建议每 6~12 个月重复 1 次体格检查以及颈部超声、血清基础降钙素与 CEA 检查。患者的血清降钙素可能保持稳定或缓慢升高，但长期生存影响不大。此时频繁重复的影像学检查（如 CT、PET 和骨骼扫描）是没有必要而且是有害的[28]。

对于术后基础降钙素>150pg/ml 或短期内降钙素水平持续升高的患者，应进行影像学评估。当降钙素水平>5 000pg/ml 时，患者存在远处转移的可能性达50%。当降钙素水平>20 000pg/ml 时，远处转移病灶的检出率为100%[43]。对于颈部病灶建议进行颈部超声检查，MRI 主要针对肝脏转移灶，MRI 和骨扫描主要针对骨转移灶[44]。使用不同示踪剂的 PET-CT（^{18}F-FDG，^{18}F-DOPA，^{68}Ga-DOTATATE 等）可能有助于定位转移病灶。为了避免对长期生存者进行重复和不必要的影像学检查，在初始评估之后，除极少数情况外，CT 扫描应不超过每年1次，并根据血清降钙素的升高趋势进行调整。

此外，降钙素和 CEA 的倍增时间（DT），尤其是降钙素的 DT[45]，是很好的生存预测指标。同时还可以用于对疾病进展的预测，当降钙素和 CEA 倍增时间一致且少于25个月时，MTC 进展的概率为94%。当降钙素和 CEA 倍增时间不一致且少于25个月时，MTC 进展的概率为56%[46]。降钙素和 CEA 的 DT 可以在 ATA 网站上在线计算，可以根据 DT 选择患者的 CT 扫描时间（www.thyroid.org/thyroid-physicians-professionals/calculators/thyroid-cancer-carcinoma）。

持续性/复发性 MTC 的治疗

通常不建议进行以治愈为目的的第二次手术治疗。事实上，只有1/3的 MTC 患者术后基础和刺激后的血清降钙素在正常范围内，而低于检测下限的更少[47,48]。如何识别可能受益于二次手术的患者非常重要。但是，尚无随机化的临床试验比较再次手术与单独观察的优劣[49,50]。颈部再次手术适用于快速进展的威胁到局部结构的淋巴结转移灶、有症状的病变以及 MTC 中不太可能发生的溃疡病变等。首次手术包膜浸润以及超过10个淋巴结转移是再次手术受益有限的重要预测指标。经过充分的诊断和治疗后，颈部淋巴结受累主要发生在转移性患者中，多数情况下可通过颈部超声随访。

与淋巴结转移灶相似，远处转移灶如果没有损害重要结构或威胁生命，不必进行手术。对于较大的肝脏单发转移灶，如果病灶持续增大，尤其合并腹痛腹泻等症状时，手术切除可能会使患者获益。其他相对安全的局部治疗手段包括射频消融、化学栓塞与经动脉放射栓塞等[28]。这些局部治疗方法也适用于骨和肺的转移病灶。局部治疗方法在一定程度上可以推迟系统性全身治疗的时间。

EBRT 建议只在合并如下症状的肺转移患者中使用：咳嗽、呼吸困难、吞咽困难等。接受肺部 EBRT 的患者有较高概率发生放射纤维化和呼吸衰竭，后者可能致死。另外，EBRT 可以缓解骨转移患者的骨痛症状。每月 1 次唑来膦酸静脉滴注或地诺单抗（denosumab）皮下给药也会减少骨骼相关不良反应的发生，对于骨多发损害的患者尤为有效。其他预防/延迟骨折的方法包括射频消融、椎体成形术或后凸成形术。

脑转移病灶也可以通过 EBRT 或立体定向放射疗法得到局部控制，以延长患者存活时间，提高生活质量。不建议手术切除无症状的脑转移灶，因为手术有风险，而患者并不受益。

对于累及多器官的多发转移病灶，如果有疾病进展的证据，应考虑全身系统治疗。这部分患者对经典的细胞毒性化疗药物反应率低（约 15%~20%），并且作用持续时间短[28]。最近的研究提示，以生长抑素受体为靶点的放射肽可能使患者获得完全或部分缓解。但尚需设计更好的样本量更大的研究以确认其治疗效果。

自 2005 年以来，针对 MTC 靶向治疗的研究兴趣不断增长[51]。这是因为在几乎所有家族性病例和大多数散发病例中都存在 *RET* 基因突变[52]。除了 *RET*，其他重要靶点［例如，血管内皮生长因子受体（VEGFR）、表皮生长因子受体（EGFR）、肝细胞生长因子受体（MET）等］也在 MTC 肿瘤中过度表达。这些发现为酪氨酸激酶抑制剂（TKI）治疗 MTC 提供了分子生物学证据。表 19.1 展示了最重要的 MTC 靶向药物和靶点。

motesanib 是第一批被评估 MTC 疗效的药物之一[53]，但在 II 期临床试验中缺乏安慰剂对照并且纳入了许多病情稳定的患者，治疗效果很差。基于上述两个原因，该药未曾面世。在随后的几年中，axitinib、pazopanib 与 lenvatinib 等多种 TKI 进行了 MTC 患者的 II 期临床试验，但这些药物均未进入 III 期临床试验[54-56]。凡德他尼（vandetanib）是第一个进行 III 期临床试验（ZETA 试验）的 MTC 靶向药物[57]。结果显示，与安慰剂相比，凡德他尼在疗效和耐受性方面均显示出较好的结果。治疗组患者获得了症状改善及无进展生存期（progression-free survival，PFS）的延长。因此，凡德他尼分别在 2011 年和 2013 年被美国食品药品管理局和欧洲药品管理局批准，用于治疗有症状、进行性的 MTC 患者。

表 19.1 针对 MTC 的靶向治疗药物临床试验

药物	靶点	临床试验	病例数（n）	部分缓解/%	病情稳定 ≥ 6 个月/%	无进展生存中位数/月	总生存中位数/月	参考文献
axitinib	VEGFR1,VEGFR3,PDGFR,cKIT	II	13	23.1	NE	9.4	18.9	Capdevila 等[54],2017
cabozantinib	VEGFR2,*RET*,MET,cKIT	III	330	28	NE	11.2	26.6	Elisei 等[58],2013
lenvatinib	VEGFR1,VEGFR3,PDGFR,cKIT,*RET*,FGFR	II	59	36	67	9	16.6	Schlumberger 等[56],2016
motesanib	VEGFR1,VEGFR3,PDGFR,cKIT,*RET*	II	91	2	48	12	NE	Schlumberger 等[53],2009
pazopanib	VEGFR1,VEGFR3,cKIT,PDGFR	II	35	14.3	>70	9.4	19.9	Bible 等[55],2014
vandetanib	VEGFR2,*RET*,FGFR,cKIT,EGFR	III	331	45	87	NE	NE	Wells 等[57],2012

EGFRE,epidermal growth factor receptor,表皮生长因子受体;FGFR,fibroblast growth factor receptor,成纤维细胞生长因子受体;KIT,v-kit Hardy-zuckerman 4 feline sarcoma viral oncogene;MET,hepatocyte growth factor receptor,肝细胞生长因子受体;PDGFR,platelet-derived growth factor receptor,血小板来源的生长因子受体;*RET*,rearranged during transfection receptor,转染重排受体;VEGFR,vascular endothelial growth factor,血管内皮生长因子受体;NE,not estimated,未评估

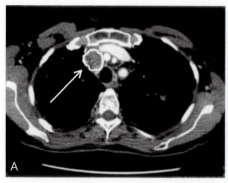
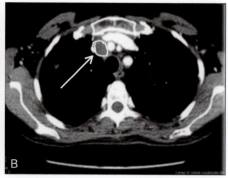

图19.5 CT 扫描显示肺门淋巴结转移。(A)治疗前和(B)TKI 治疗3个月后(白色箭头):病变大小明显缩小,由于病变去血管化,可以观察到 CT 外形的变化

卡博替尼(cabozantinib)是第二个获得美国食品药品管理局(2012年)、欧洲药物管理局(2014年)批准的用于治疗晚期进展性 MTC 的药物。卡博替尼的Ⅲ期临床试验(EXAM trial)[58]纳入了330名晚期进展性 MTC 患者,相对于安慰剂组,卡博替尼(140mg)治疗组患者的 PFS 有明显获益。这种获益不仅见于既往没接受过 TKI 治疗的患者中,而且在以往使用过其他 TKI 药物的患者中也能观察到。这说明卡博替尼可以作为晚期进展性 MTC 的一线用药,也可以作为二线用药。

虽然两种药物均具有 PFS 获益,但似乎都不能延长 MTC 患者的 OS,尽管在 M918T RET 突变的亚组中,卡博替尼治疗组 OS 优于安慰剂组(44.3个月 vs. 18.9个月)[59]。虽然两种药物只具有抑制细胞生长的能力而无细胞毒性,但经过数周/月的治疗后,目标病灶确实发生了显著的治疗作用(图19.5)。

两种药物都存在不良反应(AE),这些不良反应是这两种药物最大的缺陷(表19.2)。根据 RECIST(Response Evaluation Criteria in Solid Tumor)的标准,在疾病发生全身进展之前,都不建议对患者进行全身系统性的 TKI 治疗。这些药物的不良反应会严重影响患者的生活质量。高血压、腹泻可用药物加以控制,而 QT 间期延长、疲乏、体重减轻等则需要减少 TKI 的剂量[60]。由于 EXAM 和 ZETA 两个试验设计的差别,不能直接比较凡德他尼和卡博替尼两种药物的疗效和毒副作用。因此,用药前应综合考虑患者的合并症、药物潜在毒性、是否需要快速控制症状以及既往治疗史。值得一提的是,凡德他尼可以逆转或控制晚期 MTC 合并的异位库欣综合征,而后者提示预后不良。总之,晚期进展性 MTC 患者需要由一个经验丰富的团队来进行综合管理,团队中至少包括内分泌科、肿瘤科、心内科、皮肤科以及放射科医生。

上述不良反应多由药物的多靶点效应引起,其中最主要的是抗VEGFR效应。因此,其他直接针对 RET 基因突变的药物(如 LOXO-292、BLU-667)还在进行Ⅰ期、Ⅱ期临床试验评估中[61,62]。

表 19.2
ZETA 或 EXAM 试验发生率超过 10% 的不良反应

不良反应	凡德他尼(vandetanib)发生率/%	不良反应	卡博替尼(cabozantinib)发生率/%
腹泻	56	腹泻	56
皮疹	45	手足症候群	50
恶心	33	体重减轻	48
高血压	32	食欲减退	46
疲劳	24	恶心	43
头痛	26	疲劳	41
食欲减退	21	味觉障碍	34
痤疮	20	发色改变	34
皮肤干燥	15	高血压	33
皮炎	15	口腔炎	29
衰弱	14	便秘	27
呕吐	14	出血	25
腹痛	14	呕吐	24
QT 间期延长	14	肌炎	23
失眠	13	衰弱	21
鼻咽炎	11	发声困难	20
咳嗽	10	皮疹/干燥	19
体重减轻	10	头痛/口咽痛	18
		腹痛	17
		脱发	16
		背痛	15
		口干	13
		肌肉痉挛	12
		消化不良	11
		红斑/精神分裂	10

总结

MTC 是一种罕见的甲状腺肿瘤,但在诊断时相当比例患者的肿瘤已经是进展期了。目前,MTC 的唯一治愈机会是在早期肿瘤仅局限于甲状腺内时。MTC 可以是散发的(75%),也可以是遗传性的(25%),胚系 *RET* 基因检测可以鉴别两者。一旦患者确认携带胚系 *RET* 基因突变,家系中所有一级亲属都应接受 *RET* 基因检测。早期发现 *RET* 基因突变,携带者可以尽早接受甲状腺全切术,获得完全治愈。降钙素是 MTC 的特异性血清标志物。降钙素的 DT 是 MTC 患者生存和疾病发展最重要的预后因素之一。CEA 虽然不具有特异性,但与肿瘤负荷相关,CEA 的 DT 也是随访的重要指标。大约有 30% 的患者首次就诊时已发生 MTC 转移,可能会进入疾病进展期。在排除局部治疗的可能性之后,尤其是对进展性病灶进行充分评估与定位之后,可以考虑用凡德他尼或卡博替尼进行治疗。最后,建议由一个多学科团队来对 MTC 进行精准评估,以制订合适的用药和随访方案。

(武晓泓　叶 蕾)

参考文献

1. Hazard JB, Hawk WA, Crile G. Medullary (solid) carcinoma of the thyroid—a clinicopathologic entity. J Clin Endocrinol Metab 1959. https://doi.org/10.1210/jcem-19-1-152.
2. Melvin KE, Tashjian AH Jr. The syndrome of excessive thyrocalcitonin produced by medullary carcinoma of the thyroid. Proc Natl Acad Sci U S A 1968. https://doi.org/10.1073/pnas.59.4.1216.
3. Bergholm U, Adami HO, Telenius-Berg M, et al. Incidence of sporadic and familial medullary thyroid carcinoma in Sweden 1959 through 1981: A nationwide study in 126 patients. Acta Oncol (Madr) 1990. https://doi.org/10.3109/02841869009089985.
4. Keiser HR, Beaven MA, Doppman J, et al. Sipple's syndrome: medullary thyroid carcinoma, pheochromocytoma, and parathyroid disease. Studies in a large family. NIH conference. Ann Intern Med 1973. https://doi.org/10.7326/0003-4819-78-4-561.
5. Donis-keller H, Dou S, Chi D, et al. Mutations in the RET proto-oncogene are associated with MEN 2a and FMTC. Hum Mol Genet 1993. https://doi.org/10.1093/hmg/2.7.851.
6. Mulligan LM, Kwok JBJ, Healey CS, et al. Germ-line mutations of the RET proto-oncogene in multiple endocrine neoplasia type 2A. Nature 1993. https://doi.org/

10.1038/363458a0.
7. Ciampi R, Mian C, Fugazzola L, et al. Evidence of a low prevalence of RAS mutations in a large medullary thyroid cancer series. Thyroid 2013. https://doi.org/10.1089/thy.2012.0207.
8. GHARIB H, McCONAHEY WM, TIEGS RD, et al. Medullary thyroid carcinoma: clinicopathologic features and long-term follow-up of 65 patients treated during 1946 through 1970. Mayo Clin Proc 1992. https://doi.org/10.1016/S0025-6196(12)60923-9.
9. Kebebew E, Ituarte PHG, Siperstein AE, et al. Medullary thyroid carcinoma: Clinical characteristics, treatment, prognostic factors, and a comparison of staging systems. Cancer 2000;88(5):1139–48.
10. Romei C, Pardi E, Cetani F, et al. Genetic and clinical features of multiple endocrine neoplasia types 1 and 2. J Oncol 2012. https://doi.org/10.1155/2012/705036.
11. Trimboli P, Treglia G, Guidobaldi L, et al. Detection rate of FNA cytology in medullary thyroid carcinoma: a meta-analysis. Clin Endocrinol (Oxf) 2015. https://doi.org/10.1111/cen.12563.
12. Chang TC, Wu SL, Hsiao YL. Medullary thyroid carcinoma: Pitfalls in diagnosis by fine needle aspiration cytology and relationship of cytomorphology to RET proto-oncogene mutations. Acta Cytol 2005. https://doi.org/10.1159/000326191.
13. Papaparaskeva K, Nagel H, Droese M. Cytologic diagnosis of medullary carcinoma of the thyroid gland. Diagn Cytopathol 2000;22(6):351–8.
14. Costante G, Filetti S. Early diagnosis of medullary thyroid carcinoma: is systematic calcitonin screening appropriate in patients with nodular thyroid disease? Oncologist 2011. https://doi.org/10.1634/theoncologist.2010-0344.
15. Pacini F, Fontanelli M, Fugazzola L, et al. Routine measurement of serum calcitonin in nodular thyroid diseases allows the preoperative diagnosis of unsuspected sporadic medullary thyroid carcinoma. J Clin Endocrinol Metab 1994. https://doi.org/10.1210/jcem.78.4.8157706.
16. Niccoli P, Wion-Barbot N, Caron P, et al. Interest of routine measurement of serum calcitonin: Study in a large series of thyroidectomized patients. J Clin Endocrinol Metab 1997. https://doi.org/10.1210/jcem.82.2.3737.
17. Elisei R, Bottici V, Luchetti F, et al. Impact of routine measurement of serum calcitonin on the diagnosis and outcome of medullary thyroid cancer: experience in 10,864 patients with nodular thyroid disorders. J Clin Endocrinol Metab 2004. https://doi.org/10.1210/jc.2003-030550.
18. Vierhapper H, Raber W, Bieglmayer C, et al. Routine measurement of plasma calcitonin in nodular thyroid diseases. J Clin Endocrinol Metab 1997. https://doi.org/10.1210/jcem.82.5.3949.
19. Borchhardt KA, Hörl WH, Sunder-Plassmann G. Reversibility of "secondary hypercalcitoninemia" after kidney transplantation. Am J Transplant 2005. https://doi.org/10.1111/j.1600-6143.2005.00908.x.
20. Bevilacqua M, Dominguez LJ, Righini V, et al. Dissimilar PTH, gastrin, and calcitonin responses to oral calcium and peptones in hypocalciuric hypercalcemia, primary hyperparathyroidism, and normal subjects: a useful tool for differential diagnosis. J Bone Miner Res 2006. https://doi.org/10.1359/JBMR.051210.
21. Schuetz M, Duan H, Wahl K, et al. T lymphocyte cytokine production patterns in Hashimoto patients with elevated calcitonin levels and their relationship to tumor initiation. Anticancer Res 2006;26(6B):4591–6.

22. Pratz KW, Ma C, Aubry MC, et al. Large cell carcinoma with calcitonin and vasoactive intestinal polypeptide-associated Verner-Morrison syndrome. Mayo Clin Proc 2005. https://doi.org/10.1016/s0025-6196(11)62968-6.
23. Shi X, Liu R, Basolo F, et al. Differential clinicopathological risk and prognosis of major papillary thyroid cancer variants. J Clin Endocrinol Metab 2016;101(1). https://doi.org/10.1210/jc.2015-2917.
24. Sim SJ, Glassman AB, Ro JY, et al. Serum calcitonin in small cell carcinoma of the prostate. Ann Clin Lab Sci 1996;26(6):487–95.
25. Machens A, Haedecke J, Holzhausen HJ, et al. Differential diagnosis of calcitonin-secreting neuroendocrine carcinoma of the foregut by pentagastrin stimulation. Langenbecks Arch Surg 2000. https://doi.org/10.1007/s004230000169.
26. Mian C, Perrino M, Colombo C, et al. Refining calcium test for the diagnosis of medullary thyroid cancer: cutoffs, procedures, and safety. J Clin Endocrinol Metab 2014;99(5):1656–64.
27. Boi F, Maurelli I, Pinna G, et al. Calcitonin measurement in wash-out fluid from fine needle aspiration of neck masses in patients with primary and metastatic medullary thyroid carcinoma. J Clin Endocrinol Metab 2007. https://doi.org/10.1210/jc.2007-0326.
28. Wells SA, Asa SL, Dralle H, et al. Revised American thyroid association guidelines for the management of medullary thyroid carcinoma. Thyroid 2015. https://doi.org/10.1089/thy.2014.0335.
29. Barbosa SL-S, Rodien P, Leboulleux S, et al. Ectopic adrenocorticotropic hormone-syndrome in medullary carcinoma of the thyroid: a retrospective analysis and review of the literature. Thyroid 2005. https://doi.org/10.1089/thy.2005.15.618.
30. Romei C, Cosci B, Renzini G, et al. RET genetic screening of sporadic medullary thyroid cancer (MTC) allows the preclinical diagnosis of unsuspected gene carriers and the identification of a relevant percentage of hidden familial MTC (FMTC). Clin Endocrinol (Oxf) 2011;74(2). https://doi.org/10.1111/j.1365-2265.2010.03900.x.
31. Elisei R, Romei C, Cosci B, et al. Brief report: RET genetic screening in patients with medullary thyroid cancer and their relatives: experience with 807 individuals at one center. J Clin Endocrinol Metab 2007. https://doi.org/10.1210/jc.2007-1005.
32. Kihara M, Miyauchi A, Yoshioka K, et al. Germline RET mutation carriers in Japanese patients with apparently sporadic medullary thyroid carcinoma: a single institution experience. Auris Nasus Larynx 2016. https://doi.org/10.1016/j.anl.2015.12.016.
33. Bilezikian JP, Bandeira L, Khan A, et al. Hyperparathyroidism. Lancet 2018. https://doi.org/10.1016/S0140-6736(17)31430-7.
34. Moore S, Zaahl M. The Hirschsprung's–multiple endocrine neoplasia connection. Clinics (Sao Paulo) 2012. https://doi.org/10.6061/clinics/2012(Sup01)12.
35. Romei C, Ciampi R, Elisei R. A comprehensive overview of the role of the RET proto-oncogene in thyroid carcinoma. Nat Rev Endocrinol 2016. https://doi.org/10.1038/nrendo.2016.11.
36. Elisei R, Romei C, Renzini G, et al. The timing of total thyroidectomy in RET gene mutation carriers could be personalized and safely planned on the basis of serum calcitonin: 18 Years experience at one single center. J Clin Endocrinol Metab

2012. https://doi.org/10.1210/jc.2011-2046.
37. Essig GF, Porter K, Schneider D, et al. Multifocality in sporadic medullary thyroid carcinoma: an international multicenter study. Thyroid 2016. https://doi.org/10.1089/thy.2016.0255.
38. Machens A, Dralle H. Biomarker-based risk stratification for previously untreated medullary thyroid cancer. J Clin Endocrinol Metab 2010. https://doi.org/10.1210/jc.2009-2368.
39. Rohmer V, Vidal-Trecan G, Bourdelot A, et al. Prognostic factors of disease-free survival after thyroidectomy in 170 young patients with a RET germline mutation: a multicenter study of the Groupe Français d'Etude des Tumeurs Endocrines. J Clin Endocrinol Metab 2011. https://doi.org/10.1210/jc.2010-1234.
40. Martinez SR, Beal SH, Chen A, et al. Adjuvant external beam radiation for medullary thyroid carcinoma. J Surg Oncol 2010. https://doi.org/10.1002/jso.21557.
41. Pellegriti G, Leboulleux S, Baudin E, et al. Long-term outcome of medullary thyroid carcinoma in patients with normal postoperative medical imaging. Br J Cancer 2003. https://doi.org/10.1038/sj.bjc.6600930.
42. Franc S, Niccoli-Sire P, Cohen R, et al. Complete surgical lymph node resection does not prevent authentic recurrences of medullary thyroid carcinoma. Clin Endocrinol (Oxf) 2001. https://doi.org/10.1046/j.1365-2265.2001.01339.x.
43. Machens A, Schneyer U, Holzhausen HJ, et al. Prospects of remission in medullary thyroid carcinoma according to basal calcitonin level. J Clin Endocrinol Metab 2005. https://doi.org/10.1210/jc.2004-1836.
44. Giraudet AL, Vanel D, Leboulleux S, et al. Imaging medullary thyroid carcinoma with persistent elevated calcitonin levels. J Clin Endocrinol Metab 2007. https://doi.org/10.1210/jc.2007-1211.
45. Barbet J, Campion L, Kraeber-Bodéré F, et al. Prognostic impact of serum calcitonin and carcinoembryonic antigen doubling-times in patients with medullary thyroid carcinoma. J Clin Endocrinol Metab 2005. https://doi.org/10.1210/jc.2005-0044.
46. Giraudet AL, Al Ghulzan A, Aupérin A, et al. Progression of medullary thyroid carcinoma: Assessment with calcitonin and carcinoembryonic antigen doubling times. Eur J Endocrinol 2008. https://doi.org/10.1530/EJE-07-0667.
47. Tisell LE, Hansson G, Jansson S, et al. Reoperation in the treatment of asymptomatic metastasizing medullary thyroid carcinoma. Surgery 1986;99(1):60–6.
48. Fialkowski E, DeBenedetti M, Moley J. Long-term outcome of reoperations for medullary thyroid carcinoma. World J Surg 2008. https://doi.org/10.1007/s00268-007-9317-7.
49. Scollo C, Baudin E, Travagli JP, et al. Rationale for central and bilateral lymph node dissection in sporadic and hereditary medullary thyroid cancer. J Clin Endocrinol Metab 2003. https://doi.org/10.1210/jc.2002-021713.
50. Miccoli P, Minuto MN, Ugolini C, et al. Clinically unpredictable prognostic factors in the outcome of medullary thyroid cancer. Endocr Relat Cancer 2007. https://doi.org/10.1677/ERC-07-0128.
51. Viola D, Valerio L, Molinaro E, et al. Treatment of advanced thyroid cancer with targeted therapies: ten years of experience. Endocr Relat Cancer 2016;23(4):R185–205.
52. Romei C, Casella F, Tacito A, et al. New insights in the molecular signature of advanced medullary thyroid cancer: evidence of a bad outcome of cases with

double RET mutations. J Med Genet 2016;53(11). https://doi.org/10.1136/jmedgenet-2016-103833.
53. Schlumberger MJ, Elisei R, Bastholt L, et al. Phase II study of safety and efficacy of motesanib in patients with progressive or symptomatic, advanced or metastatic medullary thyroid cancer. J Clin Oncol 2009. https://doi.org/10.1200/JCO.2008.18.7815.
54. Capdevila J, Trigo JM, Aller J, et al. Axitinib treatment in advanced RAI-resistant differentiated thyroid cancer (DTC) and refractory medullary thyroid cancer (MTC). Eur J Endocrinol 2017. https://doi.org/10.1530/EJE-17-0243.
55. Bible KC, Suman VJ, Molina JR, et al. A multicenter phase 2 trial of pazopanib in metastatic and progressive medullary thyroid carcinoma: MC057H. J Clin Endocrinol Metab 2014. https://doi.org/10.1210/jc.2013-3713.
56. Schlumberger M, Jarzab B, Cabanillas ME, et al. A phase II trial of the multitargeted tyrosine kinase inhibitor lenvatinib (E7080) in advanced medullary thyroid cancer. Clin Cancer Res 2016. https://doi.org/10.1158/1078-0432.CCR-15-1127.
57. Wells SA, Robinson BG, Gagel RF, et al. Vandetanib in patients with locally advanced or metastatic medullary thyroid cancer: a randomized, double-blind phase III trial. J Clin Oncol 2012. https://doi.org/10.1200/jco.2011.35.5040.
58. Elisei R, Schlumberger MJ, Müller SP, et al. Cabozantinib in progressive medullary thyroid cancer. J Clin Oncol 2013. https://doi.org/10.1200/JCO.2012.48.4659.
59. Schlumberger M, Elisei R, Müller S, et al. Overall survival analysis of EXAM, a phase III trial of cabozantinib in patients with radiographically progressive medullary thyroid carcinoma. Ann Oncol 2017. https://doi.org/10.1093/annonc/mdx479.
60. Matrone A, Valerio L, Pieruzzi L, et al. Protein kinase inhibitors for the treatment of advanced and progressive radiorefractory thyroid tumors: From the clinical trials to the real life. Best Pract Res Clin Endocrinol Metab 2017;31(3). https://doi.org/10.1016/j.beem.2017.06.001.
61. Subbiah V, Velcheti V, Tuch BB, et al. Selective RET kinase inhibition for patients with RET-altered cancers. Ann Oncol 2018. https://doi.org/10.1093/annonc/mdy137.
62. Subbiah V, Gainor JF, Rahal R, et al. Precision targeted therapy with BLU-667 for RET-driven cancers. Cancer Discov 2018. https://doi.org/10.1158/2159-8290.CD-18-0338.

甲狀腺癌
Thyroid Cancer

Thyroid Cancer